Endocrine Dia

Clinical and Laboratory

Endocrine Diagnosis
Clinical and Laboratory Approach

EDITED BY

William F. Streck, M.D.

Attending Physician, Department of Medicine, Endocrine Section, Mary Imogene Bassett Hospital, Cooperstown, New York; Assistant Professor of Clinical Medicine, College of Physicians and Surgeons, Columbia University, New York, New York

Dean H. Lockwood, M.D.

Professor of Medicine and Head, Endocrine-Metabolism Unit, University of Rochester School of Medicine; Department of Medicine, Strong Memorial Hospital, Rochester, New York

LITTLE, BROWN AND COMPANY
Boston/Toronto

Contents

Contributing Authors   vii
Preface   ix
List of Diagnostic Protocols   xi

1. **Diabetes Mellitus**   1
   Dean H. Lockwood

2. **Anterior Pituitary Disorders: Hypopituitarism, Prolactin, Growth Hormone**   15
   Laurence S. Jacobs

3. **Hyperthyroidism, Hypothyroidism, and Thyroiditis; Goiters and Thyroid Nodules**   53
   Paul D. Woolf

4. **Hypercalcemia**   81
   Angelo A. Licata
   William F. Streck

5. **Hypocalcemia**   97
   Angelo A. Licata
   William F. Streck

6. **Diabetes Insipidus and SIADH**   107
   S. Zane Burday
   William F. Streck

7. **Adrenocortical Insufficiency**   125
   William F. Streck

8. **Cushing's Syndrome**   143
   William F. Streck

9. **Pheochromocytoma**   159
   Robert G. Campbell

10. **Primary Aldosteronism**   173
    Robert E. Heinig

11. **Amenorrhea**   191
    William T. Cave, Jr.
    William F. Streck

12. **Hirsutism**   209
    William T. Cave, Jr.
    William F. Streck

13. **Male Hypogonadism and Infertility**   223
    John M. Amatruda
    William F. Streck

14. **Hyperlipidemia** 247
Robert G. Brodows
William F. Streck

15. **Multiple Endocrine Neoplasia (MEN) Syndromes** 261
T. Franklin Williams
William F. Streck

16. **Hypoglycemia** 279
Dean H. Lockwood
Zachary R. Freedman

17. **Interference in Endocrine Testing** 297
Lewis B. Morrow

Index 307

Contributing Authors

John M. Amatruda, M.D.
Associate Professor of Medicine, University of Rochester School of Medicine and Dentistry; Endocrine-Metabolism Unit, Strong Memorial Hospital, Rochester, New York

Robert G. Brodows, M.D.
Associate Professor of Medicine, University of Rochester School of Medicine and Dentistry; Head, Endocrine-Metabolism Division, The Genesee Hospital, Rochester, New York

S. Zane Burday, M.D.
Clinical Associate Professor of Medicine, University of Rochester School of Medicine and Dentistry; Associate Physician, Department of Medicine, Strong Memorial Hospital, Rochester, New York

Robert G. Campbell, M.D.
Professor of Medicine and Biochemistry, University of Rochester School of Medicine and Dentistry; Director, Endocrine-Metabolism Unit, Monroe Community Hospital, Rochester, New York

William T. Cave, Jr., M.D.
Assistant Professor of Medicine, University of Rochester School of Medicine and Dentistry; Head, Endocrine Unit, St. Mary's Hospital, Rochester, New York

Zachary R. Freedman, M.D.
Assistant Professor of Medicine, University of Rochester School of Medicine and Dentistry; Endocrine-Metabolism Unit, Strong Memorial Hospital, Rochester, New York

Robert E. Heinig, M.D.
Assistant Professor of Medicine, University of Rochester School of Medicine and Dentistry; Head, Endocrine-Metabolism Unit, Rochester General Hospital, Rochester, New York

Laurence S. Jacobs, M.D.
Professor of Medicine and Director, Clinical Research Center, University of Rochester School of Medicine and Dentistry; Endocrine-Metabolism Unit, Strong Memorial Hospital, Rochester, New York

Angelo A. Licata, M.D.
Assistant Professor of Medicine, Department of Endocrinology, The Cleveland Clinic Foundation, Cleveland, Ohio

Dean H. Lockwood, M.D.
Professor of Medicine and Head, Endocrine-Metabolism Unit, University of Rochester School of Medicine and Dentistry; Department of Medicine, Strong Memorial Hospital, Rochester, New York

Lewis B. Morrow, M.D.
Professor of Medicine, Medical College of Ohio; Endocrine-Metabolism Unit, Medical College of Ohio Hospital, Toledo, Ohio

William F. Streck, M.D.
Attending Physician, Department of Medicine, Endocrine Section, Mary Imogene Bassett Hospital, Cooperstown, New York; Assistant Professor of Clinical Medicine, College of Physicians and Surgeons, Columbia University, New York, New York

T. Franklin Williams, M.D.
Professor of Medicine, University of Rochester School of Medicine and Dentistry; Medical Director, Monroe Community Hospital, Rochester, New York

Paul D. Woolf, M.D.
Associate Professor of Medicine, University of Rochester School of Medicine and Dentistry; Endocrine-Metabolism Unit, Strong Memorial Hospital, Rochester, New York

Preface

Clinical problems in medicine that are of an endocrine or metabolic nature provide unique opportunities for the integration of clinical observation and sophisticated laboratory technology. The complex array of laboratory tests available for the assessment of endocrine problems makes effective use of these tests a challenge. The expense of many of these tests makes cost-effectiveness mandatory. It is not surprising, therefore, that quite a number of books attempting to assess endocrine and metabolic problems have been published within the last several years.

This book emphasizes the *process* of diagnosis, that is, the orderly and systematic use of information to provide correct and economic solutions to endocrine diagnostic problems. This approach is somewhat different from that presented in other texts and distinguishes this book from most others. For instance, standard texts might describe the woman with polycystic ovarian disease as having elevated free testosterone levels, an LH:FSH ratio of 2:1 or greater, and an estrogen suppression test that shows decreased testosterone and/or androstenedione. This description lists the characteristics that define the polycystic ovarian syndrome, without providing a method by which they may be correctly sought or observed. However, the hirsute woman presenting for evaluation has a series of potential problems that require investigation. Therefore, this book stresses the use of methods and the sequence of investigation that will allow diagnosis of this disorder without a series of extraneous tests. Each chapter emphasizes the process by which conclusions are drawn in the assessment of endocrine disorders, and illustrates this process by means of flowcharts of Diagnostic Protocols, which are provided for each disorder. (For a list of the Diagnostic Protocols, see p. xi.)

Chapters are arranged in a standardized format, based on the premise that the physician begins with a specific clinical problem, such as hirsutism, hyperlipidemia, or hypercalcemia. From this starting point each chapter follows a format designed to complement the clinical method, in which the systematic gathering of information, selection of tests, delineation of decision points, and review of data are used to reach a diagnostic conclusion.

In the first part of each chapter, Clinical Considerations, the clinical characteristics of various disorders that enter the differential diagnosis for a given problem are discussed. Emphasis on laboratory characteristics is kept to a minimum in this section.

The second section, Diagnostic Methods, lists in sequence the major tests available for the assessment of the endocrine and metabolic disorder under discussion. Each test is discussed briefly. Limitations of the tests are touched on and normal values are provided.

The third section of each chapter, Diagnostic Protocol, incorporates some of the clinical clues and provides a systematic way to order laboratory tests and make decisions in the investigation of a given problem. It should be emphasized that these are simply proposed means to approach problems, since there are certainly few absolute ways to deal with any given problem. The suggestions in this section represent in large part the clinical approach used in the Endocrine-Metabolism Unit of the University of Rochester School of Medicine and Dentistry. We believe they are fairly comprehensive.

The fourth section of each chapter, Discussion, recognizes the variabilities in approach and the fact that there are limitations to any test in whatever sequence it has been obtained. Thus, this section reviews the limitations of the testing protocol, the pros and cons of various tests, and the rationale for the tests as provided.

Current references are provided throughout each chapter to allow the reader to seek more definitive information on the recommendations, clinical pictures, or procedures described in this book. We have included these references to provide the reader with the opportunity to enhance the practical application of knowledge that each chapter attempts to provide.

W. F. S.
D. H. L.

List of Diagnostic Protocols

Diagnostic Protocols are provided for disorders described in this book for two reasons. The first is very practical. When a clinical problem is encountered, there is often uncertainty as to the most efficient way to *initiate an evaluation*. The problem-focused protocols are designed to allow a correct, efficient, and readily accessible first step in the approach to endocrine diagnostic problems. Simply by referring to these protocols, appropriate tests may be reviewed and inappropriate or less useful tests avoided.

The initiation of an evaluation unlocks a cascade of clinical and laboratory alternatives; at each level, decisions must be made until a diagnosis emerges. Thus, the second use of the Diagnostic Protocols is to provide the framework to *complete an evaluation* of a given problem. The approaches recommended are reviewed and discussed in the corresponding text for each chapter.

Diagnostic Protocol   **Page**

Diagnostic Protocol	Page
1-1. Suspected diabetes mellitus in nonpregnant adults	7
2-1. Suspected hypopituitarism	26
2-2. Hyperprolactinemia	31
2-3. Suspected acromegaly	38
2-4. Proportionate short stature	46
3-1. Hyperthyroidism	68
3-2. Hypothyroidism	70
3-3. Solitary thyroid nodule	75
4-1. Hypercalcemia	90
5-2. Hypocalcemia	104
6-1. Polyuria	120
6-2. Hyponatremia	122
7-1. Adrenocortical insufficiency (no prior glucocorticoids)	136
7-2. Adrenocortical insufficiency (prior or current steroid therapy)	138
8-1. Evaluation of suspected hypercortisolism	151
8-2. Investigation of the etiology of Cushing's syndrome	152
9-1. Suspected pheochromocytoma	168
10-1. Initial laboratory evaluation of suspected primary aldosteronism	177
10-2. Confirmatory testing and localization in primary aldosteronism	185
11-1. Secondary amenorrhea	203
11-2. Primary amenorrhea	205

12-1. Hirsutism   217
13-1. Male hypogonadism and/or infertility   239
13-2. Suspected hypothalamic-pituitary hypogonadism   240
13-3. Eunuchoid habitus, gynecomastia, or feminization   242
14-1. Suspected hyperlipidemia   257
15-1. Suspected MEN-I   272
15-2. Suspected MEN-II   274
16-2. Suspected fasting hypoglycemia   289
16-3. Suspected insulinoma (suggestive history)   290
16-4. Suspected postprandial hypoglycemia   292

Endocrine Diagnosis
Clinical and Laboratory Approach

NOTICE

The indications and dosages of all drugs in this book have been recommended in the medical literature and conform to the practices of the general medical community. The medications described do not necessarily have specific approval by the Food and Drug Administration for use in the diseases and dosages for which they are recommended. The package insert for each drug should be consulted for use and dosage as approved by the FDA. Because standards for usage change, it is advisable to keep abreast of revised recommendations, particularly those concerning new drugs.

1   Diabetes Mellitus

Dean H. Lockwood

Diabetes mellitus is a complex metabolic disorder in which the basic defect appears to be a relative or absolute lack of insulin. Although not clearly defined, viral, immunologic, and genetic factors have been implicated as playing causal roles [2,13,17]. Because of the increased longevity and reproductive capabilities of diabetics in the past 60 years, the prevalence of this disease is continually increasing. Conservative estimates suggest that approximately 5% of the population of the United States is afflicted with this disorder. Currently, diabetes ranks fifth as a cause of death in the United States and is the major cause of blindness and loss of limb in the adult population. The economic impact of diabetes and its complications was estimated to be about 8 billion dollars per year in 1979. These grim statistics should serve to emphasize the importance of making a correct diagnosis as early as possible, with the hope that proper management will minimize morbidity and delay mortality. As will be discussed subsequently, the criteria for the diagnosis of diabetes have been revised substantially.

CLINICAL CONSIDERATIONS

Physicians have long recognized that there are two general types of diabetes which can usually be distinguished by their clinical presentation. These two categories, which were formerly termed *juvenile-onset* and *maturity-onset diabetes*, have been recently reclassified as type I, *ketosis-prone*, or *insulin-dependent diabetes*, and type II, *nonketosis-prone*, *non-insulin-dependent diabetes*.

Type I Diabetes

In patients with type I diabetes, the presenting symptoms are often dramatic because there is an associated severe insulin deficiency. These patients, who are usually less than 20 years of age, may have the rapid development of polyuria, polydipsia, and polyphagia, with associated weight loss. Lack of insulin in this situation ultimately leads to severe dehydration, ketoacidosis, and eventually coma. Studies of the etiology of type I diabetes suggest the involvement of both genetic and environmental factors [13]. Insulin-dependent diabetes is frequently associated with certain histocompatibility antigen (HLA) types and abnormal immune responses, including islet cell antibodies. Furthermore, there is mounting evidence to suggest that certain cases are the result of viral infections.

Type II Diabetes

An insidious onset usually characterizes type II diabetes mellitus, which is frequently seen in older obese patients. In fact, the diagnosis is frequently made on the basis of laboratory information obtained when the patient is without symptoms, as during a routine examination. However, some patients will develop signs and symptoms of significant insulin deficiency, especially under conditions in which pancreatic insulin output is stressed. This may occur with pregnancy, obesity, and infection and in association with certain drug therapies. The patient may complain of blurring of vision and myopia, as well as episodes of recurrent infection, such as carbuncles, furuncles, urinary tract infections, monilial vaginitis in the female, and balanitis in the male. Although these patients are considered to be partially insulin-deficient, it is becoming increasingly apparent that most type II diabetics also have insulin resistance at the level of the target tissue. In addition, some patients can present with transient postprandial hypoglycemia, and others, at the time of diagnosis, may have evidence of the chronic complications of the disease. Patients with type II diabetes may require insulin for correction of hyperglycemia, but they are not considered insulin-dependent or ketosis-prone. Genetic susceptibility is felt to be a strong etiologic factor, but unlike type I diabetes, there is no association with the HLAs.

Impaired Glucose Tolerance
Until recently, the proposed criteria for the diagnosis of diabetes based on fasting plasma glucose levels and plasma glucose levels obtained during an oral glucose tolerance test have varied widely. The differing criteria, coupled with population studies that frequently have been unable to distinguish between the upper limits of normal and mild diabetes, have led to considerable confusion concerning the appropriate diagnosis. More recently, epidemiologic studies have strongly suggested that our criteria for diagnosis have been inappropriate, and in general, physicians have overdiagnosed the disease. Epidemiologic studies of diabetes in the Pima Indians [1] have revealed a bimodal distribution for both fasting plasma glucose and the two-hour level obtained during an oral glucose tolerance test. This study convincingly demonstrates that diabetes definitely persists and is associated with the well-known complications when fasting plasma glucose is above 140 mg/dl and the two-hour sample is above 200 to 240 mg/dl. Other studies, carried out in Great Britain and the United States, support these criteria [6, 15]. Of greater interest is the observation that patients with milder degrees of glucose intolerance over time can decompensate to frank diabetes, revert to normal glucose tolerance, or remain "chemical diabetics." Because decompensation occurs at a rate of only 1 to 5% per year, a new classification termed *impaired glucose tolerance* has been established for this group.

In addition to the signs and symptoms already discussed, there are three other clinical situations that have an increased association with diabetes and may prompt the physician to pursue the diagnosis of diabetes vigorously.

Table 1-1. Commonly Used Drugs Affecting Glucose Tolerance

Hyperglycemia	*Hypoglycemia*
Amitriptyline	Biguanides
Caffeine	Ethanol
Catecholamines	Sulfonamides
Chlorthalidone	Sulfonylureas
Clonidine	
Corticosteroids	
Diphenylhydantoin	
Furosemide	
Haloperidol	
Imipramine	
Indomethacin	
Lithium carbonate	
Oral contraceptives	
Phenothiazines	
Thiazides	

Pregnancy

Several studies indicate that good control of diabetic metabolic abnormalities during the third trimester of pregnancy reduces neonatal morbidity and mortality [8]. More recently, additional evidence strongly suggests that good control beginning at conception may prevent congenital malformations [10]. Thus, diabetes mellitus should be strongly considered in pregnant women who have any of the following conditions: (1) glucosuria; (2) a family history of diabetes in a first-degree relative; (3) a history of spontaneous abortion, stillbirth, or fetal malformations in previous pregnancies; (4) previous delivery of an offspring weighing more than 9 pounds; (5) obesity; (6) a high maternal age; (7) a parity of five or more [12]. Since these high-risk factors may be absent, screening for glucose intolerance during all pregnancies is advisable.

Previous Abnormality of Glucose Tolerance

Individuals who have had documented hyperglycemia and have subsequently returned to normal glucose tolerance fit in the category of previous abnormality of glucose tolerance. Situations that may unmask a predisposition to glucose intolerance include pregnancy, the acute phase of a myocardial infarction, serious trauma, and ingestion of certain diabetogenic medications (Table 1-1).

Potential Abnormality of Glucose Tolerance

Individuals in the category of potential abnormality of glucose tolerance have not been shown to have abnormal glucose tolerance previously, but they are at an increased risk over the general population for the development of diabetes. Those who have a monozygotic twin or other first-degree relative—sibling, parent, offspring—with either type I or type II diabetes fall into this category. Persons who are obese and mothers who have delivered babies weighing more than 9 pounds also fall into this category.

DIAGNOSTIC METHODS
Tests Used for Making the Diagnosis of Diabetes
FASTING PLASMA GLUCOSE. The initial laboratory assessment for the diagnosis of glucose intolerance in adults is the fasting plasma glucose. The blood sample should be obtained in the morning, 10 to 16 hours after fasting, before noncaloric stimulants, that is, coffee and tea, are ingested and before any smoking activities. In nonpregnant adults, the demonstration on two separate occasions of a fasting plasma glucose of 140 mg/dl or greater is enough evidence to make the diagnosis of diabetes mellitus. Values of less than 115 mg/dl are considered normal. If the value is between 115 and 140 mg/dl or there are other clinical indications of diabetes, an oral glucose tolerance test is in order. Glucose values obtained from whole blood rather than plasma are approximately 15% lower, so the fasting criterion would be 120 mg/dl.

ORAL GLUCOSE TOLERANCE TEST. The oral glucose tolerance test (OGTT) should be performed in the morning. Before testing the patient must fast for 10 to 16 hours, following a period of at least 3 days of unrestricted diet containing at least 150 gm of carbohydrate per day, and during this period normal exercise should be encouraged. Also, as shown in Table 1-1, many drugs are known to influence glucose tolerance. When possible, these drugs should be discontinued for at least 3 days prior to the OGTT. It should be recognized that certain drugs are known to interfere with various laboratory tests for serum glucose (see Table 4 of [12]). During the test, the patient should remain seated and should not smoke, drink coffee, or eat food until the test is completed. For nonpregnant adults, a fasting blood sample is collected, and 75 gm of glucose dissolved in no more than 400 cc is ingested over a 5-minute period. Blood samples are collected at 30-minute intervals for 2 hours. As shown in Figure 1-1 (p. 7), a fasting plasma glucose of less than 140 mg/dl coupled with a 2-hour value of 200 mg/dl or more is diagnostic of diabetes mellitus, providing at least one value between ½ and 1½ hours is equal to or greater than 200 mg/dl. The diagnosis should not be made unless the above criteria are present on two separate occasions.

The diagnosis of impaired glucose tolerance in nonpregnant adults is indicated when the fasting value is less than 140 mg/dl and the 2-hour value during an OGTT is between 140 and 200 mg/dl. Intervening values during the glucose tolerance test must be greater than or equal to 200 mg/dl. A 2-hour plasma glucose level of less than 140 mg/dl effectively rules out the diagnosis of diabetes mellitus.

URINALYSIS. The diagnosis of diabetes mellitus should not be made as a result of the presence of glucose in the urine. The reasons for this are threefold: (1) the patient may have renal glucosuria, a nondiabetic condition; (2) use of the copper-reduction reaction (Clinitest) can be positive if reducing substances (e.g., fructose, salicylates) other than glucose are present in the urine; and (3) the correlation between urinary glucose and plasma glucose in many instances is poor. However, the finding of glucose concentrations of 1 to 2% in the urine should prompt the physician to evaluate the possibility of diabetes.

RANDOM PLASMA GLUCOSE. The presence of the well-known symptoms of diabetes coupled with a random plasma glucose of more than 200 mg/dl is considered indicative of diabetes in children. In contrast, in adults, the diagnosis of diabetes usually requires either a fasting plasma glucose or an oral glucose tolerance test. As discussed, a random plasma glucose in an adult above 200 mg/dl does not necessarily mean that the patient has diabetes mellitus. However, as for significant glucosuria, the finding of a markedly elevated random plasma glucose can be indicative of diabetes.

INTRAVENOUS GLUCOSE TOLERANCE TEST. The intravenous glucose tolerance test is reserved for those patients who have significant upper gastrointestinal problems. These include malabsorption, impaired absorption due to hyperthyroidism or hypothyroidism, and conditions that occur after upper gastrointestinal surgery such as gastrectomy. The drug history and pretest dietary management are the same as for the OGTT. The test should be conducted in the morning after an overnight fast, and conditions should be the same as for the OGTT. Glucose, at a dose of 0.5 gm per kilogram of body weight, is infused as a 25% or 50% solution and should be completed within 3 to 4 minutes. Blood determinations are obtained at 3, 5, 10, 20, 30, 40, 50, and 60 minutes after glucose infusion. The results are expressed by the k value, which is the coefficient of glucose disappearance (in percent per minute). When the glucose values (in milligrams per deciliter) are plotted against time on semilogarithmic paper, a straight line occurs, indicating that the decrease is exponential. From the graph, one then determines the time interval during which the plasma glucose has fallen from a certain level to half that level. This half-time ($t_{1/2}$) is usually obtained from values obtained between 10 and 60 minutes. The k value is then calculated as follows:

$$k = \frac{0.693}{t_{1/2}} \times 100\% \text{ per minute}$$

A k value less than 0.9 is indicative of diabetes mellitus. Values between 0.9 and 1.1 are considered borderline, but this relation to impaired glucose tolerance is not known. Values of 1.3 and above are considered normal.

PROVOCATIVE TESTS FOR THE DIAGNOSIS OF DIABETES MELLITUS. In earlier times, when the diagnosis of chemical diabetes was believed to be of extreme importance, certain provocative tests were employed to uncover very mild degrees of carbohydrate intolerance. These included the steroid provocative test and the tolbutamide tolerance test. In view of recent data clarifying the natural courses of carbohydrate intolerance, these tests are no longer considered standard practice.

THE CHLORPROPAMIDE ALCOHOL FLUSH. Recently, it has been reported that a facial flush caused by small amounts of ingested alcohol following short-term treatment with chlorpropamide occurs with an extremely high incidence in type II diabetics with a family history of diabetes mellitus [16]. The investigators further suggested that this chlorpropamide alcohol flush is a genetic marker for type II diabetes with autosomal dominant inheritance. However, data from another large study are contradictory [9], and further investigations are needed to clarify the usefulness of the chlorpropamide alcohol flush test.

Special Diagnostic Categories

ALTERED CARBOHYDRATE TOLERANCE IN CHILDREN. Usually, children present with type I diabetes, a condition that is generally manifested by classic signs and symptoms of insulin deficiency. If these are present and a random plasma glucose is greater than 200 mg/dl, the diagnosis of diabetes can safely be made.

In asymptomatic individuals, an oral glucose tolerance test may be indicated, and the requirements for testing are the same as for nonpregnant adults, except that the dose of glucose is 1.75 gm per kilogram of ideal body weight up to a maximum of 75 gm. In children, the OGTT is considered diagnostic for diabetes when *both* the fasting and 2-hour plasma glucose values are elevated. Specifically, the fasting plasma value must be equal to or greater than 140 mg/dl. As for nonpregnant adults, an elevated glucose concentration during the OGTT must be demonstrated at least once before the 2-hour value is obtained.

When the study is performed using capillary whole blood, the diagnosis of diabetes demands that the fasting value be equal to or greater than 120 mg/dl and the 2-hour value and an intervening value must be equal to or greater than 200 mg/dl. Impaired glucose tolerance in children is defined as a fasting plasma glucose value of less than 140 mg/dl and a 2-hour value of more than 140 mg/dl. If measurements are made

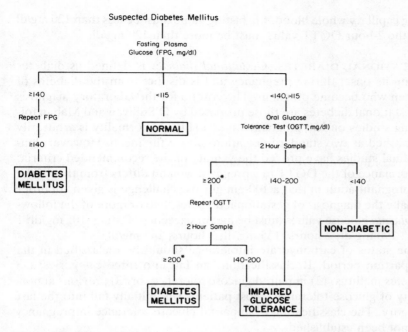

Figure 1-1. Diagnostic protocol: Suspected diabetes mellitus in nonpregnant adults. FPG, fasting plasma glucose; OGTT, oral glucose tolerance test. *At least one plasma value between administration of glucose and 2-hour sample must be ≥ 200 mg/dl.

using capillary whole blood, the fasting value must be less than 120 mg/dl
and the 2-hour OGTT value must be more than 120 mg/dl.

GESTATIONAL DIABETES. *Gestational diabetes* is defined as diabetes
having its onset during pregnancy and is distinct from the diabetes of
women who become pregnant. The criteria for the laboratory diagnosis
of gestational diabetes are those proposed by O'Sullivan and Mahan following studies on 750 pregnant women [14]. Abnormality is arbitrarily
established as two standard deviations above the mean. However, longitudinal studies have proved the validity of the recommended criteria.
Performance of the OGTT in a pregnant woman differs from that of the
nonpregnant adult in that a 100-gm glucose challenge is given. In order
to make the diagnosis of gestational diabetes, two or more of the following *plasma* glucose values must be met or exceeded: fasting, 105 mg/dl; 1
hour, 190 mg/dl; 2 hours, 165 mg/dl; 3 hours, 145 mg/dl.

The status of carbohydrate intolerance should be reclassified in the
postpartum period. Reclassification can fall into three categories: (1)
diabetes mellitus, (2) impaired glucose tolerance, or (3) previous abnormality of glucose tolerance. Most patients will initially fall into the last
category. The classification of impaired glucose tolerance in pregnancy
has not been established.

DISCUSSION

Establishment of the diagnosis of diabetes mellitus is straightforward
when the signs and symptoms of severe insulin deficiency are present, as
with ketoacidosis or the hyperglycemic, hyperosmolar, nonketotic syndrome. Fortunately, most diabetics do not present with such severe
biochemical abnormalities. This is especially true for type II diabetics,
who may be found to have glucosuria on a routine urinalysis. With the
finding of glucosuria, the physician must determine if the patient's carbohydrate tolerance is within normal limits or if an abnormality exists. In
the latter instance, the physician must decide if this is due to frank diabetes or if the patient may be more appropriately classified as having impaired glucose tolerance. As indicated in Figure 1-1 and in the accompanying text, the laboratory approach is simple and direct. However, in
order to ensure that the correct diagnosis is made, the physician must be
familiar with the protocols for performance of the fasting plasma glucose
and oral glucose tolerance tests and must be especially cognizant of drugs
that influence glucose homeostasis. As was discussed, there is currently a
new emphasis on reclassification of patients formerly diagnosed as chemical diabetics. These patients, now classified as having impaired glucose
tolerance, have a very good chance of never developing frank diabetes.
Thus these patients, correctly diagnosed, should not have to suffer the
socioeconomic sanctions that frequently accompany the diagnosis of

diabetes mellitus. Among others, these sanctions include difficulty in obtaining life insurance, decreased chances of finding new employment, and in some cases a negative perception of the patient by family and friends. Of course, those patients with impaired glucose tolerance should be reevaluated on a periodic basis or if clinical indications of diabetes develop.

Perhaps the most difficult decision the physician faces in diagnosing diabetes is whether or not to perform an oral glucose tolerance test when the fasting plasma glucose is normal. The factors in pregnancy that are associated with a high incidence of gestational diabetes have been previously delineated. The prevailing evidence concerning glucose control and complications of pregnancy indicates that good control is beneficial. In the absence of classic symptoms in the nonpregnant state, the physician must decide on the basis of the history and physical examination whether to pursue the diagnosis vigorously. Clearly, this problem arises most frequently with type II diabetics, whose disease usually has an insidious onset. It must be appreciated that although the genetics of type II diabetes are unclear, a genetic factor appears to be important in the etiology. In addition, environmental factors such as obesity and current drug therapy must be considered. Occasionally, certain diabetic complications can precede overt glucose intolerance, especially in type II diabetes. These complications may be unexplained sensory or motor neuropathies or a variety of ophthalmologic problems. If a potential diabetic complication exists that is known to benefit by improved control, the physician should be thorough in the diagnostic approach.

The newer criteria for the diagnosis of diabetes simplify the classification of the patient. Beyond this initial step of defining a diagnostic category lie the problems of identifying the severity of the carbohydrate disorder and determining methods to assess the benefits of any therapy provided. Since a given patient may move from one category to another, familiarity with the methods available for diagnosis as well as management is helpful. For these reasons, it seems appropriate to consider briefly those laboratory tests employed in the ongoing assessment and management of the patient with diabetes.

Laboratory Tests Used in the Management of Diabetes
URINE GLUCOSE. Normal individuals, free of diabetes mellitus and/or renal glucosuria, usually excrete well under 100 mg of glucose per 24 hours. The amount of glucose excreted over a 24-hour period is the only quantitative test for urine sugar in general usage. The amount of glucose excreted over a period of time can be a valuable indicator of current control and useful in planning treatment. On occasion, the physician may be surprised to learn that 24-hour glucose excretion is considerable despite apparent good control as determined by repeated plasma glucose measurements. In the past, it was said that spillage of no more than 10% of

ingested carbohydrate represents good control. Obviously, with today's emphasis on frequent urine and plasma glucose monitoring, coupled with multiple daily injections or even continuous infusions of insulin, the goal of a 24-hour glucose excretion should be a return toward normalcy. The 24-hour urinary glucose is limited by the difficulties in obtaining a 24-hour urine sample on an outpatient basis and often by poor patient compliance. The introduction of hemoglobin $A1_c$ ($HbA1_c$) as a means of measuring chronic glucose control has partially replaced the use of the 24-hour urinary glucose test.

At present, assessment of diabetic control in most patients is carried out by semiquantitative testing for urinary glucose. Insulin-dependent patients usually test their urine before each meal and at bedtime, whereas non–insulin-dependent patients may also assess urine glucose 2 to 3 hours after eating. In addition to obtaining urine specimens at the periods that have been indicated, many diabetologists recommend collecting and testing a second-voided urine specimen. The second-voided specimen is obtained 30 minutes after the bladder is emptied and immediately following ingestion of varying amounts of water. The argument for the necessity of the second-voided specimen is that it more accurately reflects the patient's metabolic status (plasma glucose) at the time that the sample is collected. In view of the extra effort required to obtain the double-voided specimen, several recent studies have questioned the usefulness of this procedure [3,5].

The methodology employed for semiquantitative measurements of urinary glucose is either the copper-reduction reaction (Clinitest) or the glucose oxidase reaction (Clinistix, Diastix, Tes-Tape). As mentioned previously, Clinitest can give false-positive results in the presence of certain reducing substances such as salicylates, ascorbic acid, and fructose. Although the glucose oxidase test is specific for glucose, false-negative results can be obtained in patients ingesting aspirin and L-dopa. The validity of semiquantitative measurements of urine glucose as an index of carbohydrate control has been questioned by Feldman and Lebovitz [4]. In their study, 513 separate urine specimens were fortified with glucose to a final concentration of ½%. When these samples were tested by the four semiquantitative methods already listed, correct estimation occurred only 40% of the time. Twenty-three percent of the samples were underestimated, especially with the use of Clinistix and Diastix. Overestimation occurred in 34% of the specimens tested and was most frequent when Clinitest was used. Tes-Tape was sensitive for detecting glucose and avoided false-negative tests, but was a poor discriminator of glucose concentrations above ½%. Furthermore, a recent large study found a poor correlation between plasma and urine glucose [11]. For these studies, quantitative and semiquantitative measurements of urinary glucose were conducted on second voided urine specimens, and blood for plasma glucose measurements was obtained 20 to 30 minutes before the second urine collection. Semiquantitative analysis for glucose was found to be negative 90% of the time when the plasma glucose was below 150 mg/dl. Also, when the urine glucose concentration was 1 to 2%, the plasma glucose was found to be above 200 mg/dl 98% of the time. The investigators concluded that the errors associated with urine glucose in the range of trace to 2 + (1%) are too great for urine glucose measurements to serve as a substitute for plasma glucose in assessing diabetic control.

CAPILLARY BLOOD GLUCOSE. Many recent studies have shown that frequent measurements of capillary blood glucose levels by diabetics at home result in improved carbohydrate control [18]. These home blood glucose monitoring programs have been made possible by the availability of glucose oxidase-impregnated paper strips, which allow the patient to make rapid determinations of blood glucose levels. Some techniques require the usage of a reflectance meter (Glucometer and StatTek), whereas others require only visual interpretation (e.g., Chemstrip bG and Visidex). Studies comparing these rapid measurements of capillary blood glucose levels with plasma glucose levels indicate an excellent correlation in most instances [19]. Thus, compliant and properly instructed patients can conveniently and at reasonable cost provide important information concerning their carbohydrate control at significant times during the day. The ability of patients to adhere to home monitoring programs for long periods of time and the actual benefits of long-term improved control are yet to be established.

GLYCOSYLATED HEMOGLOBIN. HbA1$_c$ is the stable product of a nonenzymatic reaction between glucose and the N-terminal valines of the B chains of hemoglobin A. This glycosylated hemoglobin is formed slowly and continuously throughout the 120-day life span of a red cell. The levels of HbA1$_c$ are increased in diabetics above normal (4–6%) and reflect the mean serum plasma glucose concentration over the preceding several months. The latter observation has provided diabetologists with an opportunity to evaluate the clinical utility of glycosylated hemoglobin in several settings [7]. Although high concentrations of HbA1$_c$ are specific for diabetes mellitus, this measurement is not very useful as a diagnostic test, since it is less sensitive than the OGTT. As an indicator of diabetic control, this determination seems to be most useful in type I diabetes and diabetes in pregnancy. However, during pregnancy, blood glucose levels normally fall and diabetic values must be compared to the appropriate controls. There is also a good correlation between the percentage of glycosylated hemoglobin and fasting serum glucose concentration in type II diabetes. Because the glycosylated hemoglobin level is an integration of carbohydrate control over a 3-month period, levels should not be obtained more frequently than every 4 to 6 weeks and determination should be reserved as a confirmation of apparently good control. Glycosylated hemoglobin measurements are also being employed to readdress the question of the role of carbohydrate control in the development of chronic diabetic complications.

Finally, it should be recognized that there are small amounts of labile glycosylated hemoglobins, some of which become glycoslylated following short-term exposure to elevated glucose concentrations. Some of the methodologies for determining HbA1$_c$ levels may include these labile glycosylated hemoglobins, which could influence the interpretation of the results. These unwanted components can usually be removed by dialysis prior to determination of the HbA1$_c$.

Circulating Insulin, Proinsulin, and Connecting Peptide

Radioimmunoassays have been developed for circulating insulin, the precursor molecule of insulin (proinsulin), and the noninsulin component of proinsulin, connecting peptide (C-peptide). Because impaired glucose tolerance and diabetes are observed in association with both hypo- and hyperinsulinemia, measurement of insulin levels is rarely useful clinically. Also, patients receiving exogenous insulin uniformly develop antibodies that invalidate the usefulness of the usual radioimmunoassay for insulin. Clinical use of these assays is usually reserved for diagnosing the etiology of hypoglycemia.

In reviewing these newer methodologies for the assessment and management of glucose intolerance, it should be emphasized that the diagnostic criteria for diabetes have been simplified, not made more complex. The first step is careful determination of the need for testing, followed by correct testing procedures. With the correct diagnosis in hand, it is important to acknowledge that home monitoring programs have shown that carbohydrate intolerance can be significantly improved over the initial months. It appears that many insulin-dependent diabetics will be receiving continuous insulin infusions as outpatients within this decade. Both of these regimens require greater laboratory surveillance on the part of both the physician and the patient, and recent studies indicate that measurements of blood glucose are far superior to those that assess urinary glucose. Since these new programs are in their infancy, it is important that the physician continue to be knowledgeable about both the safety and the efficacy of the treatment programs and the laboratory procedures used in treatment planning as well as diagnosis.

REFERENCES

1. Bennett, P. H., et al.   Epidemiologic studies of diabetes in the Pima Indians. *Recent Prog. Horm. Res.* 32:333–371, 1976.
2. Craighead, J. E.   Viral diabetes mellitus in man and experimental animals. *Am. J. Med.* 70:127–134, 1981.
3. Davidson, M.   The case for routinely testing the first-voided urine specimen. *Diabetes Care* 4:443–444, 1981.

4. Feldman, J. M., and Lebovitz, F. L.   Tests for glucosuria. An analysis of factors that cause misleading results. *Diabetes* 22:115–121, 1973.
5. Guthrie, D. W., Hinnen, D., and Guthrie, R. A.   Single-voided vs. double-voided urine testing. *Diabetes Care* 2:269–271, 1979.
6. Jarett, R. S., and Keen, H.   Hyperglycemia and diabetes mellitus. *Lancet* 2:1009–1012, 1976.
7. Jovanovic, L., and Peterson, C. M.   The clinical utility of glycosylated hemoglobin. *Am. J. Med.* 70:331–338, 1981.
8. Karlsson, K., and Kjellmer, I.   The outcome of diabetic pregnancies in relation to the mother's blood sugar level. *Am. J. Obstet. Gynecol.* 112:213–220, 1972.
9. Kobberling, J., et al.   The chlorpropamide alcohol flush. Lack of specificity for familial non-insulin dependent diabetes. *Diabetologia* 19:359–363, 1980.
10. Miller, E., et al.   Elevated maternal hemoglobin $A1_c$ in early pregnancy and major congenital anomalies in infants of diabetic mothers. *N. Engl. J. Med.* 304:1331–1334, 1981.
11. Morris, L. R., McGee, J. A., and Kitabchi, A. E.   Correlation between plasma and urine glucose in diabetes. *Ann. Intern. Med.* 94:469–471, 1981.
12. National Diabetes Data Group.   Classification and diagnosis of diabetes mellitus and other categories of glucose intolerance. *Diabetes* 28:1039–1057, 1979.
13. Nerup, J., and Lernmark, A.   Autoimmunity in insulin-dependent diabetes mellitus. *Am. J. Med.* 70:135–141, 1981.
14. O'Sullivan, J. M., and Mahan, C. M.   Criteria for the oral glucose tolerance test in pregnancy. *Diabetes* 13:278–285, 1964.
15. O'Sullivan, J. M., and Mahan, C. M.   Prospective study of 352 young patients with chemical diabetes. *N. Engl. J. Med.* 278:1038–1041, 1968.
16. Pyke, D. A., and Leslie, R. D.   Chlorpropamide-alcohol flushing: A definition of its relation to non-insulin dependent diabetes. *Br. Med. J.* 2:1521–1522, 1978.
17. Rotter, J. I., and Rimoin, D. L.   The genetics of the glucose intolerance disorders. *Am. J. Med.* 70:116–126, 1981.
18. Symposium on Home Blood Glucose Monitoring.   *Diabetes Care* 3:57–186, 1980.
19. Symposium on Blood Glucose Self-Monitoring.   *Diabetes Care* 4:392–426, 1981.

2 Anterior Pituitary Disorders: Hypopituitarism, Prolactin, Growth Hormone

Laurence S. Jacobs

The hypothalamic-pituitary unit is a major component of the body's control systems for regulating many vital functions. The hypothalamus serves as an integrative way station for temperature regulation, control of feeding behavior, satiety, and water balance; sympathetic nervous system outflow; and the body's integrated responses to stress. Further, the neurosecretions of the hypothalamus traverse the hypophyseal portal vessels to regulate the pituitary [5].

The pituitary gland secretes six hormones of major clinical interest: luteinizing hormone (LH) and follicle-stimulating hormone (FSH), thyroid-stimulating hormone (TSH), adrenocorticotropic hormone (ACTH), growth hormone (GH), and prolactin (PRL). In most instances, secretion of these hormones from the pituitary follows the stimulus of hypothalamic releasing factors acting on the pituitary. For gonadotropins and TSH, clinical studies using releasing hormones have indicated that negative feedback operates primarily at the level of the pituitary gland. Systemic treatment with sex steroid and thyroid hormones leads to blunting of the pituitary secretory responses to the respective exogenous releasing hormone. The positive and negative feedback effects of estradiol on gonadotropin secretion have also been demonstrated to occur directly on the pituitary gland. A recent finding of major importance for the pituitary-adrenal axis has been the characterization of a corticotropin-releasing factor from the hypothalamus [61]. This 41-amino acid peptide releases ACTH and β-endorphin [15] from isolated adenohypophyseal cells. Since these actions can be inhibited by prior glucocorticoid treatment in vitro, the pituitary may turn out to be a major negative feedback site in vivo for this system as well [43,61].

In addition to the regulation of classic hormonal peripheral target organs such as the adrenal cortex, the thyroid, and the gonad, the pituitary directs growth in the child and lactation in the adult woman via the secretion of GH and PRL. The regulation of GH and PRL may require dual hypothalamic influences. For GH, a large number of physiologic studies have supported the separate existence of a GH-releasing factor, and one has now been isolated and characterized [25a]. In addition, somatostatin has been shown by a number of investigators to participate in the regulation of GH and thyrotropin [4,17,58]. For PRL, the major hypothalamic influence has long been acknowledged to be inhibitory [45]. Although some controversy still continues in this area, many investigators now believe that dopamine is the major functionally relevant hypothalamic PRL-inhibiting factor.

The investigation of anterior pituitary disease necessarily focuses on these six hormones and their disordered secretion or production. The discussion in this chapter will first deal with hypopituitarism, the clinical state characterized by deficiencies in various pituitary hormones. Second, discussion will focus on the consequences of excessive production of two hormones, PRL and GH. Finally, a fourth section will address the relationship between short stature and possible GH deficiency.

Hypopituitarism

CLINICAL CONSIDERATIONS

This discussion will focus on hypopituitarism in the adult, since hypopituitarism in the child commonly leads to retarded growth and development. A wide spectrum of disorders may cause hypopituitarism, the neoplastic, vascular, and idiopathic categories being the most prevalent. A listing is provided in Table 2-1.

Processes that raise intracranial pressure or create mass effects often result in deficient secretion of GH and gonadotropins. For obscure reasons, the secretory integrity of GH and the gonadotropins is more labile than that of the other pituitary hormones. As a result, deficiency of GH and hypogonadism occur 60 to 80% of the time with mass lesions [47], whereas clinical deficiency of TSH and/or ACTH with resulting target organ hypofunction occurs only about 15% of the time [55]. In roughly twice as many instances (30%), basal thyroidal and adrenal function is normally maintained, but deficient secretory reserve of TSH or ACTH can be demonstrated by thyrotropin releasing hormone (TRH) tests or with metyrapone [55]. Reduction of the secretory reserve of PRL occurs only about 5 to 10% of the time with nonfunctional adenomas. Diabetes insipidus and other evidence of disordered hypothalamic function such as disordered regulation of sleep, appetite, or temperature are very rarely seen with pituitary adenomas. These manifestations, along with evidence of increased intracranial pressure, usually herald the presence of structural hypothalamic disease.

Pituitary Tumors

Pituitary adenomas are benign tumors that represent 8 to 10% of all adult intracranial neoplasms. They occur primarily in the middle decades of life, with a roughly equal sex incidence. The great majority of these tumors store little secretory product and therefore appear "chromophobic" by light microscopy whether they are functionless or produce GH or PRL in excess. The natural history of these tumors is not known with certainty, but most observers agree that those causing clinical dis-

Table 2-1. Etiologies of Hypopituitarism

Hypothalamic tumors
  Chordoma
  Craniopharyngioma
  Glioma
  Meningioma
Idiopathic
Infections
  Viral
  Fungal
  Tuberculosis
Infiltrations
  Hemochromatosis
  Histiocytosis (Hand-Schüller-Christian syndrome)
  Sarcoidosis
Metastatic tumors
  Breast
  Lung
Obstructive (Hydrocephalus)
Pituitary tumors
  Functional
    Cushing's disease
    Prolactinoma
  Nonfunctional
Radiotherapy
Surgical Ablation
Trauma
Vascular
  Carotid aneurysm
  Cavernous sinus thrombosis
  Postpartum necrosis (Sheehan's syndrome)
  Temporal arteritis

ease probably evolve slowly over many years. Accordingly, their effects develop insidiously and may be apparent only in retrospect. The major exceptions to this general rule are the locally aggressive, recurring tumors occurring after total bilateral adrenalectomy for Cushing's syndrome (Nelson's syndrome). A high prevalence and an indolent growth rate for most pituitary adenomas are consistent with the fact that carefully performed autopsy studies have revealed such adenomas as apparently incidental findings in 10 to 40% of unselected autopsies. Most of these adenomas, like the majority of those that come to clinical attention during life, contain and presumably secrete PRL. Whether those that go undetected until after death represent a biologically distinct entity as compared with those that come to clinical attention during life is not known.

Hypopituitarism complicating pituitary adenomas is more often partial than complete. It is rare for pituitary adenomas to compress the stalk, infundibulum, or roof of the third ventricle or to cause diabetes insipidus. The severity of the target gland hormone and related chemical abnormalities tends to be somewhat less in hypopituitarism than in primary disease of the thyroid, adrenal, or gonad. Clinical manifestations may also be less severe.

Functional pituitary adenomas, in addition to mass effects, may influence extratumorous hormone secretion by hormonal mechanisms. The suppression of gonadotropin secretion by hyperprolactinemic states is well known (see the subsequent discussion), and cortisol excess is associated with suppression of GH, gonadotropins, PRL, and TSH. Hypothyroidism does not generally ensue, but amenorrhea is very common in Cushing's syndrome and Cushing's disease.

Since pituitary adenomas make up such a sizable portion of the adult hypopituitary population, it is useful to put the spectrum of these adenomas into perspective. The prevalence of the various types is given in Table 2-2. The great majority overproduce PRL or GH, with a small group having Cushing's disease and about one-fifth of the total having nonfunctional tumors. It has become clear from recent studies [52,60] that ACTH-producing microadenomas (less than 10 mm in diameter) are the most common cause of Cushing's syndrome. In the nonfunctional tumors, which make their presence known by producing neurologic or hormonal deficiency symptoms, the size at the time of clinical detection tends to be larger than that of hormone-producing adenomas that cause distinct clinical syndromes. It is not known whether growth rates of functional tumors differ from those of nonfunctional tumors. At least some patients with nonfunctional tumors can be shown to have elevated serum concentrations of free alpha subunit, the common peptide chain in LH, FSH, TSH, and human chorionic gonadotropin (hCG) [37,49]. Insufficient data make it impossible to know in what proportion of such patients the alpha subunit is high; at present, assay capability for alpha subunit is not widespread.

Not all enlargement of the sella turcica is neoplastic, perhaps the best example of hyperplasia being the lactotrope hyperplasia and sellar enlargement that occur during normal pregnancy, primarily under estrogen influence. Another example that may cause transitory confusion by simulating a pituitary adenoma is the reversible sellar enlargement and

Table 2-2. The Spectrum of Pituitary Adenomas

Adenoma	Incidence
Hormone producing	
Hyperprolactinemia	60–65%
Acromegaly	15%
Cushing's disease	2–5%
Glycopolypeptides	Rare
Nonfunctional	15–20%

Table 2-3. Primary Empty Sella: Clinical and Pathologic Features

Feature	Incidence
Clinical	
Obesity	90%
Female sex	85%
Headache	70%
Pseudotumor cerebri	15%
Serendipitous finding	Often
Cerebrospinal fluid rhinorrhea	Rare
Visual impairment	None
Partial hypopituitarism	10%
Pathologic	
Structural defect in diaphragma sellae at postmortem	20–40%
Empty sella at postmortem	5%

thyrotrope cell hyperplasia that infrequently occur in primary hypothyroidism. This condition, which probably is rarer in adults than in children, is quickly identified with the clinical appreciation of a goiter and the finding of an elevated TSH value [62].

Empty Sella Syndrome

Another entity that may mimic a pituitary adenoma is the primary empty sella syndrome [32,40,65]. Generally coming to medical attention via an abnormal skull x-ray that is obtained because of persistent headaches, this syndrome occurs predominantly in obese women and only very rarely is accompanied by convincing evidence of pituitary hormonal deficiency. The main characteristics of this fairly common entity are outlined in Table 2-3. It is thought that obesity or other unknown factors predispose a subgroup of these patients, with presumably congenital defects in the diaphragma sellae, to tissue loss in the pituitary due to persistent cerebrospinal fluid pressure against the adenohypophysis.

Primary empty sella requires clear differentiation from a sella that is empty as a result of the course or treatment of a preexistent disease, such as hypophysitis, adenoma with infarction, or radiotherapy. The most efficient method of discriminating between primary empty sella and pituitary adenoma is by the use of modern computed tomography (CT) scanners, which can reliably detect cerebrospinal fluid density within the confines of the sella turcica.

Postpartum Necrosis of the Pituitary

A major discrepancy in etiologies of hypopituitarism between the sexes is the occurrence of postpartum necrosis of the pituitary. Although lactational failure may be the first hormonal symptom following such an event, this is only one of many presentations. Galactorrhea may also occur, probably due to relatively high infarction near or in the infundibulum, thereby creating a functional stalk section. The patterns of vascular supply from the hypothalamus to the pituitary are highly variable in experimental animals, and there is reason to think that this variability applies to women as well. It is not necessary for major external blood loss to occur for pituitary necrosis to take place. The vessels of the stalk are thought to be prone to vasospasm at the time of delivery, either because of estrogen sensitization or some pressor factors. Complete pituitary infarction is the exception rather than the rule, and many combinations of hormone deficiencies have been described.

Other Causes of Hypopituitarism
Iatrogenic hypopituitarism may be induced surgically or radiotherapeutically in the course of treatment of breast or prostatic carcinoma in adults or following radiotherapy directed at nasopharyngeal cancers. Basal skull meningitides are happily much less common now than they were 25 years ago, and the infectious, infiltrative, and metastatic etiologies listed in Table 2-1 together make up only a small fraction of total adult cases. Substantial histopathologic and biochemical evidence suggests that histiocytosis and sarcoidosis interfere with hypothalamic function, whereas hemochromatosis affects the pituitary directly. The influence of metastatic tumors on the hypothalamic-pituitary unit is primarily exerted via hypothalamic deposits, the pituitary not being a common metastatic site [66].

Hypopituitarism following radiotherapy, usually partial, may occur 10 years or more after the delivery of ionizing radiation [14]. In some cases, it is thought that vasculitis in the portal vessels may be the proximate cause of such hypopituitarism; in others, the effects are probably produced directly on the adenohypophysis. The efficacy of radiotherapy in limiting the growth of pituitary adenomas is reflected by the fact that the radiologic and symptomatic recurrence rate over about 15 years was halved in patients with seemingly nonfunctional adenomas who received postoperative radiation treatment.

A form of reversible hypothalamic hypopituitarism has been reported in patients with traumatic comas, generally from motor vehicle accidents [50]. Finally, although clinicians often wonder about the adequacy of pituitary function in patients with anorexia nervosa, the hormonal abnormalities in these patients are usually restricted to those related to reproductive function.

DIAGNOSTIC METHODS
The diagnostic approach to the patient with a suspected pituitary tumor and/or hypopituitarism has two components: neuroradiologic and en-

docrine [59,69]. The neuroradiologic evaluation attempts to define the presence or absence of a mass lesion, extension of tumor beyond the sella turcica, and involvement of the optic chiasm or adjacent structures— in sum, the anatomic characteristics of the disorder. The endocrine evaluation attempts to identify hormonal hypersecretion, if present, and to assess the pituitary reserves of the other hormones.

Neuroradiologic Evaluations

PLAIN SKULL X-RAYS. As a first step, skull films may provide evidence of pituitary enlargement suggestive of tumor. Various methods have been advocated to measure sella size or volume. In practical terms, however, the presence of clear distortion requires further evaluation; a normal film with a strong clinical suspicion of tumor is an indication for polytomography.

POLYTOMOGRAPHY OF THE SELLA. Microadenomas may cause focal bulging or distortion of the sella floor that may be detected by multidirectional polytomography.

COMPUTED TOMOGRAPHY. With improved technology, CT scanning has emerged as a reliable and important tool in the management of pituitary tumors. Microadenomas have even been detected in some series. One modification has utilized metrizamide cisternography in combination with CT scanning to delineate further the extent of tumor.

PNEUMOENCEPHALOGRAPHY. Pneumoencephalography (PEG) has been largely supplanted by CT scanning, although it is still used by some. In ambiguous cases, this procedure may prove necessary to confirm an empty sella syndrome.

CAROTID ANGIOGRAPHY. Angiography may be required to exclude aneurysmal lesions in the pituitary. Such studies also prove helpful in defining major vessel involvement with tumor and the extent of suprasellar or parasellar tumor extension.

Other Neurologic Evaluations

VISUAL FIELDS. Assessment of visual fields using Goldmann perimetery provides an indirect assessment of the extent of tumor impingement on the optic chiasm.

Endocrine Evaluation

GROWTH HORMONE. L-dopa and exercise may not be as reliable in adults as in children in provoking GH secretory responses. Normal serum values in adults are generally below 5 ng/ml in the fasting state and frequently are below the sensitivity limits of the assay (0.2–1.0 ng/ml).

The various provocative tests for GH are described in the section on short stature.

PROLACTIN. Normal PRL values in men are below 20 ng/ml and in women are below 25 ng/ml. Concentrations are higher between 3 and 7 AM than at any other time during the day and tend to fall during the morning. The normal values given are based on sampling between 8 and 10 AM. Values are very rarely undetectable and may be well within the normal range in patients with no other identifiable pituitary function. Secretion may be provoked by insulin hypoglycemia in about two-thirds of normal adults. If the dose of insulin is raised so that the attained hypoglycemia is profound (0.2 units/kg, with blood sugar frequently below 20 mg/dl), PRL responses occur in most subjects.

Other provocative tests include administration of chlorpromazine, TRH, and metoclopramide. Dopamine antagonism is probably the mechanism whereby chlorpromazine and metoclopramide are effective. Chlorpromazine may be given intramuscularly in a dose of 0.7 mg/kg up to a maximum of 50 mg, and samples obtained at 0, 15, 30, 60, 120, and 180 minutes. Postural hypotension and sedation are major side effects, and since a normal response is only a doubling of PRL, it may sometimes be hard to know when one is dealing with a reduced secretory reserve. This test is not recommended for diagnostic use.

Metoclopramide, a much more potent PRL secretagogue, is given intravenously in a standard 10-mg dose, and samples are taken at 0, 15, 30, 60, and 120 minutes. The normal response is an approximately six-fold rise in PRL. The drug may be given orally in the same dose, which results in peak values nearly as high, but with a delayed and prolonged time course. Values may remain elevated for 4 to 6 hours after intravenous administration and for 9 to 12 hours after oral administration of metoclopramide.

TRH elicits peak PRL responses about 30% lower than those seen with metoclopramide. In women, secretory responses are roughly double those of men [29,31].

LUTEINIZING HORMONE AND FOLLICLE-STIMULATING HORMONE STIMULATION. Secretory reserve of LH and FSH is assessed after intravenous administration of gonadotropin-releasing hormone (GnRH). The most commonly employed dose is 100 μg. Samples may be obtained at 0, 15, 30, 60, and 120 minutes; peak responses usually occur at 30 minutes. In men, responsivity declines with age [56]. In women, responsivity varies substantially during the menstrual cycle, the largest responses occurring at midcycle. Except immediately postpartum, FSH responsivity to GnRH is much less than LH responsivity. A normal LH response up to age 60 is a minimum twofold increase over basal values. The average normal increase in young men is nearly sevenfold, and in old men threefold.

Clomiphene activates LH and FSH secretion by blocking estrogen receptor sites, thus interfering with normal negative feedback. It is generally accepted that the major site of clomiphene action in vivo is the hypothalamus. Clomiphene is given orally at a dose of 50 mg twice daily or 100 mg twice daily for 5 days, and the LH and FSH values are determined on the last day of treatment and again 2 to 3 days thereafter. Normal individuals demonstrate increments over baseline of two- to fourfold.

THYROID-STIMULATING HORMONE STIMULATION. TSH increases promptly after intravenous administration of TRH, rising to a peak in 15 to 20 minutes. The normal responses have been studied extensively [29]. The minimum normal response is a TSH increment of 5μU/ml, except in older men, who may normally show rises as small as 2 μU/ml. Any increases to values exceeding 40 μU/ml should be considered abnormal.

ADRENOCORTICOTROPIC HORMONE. Interpretation of ACTH measurements is beset by difficulties that derive from the heterogeneity of circulating ACTH, its lability, and the fact that it is frequently within the normal range in patients with Cushing's disease. Normal values are generally between 20 and 80 pg/ml in the fasting state in the morning. ACTH measurements are useful in Addison's disease and Nelson's syndrome, in which values ordinarily exceed 300 pg/ml. The evaluation of suspected adrenocortical insufficiency is outlined in Chapter 7.

COMBINED TESTING. The evaluation of suspected hypopituitarism and the definition of normal reserve may be facilitated by administering insulin, GnRH, and TRH simultaneously and obtaining appropriately timed samples. In this fashion, a fairly complete hormonal profile may be obtained, including responses to stimulation of GH and cortisol (insulin hypoglycemia), PRL and TSH (TRH), and LH and FSH (GnRH). A suggested protocol would include the following:

Time (min)	Glucose	GH	Cortisol	TSH	PRL	LH	FSH
0	x	x	x	x	x	x	x

Administer:
500 μg TRH
100 μg GnRH
0.05—0.10 unit/kg insulin

15	x			x	x	x	x
30	x		x	x	x	x	x
45	x	x	x	x	x		
60	x	x	x	x	x	x	x
90	x	x	x				
120						x	x

DISCUSSION
Although the focus of the initial work-up will vary from patient to patient, depending on the presenting symptoms and signs, most if not all patients suspected of having hypopituitarism should undergo both neuroradiologic and neuroendocrine evaluation. The clinical decision-making process usually involves a judgment as to how much of each is ideal for any given patient. Since polytomography of the sella turcica is useful primarily for detection of subtle abnormalities not appreciable on standard skull x-rays, it is of limited utility in patients with large sellar or parasellar masses and evident bone destruction or sellar expansion on routine x-rays. CT scans are useful in this setting because an appreciable percentage of pituitary adenomas (>50%) demonstrate contrast enhancement, and for delineation of suprasellar, lateral, and infrasellar (sinus) adenoma extension when these features are present.

In those patients whose primary presenting symptoms reflect neurologic problems related to a mass lesion, it is quite common for the initial history and physical examination to uncover evidence that is suggestive of hypopituitarism. The major reasons for the frequent failure of patients to highlight their endocrine-related symptoms appear to be two: first, they commonly have much more dramatic and disabling neurologic symptoms; second, the clinical endocrine manifestations of hypopituitarism are commonly milder than those of primary target organ disease. The latter distinction carries over into the biochemical quantitation of organ hypofunction as well. It is relatively common to find only marginally abnormal values for total serum thyroxine or cortisol in patients with hyposecretion of TSH or ACTH, respectively. Accordingly, the clinician's index of suspicion must remain high in the appropriate neurologic setting, and measurements of tropic and target organ hormones must be carried out.

Because excessive secretion of PRL is common in pituitary adenomas, and because it frequently occurs with hypothalamic disease (due to interference with the normally tonic inhibition of PRL), measurement of PRL is given a central position in the endocrine evaluation of hypopituitarism. Although rare in organic hypopituitarism, PRL deficiency may have a genetic basis and may be linked with pseudohypoparathyroidism [7].

In the evaluation of suspected thyroidal insufficiency, the serum thyroxine (T_4) is far more useful than the serum triiodothyronine (T_3) concentration. The finding of a TSH concentration within the normal range in the face of hypothyroxinemia and compatible clinical symptoms mandates the testing of TSH responsivity to TRH if a precise endocrine diagnosis is to be made. One of the significant pitfalls in this area is the common occurrence of low levels of total T_4 in accutely ill patients with a variety of nonendocrine diseases [34]. This so-called euthyroid sick syndrome is ordinarily accompanied not only by normal TSH measurements but also normal free T_4 measurements. The truly hypothyroid individual will have a depressed free T_4 concentration and elevated TSH if the disease is thyroidal (see Chap. 3).

The finding of a lowered serum cortisol value in a patient suspected of having hypopituitarism should lead first to a short ACTH stimulation test (see Chap. 7). If the adrenal response is normal, one may consider early ACTH deficiency to be the cause of the hypocortisolemia. It is both unnecessary and dangerous to test ACTH secretory reserve with metyrapone if the ACTH stimulation test is abnormal. In this instance, secretory reserve has already been challenged by cortisol deficiency and has demonstrated its failure to respond. Administration of metyrapone to such individuals may precipitate clinical shock.

It is rare for normally developed adult males to note significant changes in body hair, shaving frequency, or testicular size when gonadotropin deficiency is acquired in adult life. In fact, there may be few or no symptoms, including relatively good maintenance of potency. The depression of serum testosterone must be profound for deficient sexual function to occur. Even then, because the majority of testicular volume is composed of tubular elements, often no clinically appreciable change in testicular size may be noted. With profound gonadotropin deficiency, however, testicular atrophy is the rule.

Estrogen deficiency in hypopituitary women may be associated, if severe enough, with vaginal mucosal changes, uterine atrophy, and, rarely, a decrease in breast size. Much more subtle aberrations in hormonal status may be sufficient to disrupt the menstrual cycle and cause oligomenorrhea or amenorrhea.

It is usually true that pituitary tropic hormone responses to hypothalamic-releasing hormone injection can be used to discriminate the locus of disease, so long as adequate neuroradiologic localization studies have been carried out. However, the argument can be made that such precise endocrine localization is academic, since replacement therapy will ordinarily not be altered as a result of these studies. Further, so long as the patient is treated with supraphysiologic doses of glucocorticoids during stressful diagnostic or therapeutic procedures, the argument can be made that careful endocrine evaluation is relatively academic if neurosurgery is required, since reevaluation postoperatively will be necessary in any case.

Occasionally, the situation is not quite so simple diagnostically, as has been outlined in Figure 2-1, since values for TSH are not always normal or low when pituitary disease is present [28,42]. It is presumed that the occurrence of hypothyroidism in the face of apparently adequate TSH secretion may be best explained on the basis that some or most of the TSH produced may have been an altered molecule with impaired biologic reactivity [28].

This discussion has totally omitted mention of GH measurements. The

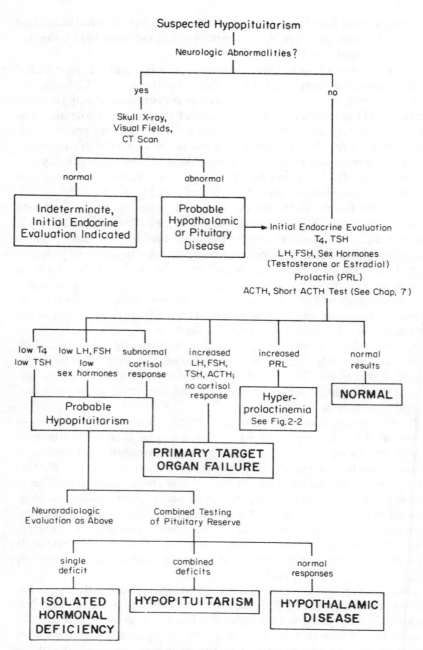

Figure 2-1. Diagnostic protocol: Suspected hypopituitarism. T₄, thyroxine; TSH, thyroid-stimulating hormone; LH, luteinizing hormone; FSH, follicle-stimulating hormone; ACTH, adrenocorticotropic hormone.

reasons are not very obscure; GH deficiency in the adult is not associated with any known clinical illness. Accordingly, delineation of GH secretory status is not immediately relevant to clinical health or disease, but rather serves as a marker for very subtle degrees of pituitary impairment in those circumstances in which most if not all other pituitary tropic hormonal functions are maintained intact. Accordingly, one can make the argument that estimation of GH secretory status in the adult with hypopituitarism is unnecessary except when systematic studies are being carried out.

Hyperprolactinemia

CLINICAL CONSIDERATIONS

One of the unexpected pieces of new information that resulted from the establishment of satisfactory radioimmunoassays for human PRL was the discovery that many apparently nonfunctional pituitary tumors secrete PRL.

The predominant hypothalamic control over PRL secretion is inhibitory; therefore, it is common for hyperprolactinemia to occur in settings of disease of the hypothalamus or interruption of the stalk, so long as the adenohypophysis does not totally infarct. Since the major physiologic inhibitor of PRL is probably dopamine, drugs that interfere with dopamine neurotransmission or deplete the hypothalamus of dopamine often result in hyperprolactinemia [20]. The drugs most commonly associated with hyperprolactinemia are listed in Table 2-4.

PRL secretion readily responds to a variety of psychic as well as physical stresses with increases in the secretion rate. Thus, not only the stress of insulin hypoglycemia but also the stresses of endoscopic procedures and even the anticipation of anesthesia or surgery may be associated with increases in PRL. The latter information has practical relevance in the interpretation of measurements performed on patients who are anxious

Table 2-4. Drugs Associated with Hyperprolactinemia

Individual Agent	Drug Class
Reserpine	Catechol depletor
Alpha-methyldopa	False neurotransmitter
Haloperidol	Butyrophenone*
Metoclopramide	Benzamide derivative*
Chlorpromazine	Phenothiazine*
Oral contraceptives	Estrogens

*Dopamine antagonists. Thiothixenes also fall into this category.

because of a probable diagnosis of pituitary tumor, an invasive procedure, or impending surgery.

Estrogens, including the relatively small amounts present in many oral contraceptives, are sufficient to stimulate PRL secretion in many women. Amenorrhea following the use of oral contraceptives may sometimes be associated with hyperprolactinemia. Not all hyperprolactinemia occurring in women who have just finished a course of oral contraceptives may be attributed to oral contraceptive medication; rather, in a significant fraction (50%) of such women, the oral contraceptive serves as the trigger that brings a preexistent microadenoma of the pituitary to the threshold of clinical detection. Alternatively, estrogens may serve as an etiologic factor in adenoma development [53]. Aberrations in the central nervous system (CNS) dopamine control of the lactotrope cell have been identified [18] and may conceivably play a separate role.

Because of the substantial number of women who remain amenorrheic for several months after discontinuation of chronic oral contraceptive therapy, it is now generally agreed that significant clinical concern is probably unwarranted unless menses have failed to resume after a minimum of 6 months after such therapy has ended. The coincident presence of galactorrhea in such post-pill amenorrheic women, however, should raise the clinical index of suspicion that hyperprolactinemia may exist.

The observation that TRH could stimulate PRL secretion has raised a host of questions about the relationship between PRL secretion and thyroid function. Mild PRL cell hyperplasia, with its concomitant hyperresponsiveness to provocative stimuli, probably exists in hypothyroidism, and the reverse (that is, suppressed PRL secretion) in thyrotoxicosis. In contrast to TSH secretion, however, PRL secretion is less tightly regulated by thyroid hormones, although the qualitative secretory dynamics are similar. The literature contains a number of case reports of galactorrhea with precocious puberty occurring in young girls with hypothyroidism [62]. Galactorrhea also may occur occasionally in adult women with this disorder. The exact reasons for the greater sensitivity of girls and women than of men and boys for this complication of hypothyroidism are not clear, but presumably the estrogen secretory status has a great deal to do with it.

Reserpine, a catecholamine depletor, alpha-methyldopa, a false neurotransmitter, and phenothiazines, butyrophenones, and benzamides such as metoclopramide, all dopamine antagonists, cause hyperprolactinemia. It appears likely that all major neuroleptics, which probably act by antagonizing dopamine action in the mesolimbic and mesocortical systems, also cause hyperprolactinemia by antagonism of dopamine in the tuberinfundibular dopamine system.

Other clinical conditions in which hyperprolactinemia occurs include hepatic cirrhosis and uremia. In both, immunocytochemical techniques have indicated pituitary PRL cell hyperplasia. To what extent PRL cell hyperplasia may precede or coexist with PRL adenomas during the natural history of tumor development is not known at present.

In considering the range of etiologies of hyperprolactinemia, by far the most common clinical circumstances encountered in which such an evaluation is needed are those in which oral contraceptives have been recently discontinued, other drugs such as neuroleptics have been administered, and the driving clinical consideration is amenorrhea, galactorrhea, or infertility.

It is worth emphasizing that 15 to 20% of women with proven PRL-secreting pituitary adenomas do not have galactorrhea as one of their presenting features. The estrogen deficiency that many such women experience probably plays an important role in determining breast responses to PRL excess. As a consequence, secondary amenorrhea alone without obvious cause is a good indication for measurement of PRL; about 35% of such patients are found to be hyperprolactinemic. If galactorrhea and amenorrhea (or oligomenorrhea) occur together, hyperprolactinemia coexists about 80% of the time. In contrast, galactorrhea with normal menses is usually associated with normal serum PRL concentrations [35].

DIAGNOSTIC METHODS
Endocrine Evaluation
PROLACTIN. Estimation of the average fasting PRL concentration remains the best practical discriminator between tumor and other causes of hyperprolactinemia. Due to the temporal variability in values, it is wise not to depend entirely on a single determination. Two to four samples obtained 20 to 30 minutes apart, preferably from an indwelling intravenous needle, should suffice. There is no evidence that PRL values measured by radioreceptor assay differ from radioimmunoassay values.

Normal PRL values in women range up to 25 ng/ml and in men up to 20 ng/ml.

STIMULATION AND SUPPRESSION TESTS. Unfortunately, none of the stimulation or suppression tests of PRL have proved useful in diagnostic discrimination between tumorous and nontumorous hyperprolactinemia. Although most patients with hyperprolactinemia due to tumor do not respond acutely to either TRH or chlorpromazine, this is also true of many patients with hyperprolactinemia not due to tumor. Administration of the standard test dose of L-dopa (0.5 gm) results in PRL suppression to less than 50% of baseline values in almost all patients with PRL-secreting tumors as well as in those with nontumorous hyperprolactinemia. Although it is not a practical diagnostic test for many reasons, dopamine infusion at several dose levels [2] does show a shifted dose-response relationship in hyperprolactinemia, and may offer a means to the biochemical discrimination of tumor from other causes as additional experience with the technique is accumulated.

Neuroradiologic Evaluations
Plain Skull X-Rays
Polytomography of the Sella
Computed Tomography
Pneumoencephalography
Carotid Angiography
(See the section on neuroradiologic evaluations of hypopituitarism, page 21.)

DISCUSSION
Evaluation of the patient with hyperprolactinemia begins with a careful history that pays special attention to medications and drug ingestion (Figure 2-2). Unless there are thyroidal, neurologic, or visual manifestations from a large pituitary adenoma, the physical examination is not often a source of important differential information. Neither the presence/absence nor the laterality of galactorrhea allows useful diagnostic inferences.

A serum thyroxine level should always be obtained in patients with hyperprolactinemia. Clinical experience has demonstrated that even experienced endocrinologists may sometimes be misled in young adults as well as in the elderly, in whom clinical manifestations of thyroid disease are known to be often subtle and occasionally virtually absent. Further, galactorrhea may occur in a setting of mild to moderate hypothyroidism; profound myxedema is not a prerequisite for galactorrhea or hyperprolactinemia. For entirely obscure reasons, thyrotoxicosis is occasionally associated with galactorrhea; as with hypothyroidism, appropriate thyroidal therapy is curative.

Most patients with PRL concentrations in excess of 100 ng/ml will be shown to have pituitary PRL-secreting adenomas. That diagnosis becomes virtually certain if the PRL is in excess of 250 ng/ml. A substantial fraction of patients with PRL concentrations between 25 and 100 ng/ml will also have tumors, but in this range, most of the drug-related and other etiologies are also found. In the spectrum of PRL values in patients with adenomas, only about 10% are below 40 ng/ml; nonetheless, marginally elevated values by no means rule out adenoma.

Many patients who harbor demonstrable pituitary adenomas have normal lateral skull x-rays. In this context, the notion of pituitary microadenoma (a pituitary adenoma less than 1 cm in diameter) has achieved widespread recognition. Such tumors may be recognized by subtle abnormalities on polytomographic examination of the sella turcica. Slight irregularities in the contours of the bony cortex of the sella, resulting in a double floor or a slight blistering appearance of the sella, are the charac-

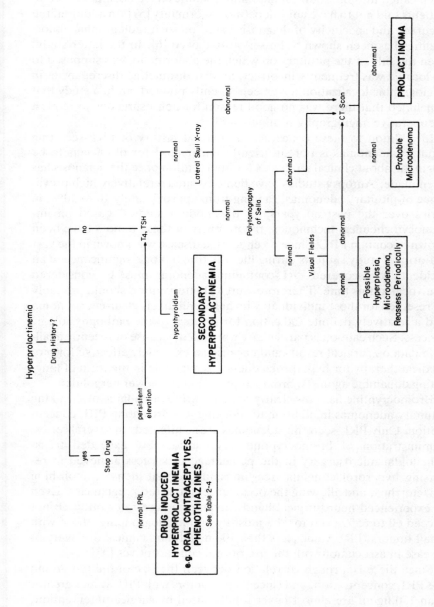

Figure 2-2. Diagnostic protocol: Hyperprolactinemia. PRL, prolactin; T₄, thyroxine; TSH, thyroid-stimulating hormone.

teristic hallmark of such microadenomas when they are strategically located close to the bony rim of the sella [63]. It should be clear that a microadenoma located entirely within the substance of the gland is unlikely to present with any recognizable radiographic abnormality.

Even the specificity of these subtle radiographic abnormalities has been called into question. Similar abnormalities have been described in patients said not to have any endocrine abnormality [57]. In addition, the accuracy and specificity of diagnosis based on such radiographic abnormalities has been shown to be seriously flawed [6]. In the latter study, even the side of the pituitary on which the abnormality was supposed to be located was frequently incorrect. Similar disquieting discrepancies in angiographic localization have been recently pointed out in a study that concluded that there was no good reason for neurosurgeons to request preoperative angiography routinely [48].

In addition to these concerns, the natural history of PRL-secreting pituitary adenomas is not sufficiently understood for physicians to be dogmatic about clinical strategies for intervention once the diagnosis has been made. Autopsy studies have demonstrated a relatively high prevalence of pituitary adenomas, ranging from approximately 10 to 30%, in series over the past 50 years. In the modern studies, based on immunocytochemical techniques, the majority of these tumors have been shown to contain PRL. Since no endocrine disease was known in the vast majority of study subjects during life, the true biologic significance of an incidentally discovered PRL-containing adenoma must be considered equivocal at this time. Therefore, surgical intervention should probably be reserved for those individuals who have a relatively clear-cut adenoma and a relatively definite indication for reversal of the pathophysiologic process. Such caution is particularly warranted because of recently available data on surgical results and because an extremely effective form of medical therapy for hyperprolactinemia is available in the form of long-acting dopamine agonists, bromocryptine and the newer pergolide.

Bromocryptine has now clearly been shown to be capable of shrinking pituitary adenomas in addition to reducing the circulating PRL concentration. Only PRL-secreting adenomas are so affected. In several series, administration of bromocryptine has considerably exceeded trans-sphenoidal microsurgery in the percentage of success achieved in reversing hyperprolactinemia, reestablishing normal menses, abolishing galactorrhea, and allowing the occurrence of desired pregnancies. Even in experienced neurosurgical hands, long-term cure rates often do not exceed 60 to 65% even for the most favorable subgrouping, those with small tumors, PRL values less than 100 ng/ml, and clinical discovery of disease in association with the use of oral contraceptives [53].

Since there is a rough correlation between the size of the tumor and the PRL concentration, and since larger tumors with PRL values greater than 150 ng/ml are almost never totally cured by surgical intervention, even in the best of hands, one can make a persuasive case that long-acting dopamine agonists should perhaps be the therapy of choice in all PRL-secreting tumors in which no pressing neurologic indication for surgical intervention exists. The major difficulty with this view is the uncertainty and concern regarding the possible need in these patients for lifelong treatment.

For reasons that may relate primarily to the psychologic threshold for seeking help related to sexual and/or reproductive function, most men with PRL-secreting pituitary tumors have larger tumors and higher PRL concentrations at the time of diagnosis than do most women. Impotence is commonly a major clinical feature and on occasion appears not to be reversed even with apparent surgical cure, but requires bromocryptine treatment for successful reversal [8]. The significance of this unexpected clinical observation is not known, but certainly the possibility exists that bromocryptine may have effects on the parasympathetic autonomic outflow in addition to its known major mechanism and site of action.

Increased recognition of the occurrence of PRL-secreting pituitary adenomas has served to focus attention on the inhibitory effects of hyperprolactinemia on the reproductive axis in both sexes. Although pituitary adenomas may inhibit gonadotropin secretion by virtue of their mass effect, in most cases gonadotropic cell secretory capacity is only suppressed, not abolished. PRL appears to act principally by inhibiting positive estrogen feedback effects on gonadotropins; thus, the mechanism by which the normal midcycle ovulatory LH and FSH surges are produced is suppressed [23]. In addition, other effects on cells from corpora lutea have been demonstrated in vitro, suggesting that ovarian responsivity to secreted gonadotropins may also be deficient when hyperprolactinemia prevails.

Acromegaly

CLINICAL CONSIDERATIONS

The diagnosis of acromegaly rests on a high index of suspicion, since the line is very fine between genetically inherited features that may be somewhat coarse and the abnormally coarse features associated with GH excess. There is no chemical screening test that will allow the reliable early determination of acromegaly prior to changes in acral and facial features. Perhaps partly as a consequence of this factor, and perhaps as a result of the biology of the disease, virtually all patients with acromegaly have identifiable pituitary tumors at the time of clinical detection. Generally, these are not subtle tumors but are readily detectable on plain

Table 2-5. Common Manifestations of Acromegaly

Due to excessive GH secretion
  Acral enlargement
  Bone overgrowth—hands, feet, prognathism, supraorbital ridges
  Soft tissue thickening—hands, feet, nose, lips, skin
  Excessive sweating
  Heat intolerance
  Degenerative joint disease
  Visceral enlargement
Due to pituitary enlargement
  Headache
  Sellar enlargement
  Visual field loss

---

roentgenograms of the skull; there is no need to resort to polytomography. Only a very small minority, however, have tumors so large or invasive as to interfere with neurologic functions or compromise the normal functions of the remainder of the pituitary. Thus, only a minority of patients with untreated acromegaly have concomitant hypogonadism or hypothyroidism. Hypoadrenocorticism is even more rare, but limitation in PRL secretory reserve is well documented [30].

The common clinical features of acromegaly are presented in Table 2-5. As indicated, they may be broadly considered as due to GH oversecretion or pituitary enlargement. In addition to the acral and facial bone and soft tissue changes and the visceral enlargement, multinodular goiter is a common finding in acromegalics. Soft tissue changes at the wrist frequently lead to median nerve entrapment and carpal tunnel syndrome. The coarsened features, thickened skin, and carpal tunnel syndrome may suggest hypothyroidism, whereas the heat intolerance and excessive sweating may suggest hyperthyroidism. Since ring, glove, and shoe size may all increase with weight gain, increasing obesity occasionally misleads the clinician to perform a laboratory evaluation for acromegaly.

This is an insidiously progressive, chronic illness that frequently can be retrospectively determined to have been present, undiagnosed, for years or even decades. One of the best clinical diagnostic tools, if available, is a series of photographs spanning 10 to 20 years. The prolonged clinical course is marked by steady, progressive changes, true remission due to tumor infarction being very rare. Since the bones and soft tissues have a finite capacity to respond to GH-mediated stimuli, cessation of the apparent progression of clinical deformity does not usually indicate any lessening of the biochemical severity of the disease process. The complications of the disease, listed in Table 2-6, usually continue to progress as well. The overall mortality rate in acromegaly is roughly twice that in the general population [67]. Most of the excessive mortality is attributable to accelerated cardiovascular disease in acromegaly, especially atherosclerosis. It seems likely that the tendency toward hypertension and

Table 2-6. Complications of Acromegaly

Heart and vascular disease
Hypertension
Glucose intolerance
Myopathy
Neuropathy
Parasellar catastrophe
Associations
   Hyperparathyroidism
   Islet cell tumors
   Hyperprolactinemia

the vascular disease associated with glucose intolerance both contribute to the very high mortality.

As noted in Table 2-2, roughly 15% of all pituitary adenomas hypersecrete GH. Of these, about four-fifths appear to be composed of somatotrope cells only, and excessive GH production is the sole abnormality in these patients. The other one-fifth demonstrate concomitant hypersecretion of PRL, which probably represents tumors of mixed cellular types. Although production of both GH and PRL from the same cell type has been postulated, few hard data in support of this notion exist, and if they do exist, they are probably very rare.

Acromegaly may occasionally occur as part of one of the multiple endocrine neoplasia (MEN) syndromes, so-called MEN-I, in which parathyroid and/or pancreatic adenomas also occur. There is no reason to think that the distribution of pituitary tumor types and functions in MEN-I differs from the overall distribution outlined in Table 2-2.

DIAGNOSTIC METHODS
Endocrine Evaluation
The chemical diagnosis of acromegaly rests on the failure of GH concentrations to suppress to less than 2 ng/ml after oral glucose administration.

BASAL GROWTH HORMONE. Since GH, like other pituitary hormones, is secreted episodically, it is good diagnostic practice to obtain several blood samples for estimation of the average resting GH concentration in the suspected acromegalic. Even though the degree of variation does not usually confuse the diagnosis by including both normal and abnormal values, this does happen occasionally. Perhaps more important is the desirability of obtaining an accurate average pretreatment estimate of resting GH. This can be accomplished by evaluating three or four separate blood samples, which can be obtained on different days or at 20- to 30-minute intervals on the same day.

ORAL GLUCOSE TOLERANCE TEST. The standard dose of glucose that has been employed for such studies derives from the time when virtually all standard oral glucose tolerance tests (OGTTs) were carried out with 100 gm; hence, most of the reliable data in the literature regarding the suppressibility of GH in both normal and acromegalic subjects rest on the administration of 100 gm of glucose. For this reason, it is recommended that the standard dose of glucose employed be 100 gm. Blood samples should be obtained prior to and at 1 and 2 hours following glucose administration as a routine. Other samples may be obtained if desired.

Contemporary GH assays have detection limits sufficiently low that 2 ng/ml is an appropriate diagnostic cutoff point [3,54]. When glucose tolerance testing is performed, about 60% of acromegalics show no GH response. Of the remainder, roughly 25% suppress, a qualitatively normal response, but do not reach the normal range; the rest, 12 to 15% of the total, demonstrate a paradoxical elevation in GH concentration [12]. Although the basis for this response is not known, the medial basal hypothalamus has been implicated as possessing glucose-sensitive cells and mediating responses to glucose. Qualitatively abnormal secretory responses of GH also occur in uremia, cirrhosis, depression, and anorexia nervosa, and some patients with widespread metastatic carcinoma.

THYROTROPIN-RELEASING HORMONE. The usual dose and sampling intervals are used, that is, 400 to 500 μg of TRH and samples at 0, 15, 30, 45, and 60 minutes. When an aberrant GH response to TRH does occur, it is usually noted at the earliest sampling times. Roughly 70% of acromegalics have GH secretory responses to TRH [16,29]; such responses almost never occur in normal subjects. Depressed patients and those with renal failure, cirrhosis, and anorexia nervosa may also display such anomalous GH rises.

LEVODOPA TEST. The usual L-dopa protocol for adults is followed, with an oral dose of 500 mg and samples at 0, 30, 60, 90, 120, 180, and 240 minutes. In contrast to the usual GH increase, many acromegalics display a suppression of GH. There is a strong concordance between aberrant TRH responses and aberrant suppression with L-dopa or other dopamine agonists such as bromocryptine.

OTHER PROCEDURES. Ancillary diagnostic procedures such as the radiographic examination of the foot for the estimation of thickness of the heel pad may occasionally be of confirmatory value but are generally unnecessary in the diagnosis of the disease. The sine qua non of the diagnosis consists of the unregulated hypersecretion of growth hormone. Recently, the radioimmunoassay of somatomedin-C has been advocated as an even more sensitive and satisfactory biochemical indicator of GH excess [9]. However, the details of the individual cases have not been reported.

Nonetheless, it should be recognized that there is a gray zone in which the diagnosis can be biochemically marginal despite suggestive clinical features. In such instances other, perhaps more subtle, indicators of hypersecretion of GH may be sought. These include failure of acromegalics to demonstrate the normal nocturnal sleep-associated bursts of GH secretion or deranged regulatory responses to stimuli other than glucose, including TRH [29] and dopamine agonists.

Neuroradiologic Evaluations
Plain Skull X-Rays
Computed Tomography
Pneumoencephalography
Carotid Angiography
(See the section on neuroradiologic evaluations of hypopituitarism, page 21.)

DISCUSSION
Acromegaly comprises roughly 15% of all pituitary adenomas [69] and is therefore uncommon but not rare. A number of large series have delineated major clinical and chemical characteristics of the disease [3,12,27,38]. A slowly progressive and insidious disease, its therapeutic outcomes are far from ideal [1,16,22,33,39,54]. It seems probable that we could improve our therapeutic efficacy by making the diagnosis and initiating treatment at the earliest possible stage of clinical disease. Early diagnosis, however, hinges on a high index of clinical suspicion.

When the diagnosis is suspected, a lateral skull film and a glucose tolerance test (GTT) should be carried out, with GH measurements at 0, 1, and 2 hours (Fig. 2-3). Most acromegalics have abnormal skull x-rays at the time of initial diagnosis, and polytomes are rarely if ever needed. If the GH values during GTT are nondiagnostic but clinical suspicion of the disease is strong, TRH testing should be carried out to assess the GH response to TRH. Although the protocol indicates that L-dopa testing can also be done, in most circumstances it is not likely to add useful information if TRH results are available.

If, despite the failure of any of these maneuvers to yield biochemically diagnostic information, clinical suspicion still persists, the safest course is careful serial follow-up, including periodic lateral skull x-rays, assuming that the initial x-rays were negative. In intermediate circumstances — for example, abnormal x-rays but no diagnostic biochemical information — decisions regarding diagnosis and therefore therapeutic intervention need to be left to the discretion of the experienced clinician. Such

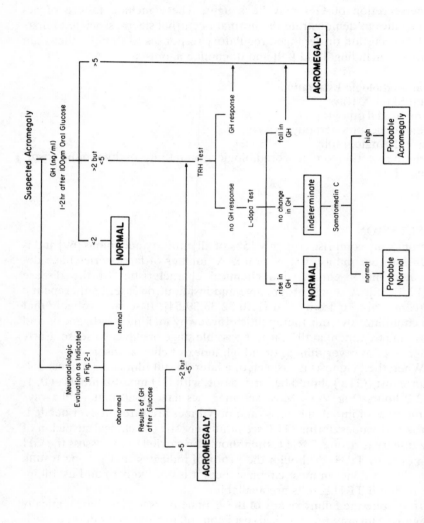

Figure 2-3. Diagnostic protocol: Suspected acromegaly. GH, growth hormone; TRH, thyrotropin releasing hormone.

decisions will also depend upon the expertise available within the given institution in transsphenoidal neurosurgical techniques. Unless extenuating circumstances exist, such as very mild GH hypersecretion in an elderly individual with severe complicating or independent illness that precludes general anesthesia, acromegaly once discovered should be treated. Especially in the relatively young patient, the sometimes disabling complications and the excess mortality of untreated acromegaly mandate cure of the disease if feasible, totally apart from cosmetic indications.

Short Stature

CLINICAL CONSIDERATIONS

When confronted with a child who has short stature, the first task of the clinician is to determine whether the condition is real or imagined. In most circumstances, evaluation beyond a careful history and physical examination may be limited to reassurance of the patient, parents, and/ or referring physician unless the child falls below the third percentile in height for age and sex. A most important procedure is to obtain an accurate growth history and plot the child's height on a relevant growth chart so that changes in growth rate and the overall pattern can be viewed in perspective. A family history and estimation of the growth rate will aid in the evaluation of genetic short stature and constitutional delay in growth and development. Neither of these conditions is associated with measurable endocrine abnormalities.

The decision to evaluate GH secretion in a short child should be predicated on a subnormal growth rate as much as, or more than, the absolute height. A subnormal rate will result in progressive deviation from the normal growth curves, which are based on observed average height increments of 5 to 8 cm a year from ages 3 to 12. Even among those children whose height is below the third percentile, less than 1% have demonstrable GH deficiency. If one selects only that group with the very slowest growth rate, or the group showing progressive deviation from the normal curves, or if one preselects on the basis of other typical clinical characteristics, that percentage can be appreciably increased. In addition to usually being chubby, the GH-deficient child also often has a rather high-pitched voice due to laryngeal hypoplasia; some GH-deficient boys demonstrate micropenis, and in rare cases fasting hypoglycemia has been reported.

Although most children with short stature will prove to have either genetic short stature or constitutional delay in growth, an awareness of this fact does not obviate the need for more extensive testing of GH levels in many of these individuals. These two disorders often become

Table 2-7. Differential Diagnosis of Short Stature

Chronic systemic disease	Chromosomal disorders
Malabsorption syndromes	Gonadal dysgenesis
Uremia	Trisomy 21 and others
Hepatic insufficiency	
Pulmonary insufficiency	
Cardiac malformation with	Congenital disorders
systemic hypoxia	Prematurity
Chronic infections	Birth trauma
	Intrauterine infection
Endocrine disorders	Intrauterine growth
Diabetes mellitus	retardation
Addison's disease	Placental insufficiency
Hypothyroidism	Thyroidal aplasia
Cushing's syndrome	
Sexual precocity and	
early epiphyseal fusion	Skeletal disease
Pseudohypoparathyroidism	Chondrodystrophies
Hypopituitarism	Osteogenesis imperfecta
Laron dwarfism	Kyphoscoliosis
(GH receptor deficiency)	Rickets
Mutant GH molecules with	Pseudo-pseudohypo-
diminished biologic activity	parathyroidism
Constitutional delay in growth	Metabolic disorders
and development	Renal tubular
	acidosis
Genetic short stature	Deranged amino
	acid metabolism
Central nervous system disease	or transport
Midline craniofacial defects	Vitamin D–resis-
Septo-optic dysplasia	tant rickets
Psychosocial dwarfism	Glycogen storage
Elevated intracranial	diseases
pressure	Lipidoses
Craniopharyngioma; other	
hypothalamic or	
diencephalic tumors	
Basal encephalitis	
Histiocytosis	

diagnoses of exclusion, dependent upon adequate documentation of GH levels, recognition of typical growth curves, and the exclusion of other endocrine disorders or systemic diseases (Table 2-7).

Other Endocrine Disorders

In addition to GH deficiency, other endocrine disorders may be associated with short stature. These include hypothyroidism, diabetes mellitus, hypopituitarism, and glucocorticoid excess or deficiency. The short stature that occurs in patients with pseudo-pseudohypoparathyroidism is more accurately considered to be due to skeletal rather than endocrine dysfunction.

Patients with hypothyroidism may present with short stature, obesity, and a low growth velocity resembling GH deficiency. Hypothyroidism often results in greater retardation of bone age than height age and occasionally causes the diagnostic radiologic changes of epiphyseal dysgenesis. Similarly, severe retardation of dentition may parallel the bone changes. (In contrast to these changes in hypothyroidism, bone age and height age retardation usually are comparable in hyposomatotropism.) It is worth noting that acquired hypothyroidism is not always associated with mental dullness in children; placidity and "good" behavior commonly accompany acquired hypothyroidism, resulting in very positive teacher evaluations in the classroom setting.

GH deficiency may be accompanied by deficiency of other pituitary hormones. In such cases of multiple pituitary hormone failure, the most common extra deficiency is of gonadotropins and the next most common involves thyrotropin. GH deficiency as a component of hypopituitarism may be due to idiopathic pituitary dysfunction or structural lesions. Neurologic features are usually the first sign of structural disease, whereas growth failure is the most common presentation of the idiopathic form. TSH responses to TRH are often adequate in the latter case [11,19].

Endogenous and exogenous glucocorticoid excesses are associated with short stature; proposed mechanisms include suppression of both GH and somatomedin production. Hypoglycemia as a consequence of GH deficiency may be even more pronounced in the setting of hypoadrenalism.

When short stature is accompanied by diabetes insipidus or neurologic symptoms, especially headache or visual field loss, a mass lesion with organic hypopituitarism is the probable cause. Craniopharyngiomas predominate, but other tumor types such as optic gliomas or, rarely, more destructive chordomas may be found at surgery. On occasion, short stature may be an important feature in the clinical presentation of a child with hypothalamic dysfunction secondary to increased intracranial pressure. More often, elevated intracranical pressure causes other neurologic symptoms that dominate the clinical picture. Pituitary adenomas are quite rare in childhood.

Systemic Illnesses

Any of a variety of major organ system chronic diseases can result in failure to thrive in the neonate and growth retardation in the child. Intrauterine growth retardation may limit attained stature despite subsequently normal growth rates and should be considered if the birth weight is less than 2.5 kg in a nonpremature infant. Impaired tissue responsivity to normal concentrations of circulating hormones may prevail in the systemic hypoxia of cardiopulmonary disease. Somatomedin levels may be subnormal with severe liver disease, and circulating somatomedin inhibitors may be present in renal disease and in poorly controlled diabetes mellitus. Poor nutrition may contribute to deficient somatomedin production and limited tissue responsivity in many chronic, severe illnesses. An unusual and reversible form of functional hypopituitarism known as *psychosocial dwarfism* is characterized by abnormal parent-child relationships, disordered eating behaviors, and improved growth away from the home setting.

Although many of the disease entities mentioned should be readily diagnosable after a careful history and physical examination, certain exceptions warrant explicit mention. Renal tubular acidoisis or even advanced uremia may sometimes be discovered, despite a paucity of symptoms and findings, but should be suspected when nocturia, hyposthenuria, or urine of alkline pH is noted. Malabsorption syndromes, particularly celiac disease, may sometimes be clinically occult, requiring microscopic examination of the stool and specific testing of absorptive functions for diagnosis.

Other Disorders
Most of the chondrodystrophies and skeletal aberrations that cause short stature lead to disproportionate dwarfism, which can be evaluated by measurement of arm span and upper/lower body segment ratios. X-rays are often characteristic in these conditions, as for example in achondroplasia and the mucopolysaccharidoses. Most short children are not disproportionate.

Chromosomal abnormalities often have characteristic phenotypic features; Turner's syndrome and mongolism predominate in this group since other chromosomal aberrations are usually not compatible with prolonged survival. Anomalies diagnosable at or shortly after birth may herald an associated hypothalamic-pituitary dysfunction with hyposomatotropism; disorders in this category are septo-optic dysplasia, and various midline craniofacial defects.

DIAGNOSTIC METHODS
The evaluation of the child with short stature requires investigation for possible systemic disease. As general screening studies, the following are recommended in addition to careful growth history and examination:

Hematocrit
Urinanalysis
Creatinine/blood urea nitrogen/electrolytes
Lateral skull film
Wrist films for bone age
Thyroid function tests

If these studies provide no indication of a reason for short stature, tests related to GH secretion and action should be employed.

Growth Hormone Determination

GH deficiency cannot be determined from single random or fasting blood specimens, since many normal children (and adults) have GH concentrations at or below the limit of detection in standard assays. Therefore, provocative testing usually must be carried out to confirm GH deficiency. In contrast, a random GH value greater than 7 ng/ml indicates probable normality.

Growth Hormone Provocative Tests

EXERCISE. Exercise has been advocated as a simple outpatient screening test for deficiency. Neither the duration nor the intensity of the exercise has been well standardized. A representative exercise study consists of asking the child to run up and down several flights of stairs for 10 minutes, followed by the drawing of one or more blood samples 10 to 20 minutes after the completion of the exercise. Any value greater than 7 ng/ml indicates probable normality of GH secretion in this and other provocative tests. Values between 5 and 7 ng/ml are considered borderline.

SLEEP. A surge of GH secretion normally occurs in children and young adults within 60 to 120 minutes after sleep onset, defined by electroencephalographic (EEG) criteria. Although bood sampling without EEG monitoring may yield falsely positive abnormal results when sleep patterns are disturbed or disrupted, sampling about 90 minutes after visually defined sleep onset may be used to assess the adequacy of GH secretion. A theoretical advantage of this procedure is that sleep, like exercise, is a physiologic stimulus to GH secretion and might therefore provide results that correlate better with disease states than the results of pharmacologic stimuli. Values above 7 ng/ml at any time should be regarded as a normal response.

INSULIN TOLERANCE TEST. The insulin tolerance test (ITT) is the oldest of the standard GH provocative tests. Insulin is administered intravenously, via an indwelling needle or catheter, by bolus injection. Doses of either 0.10 U/kg or 0.15 U/kg of regular or crystalline zinc insulin are generally used. When there is strong clinical suspicion of hypopituitarism, the dose of insulin should be limited to 0.05 U/kg. Blood specimens are obtained just before the insulin injection (zero time) and at 15, 30, 45, 60, 90, and 120 minutes thereafter. Specimens may be drawn via the same line used for the injection, provided the known volume of the intravenous tubing is first withdrawn and discarded. Other sampling protocols (e.g., 0, 20, 40, 60, and 90 minutes) may also be satisfactory. Blood glucose as well as GH should be determined at each time point, since failure to produce absolute hypoglycemia or to reduce the glucose to less than one-half of its starting value may not stimulate GH secretion in normal subjects. Tachycardia, diaphoresis, drowsiness, or anxiety should probably not constitute grounds for terminating the test; diminished rousability or confusion should, but these conditions occur in less than 2% of ITTs in children. Ampules of glucose for injection should be available at the bedside.

ARGININE PROVOCATIVE TEST. Arginine is the most potent of the amino acid GH secretagogues. It is given intravenously over 30 minutes. Although some centers have routinely employed a total dose of 30 gm, it is probably preferable to give 0.5 gm per kilogram of body weight up to a maximum dose of 40 gm. Sampling intervals are 0, 15, 30, 45, 60, 90, and 120 minutes. The GH rise does not depend on changes in blood glucose; these usually rise modestly (10–15 mg/dl) and transiently soon after arginine infusion; this is related to arginine-evoked increases in glucagon and insulin.

LEVODOPA TEST. L-dopa is given orally; 125 mg is used for children weighing less than 15 kg, 250 mg up to 30 kg, and 500 mg for children over 30 kg. Blood samples for GH are obtained 0, 30, 60, 90, 120, 180, and 240 minutes. The absorption of the drug varies greatly among individuals both in timing and in completeness; hence, there is a need for relatively prolonged observations. Children tolerate L-dopa quite well, with little nausea or vomiting, and seem to mount reproducible GH responses [64].

GLUCAGON TEST. Parenteral glucagon (0.5 mg), which sometimes causes nausea and vomiting, may elicit GH responses as a result of the rise and subsequent fall in blood sugar or the stress of its side effects. It is frequently given in combination with propranolol [41], a drug that augments all GH secretory responses except those that occur during sleep. It is perhaps surprising that standard insulin-propranolol or L-dopa-propranolol protocols have not come into wide use. Glucagon test sampling may be done at 0, 60, 120, 150, and 180 minutes. When propranolol is used, 40 mg is given orally 2 hours prior to glucagon.

APOMORPHINE TEST. Intramuscular or subcutaneous apomorphine (0.75 mg) elicits GH responses in most normal subjects. Some become nauseated and vomit with this dose. Samples are obtained at 0, 60, 90, 120, and 180 minutes.

COMBINED TESTS. Sequential use of rapidly acting stimuli (insulin and arginine [44]) and simultaneous use of additive stimuli (L-dopa and arginine [64]) have been described. The former method saves one hospital day and the latter results in greater GH stimulation, but at the expense of rendering uncertain the appropriate lower limit of normality.

Estimation of the Growth Hormone Secretion Rate
Estimation of the GH secretion rate is a research procedure that requires independent determination of the integrated GH concentration over time and the GH metabolic clearance rate. It is unnecessary for diagnostic purposes.

Growth Hormone Radioreceptor Assay
Competitive binding assay methods using receptor preparations may be applied to any specimen on which a radioimmunoassay is performed. Receptor assays react with the portions of the GH molecule required for biological activity, whereas antibodies may not. The quantitation obtained in receptor assays is not the same as that from radioimmunoassays, but rather is systematically somewhat lower [26].

Measurement of Somatomedin-C
Somatomedin-C, a small peptide produced in the liver in response to GH, can be measured by radioimmunoassay [21,46]. Interpretation of values requires age adjustment, since levels rise throughout childhood. Assay is complicated by the existence of binding proteins in serum. Nonetheless, this is an important measurement since it is the primary mediator of GH action in cartilage.

In addition to baseline somatomedin-C determination, its assay after administration of exogenous GH can provide critical evidence bearing on the biologic activity of endogenous secreted GH. Thus, short children with normal immunoreactive GH and low basal somatomedin-C may be presumed to have a mutant GH molecule if their somatomedin-C values rise normally with exogenous GH and if their growth rate is accelerated over time with GH therapy. Short children with elevated basal GH whose low somatomedin-C fails to rise when exogenous GH is given, and who fail to exhibit growth response to exogenous GH, may be presumed to have GH receptor deficiency. The high basal immunoreactive GH is thought to be caused by failure of the normal somatomedin-C-mediated negative feedback.

DISCUSSION
Once a child has been determined to be significantly short, the initial laboratory evaluation should include a buccal smear in all girls. Since the phenotypic manifestations of gonadal dysgenesis are variable, in part due to mosaicism, this practice will obviate the need to make the diagnosis somewhat later in adolesence, when the problem of the moment may be primary amenorrhea rather than short stature.

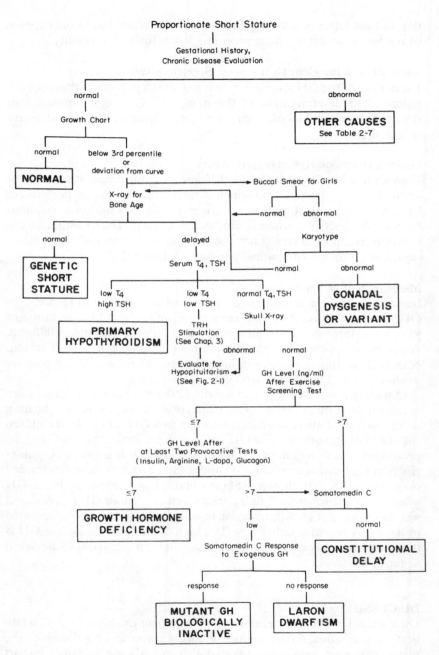

Figure 2-4. Diagnostic protocol: Proportionate short stature. TRH, thyrotropin releasing hormone; TSH, thyroid-stimulating hormone; GH, growth hormone; T_4, thyroxine.

That portion of Figure 2-4 dealing with the child who has a low T_4 and TSH in the face of a delayed bone age is not meant to indicate that all such children will turn out to have structural CNS disease. Since pituitary adenomas are rare in childhood and since isolated functional TSH deficiency is rarer still, however, the chances of structural CNS disease in such a setting are increased. In addition to tumors, histiocytosis must be considered, especially if diabetes insipidus accompanies the growth retardation. When suprasellar calcifications are present, craniopharyngioma will be the correct diagnosis most of the time. Extensive bone destruction in the sellar area and the clivus should bring to mind the possibility of a chordoma. Although not a frequent cause of short stature, a mass with obstruction near the aqueduct might suggest a dysgerminoma. Occasionally, a typical enhancement pattern on CT scan with dye injection may allow the correct diagnosis to be made and radiotherapy begun without a tissue diagnosis. These radiosensitive tumors may also present more anteriorly in the suprasellar region, where biopsy is less dangerous; in this location, they are sometimes referred to as ectopic.

The evaluation of GH secretion is often not a simple matter. Unless a random specimen shows a value above 7 ng/ml, provocative testing must be carried out to assess GH secretory reserve. Interpretation of results is clouded by the fact that roughly 10 to 15% of normal children fail to respond to a standard stimulus on any single occasion. Those who fail to respond to one will respond to others, and may in fact respond to the initial stimulus if retested on another occasion. Because of such considerations, it is wise to insist that the diagnosis of hyposomatotropism not be made unless the patient has failed to respond to at least two separate provocative stimuli [25,64,68]. The ITT appears to be associated with fewer false-negative results than the other test procedures and tends to yield higher average peak responses as well.

The syndrome of Laron dwarfism, with all the typical clinical manifestations of GH deficiency, is surprisingly associated with elevated random GH but low somatomedin values. Treatment with exogenous GH acutely does not increase somatomedin, and chronic GH therapy does not result in significant nitrogen retention or growth acceleration. Examination of the circulating GH of these children immunochemically with a number of antisera and with the radioreceptor assay has not revealed any detectable abnormality in the molecule. Recent observations support the view that Laron dwarfism represents a GH receptor deficiency state [24].

Heretofore, severe growth retardation has almost always been associated with readily demonstrable deficiency of immunoreactive GH. Very few children have been identified with normal immunoreactive GH secretory responses despite markedly slowed rates of growth. More recently, diminished somatomedin has been found in such children. The demonstration of somatomedin responsivity to short-term exogenous GH, and of growth acceleration to longer-term treatment, have served to buttress the interpretation that the deficient growth in some cases is due to a biologically inactive GH molecule that is immunologically intact [36]. Recent controversial observations have suggested that this type of abnormality may account for about one-third of severely short children (growth rates less than 2.5 cm per year) [51]. The implication is that a normal immunoreactive GH response in a conventional provocative test does not rule out functional GH deficiency that can benefit by the administration of exogenous GH. However, the experience of many investigators has been different; at other centers, most children with such severe growth retardation without other obvious causes do not have normal GH secretion as conventionally measured. Nonetheless, the recommendation that good somatomedin-C responses to short courses of GH administration be used to indicate the likelihood of long-term growth response to GH treatment seems reasonable and will probably be tried by many pediatric endocrinologists and pediatricians.

Not all examples of conventional GH deficiency are clear-cut quantitatively. Careful study of children with marginal GH secretory responses to the usual stimuli has shown that they respond to long-term GH therapy less vigorously than patients with virtually absent GH but much more than normal children or those with nonhormonal causes of short stature such as gonadal dysgenesis.

As GH therapy proceeds, a special diagnostic dilemma may sometimes arise. A child with previously normal thyroid function tests may develop chemical evidence of hypothyroidism during GH treatment. Diminished TSH secretory reserve and occasional frank hypothyroidism [13] have been reported in such circumstances. These phenomena are thought to be due to increased somatostatin secretion stimulated by the exogenous GH; the somatostatin, in turn suppresses TSH secretion. When chemical evidence of hypothyroidism develops in such a setting, replacement therapy with the usual doses of T_4 for the duration of the GH administration seems sensible. The effect of GH on TSH secretory reserve is also seen in adults [10].

REFERENCES

1. Arafah, B. M., et al. Transsphenoidal microsurgery in the treatment of acromegaly and gigantism. *J. Clin. Endocrinol. Metab.* 50:578–585, 1980.
2. Bansal, S., Lee, L., and Woolf, P. D. Abnormal prolactin responsivity to dopaminergic suppression in hyperprolactinemic patients. *Am. J. Med.* 71:961–966, 1981.
3. Beck, P., et al. Correlative studies of growth hormone and insulin plasma concentrations with metabolic abnormalities in acromegaly. *J. Lab. Clin. Med.* 66:366–379, 1965.

4. Berelowitz, M., et al. Somatomedin-C mediates growth hormone negative feedback by effects of both the hypothalamus and the pituitary. *Science* 212:1279–1281, 1981.
5. Bergland, R. M., and Page, R. B. Pituitary-brain vascular relations: A new paradigm. *Science* 204:18–24, 1979.
6. Burrow, G. N., Wortzman, G., and Rewcastle, N. B. Microadenomas of the pituitary and abnormal sella tomograms in an unselected autopsy series. *N. Engl. J. Med.* 304:156–158, 1981.
7. Carlson, H. E., Brickman, A. S., and Bottazzo, G. H. Prolactin deficiency in pseudohypoparathyroidism. *N. Engl. J. Med.* 296:140–144, 1977.
8. Carter, J. N., Tyson, J. E., and Tolis, G. Prolactin-secreting tumors and hypogonadism in 22 men. *N. Engl. J. Med.* 299:847–852, 1978.
9. Clemmons, D. R., et al. Evaluation of acromegaly by measurement of somatomedin-C. *N. Engl. J. Med.* 301:1138–1142, 1979.
10. Cobb, W. E., Reichlin, S., and Jackson, I. M. D. Growth hormone secretory status is a determinant of the thyrotropin response to thyrotropin-releasing hormone in euthyroid patients with hypothalamic pituitary disease. *J. Clin. Endocrinol. Metab.* 52:324–329, 1981.
11. Costow, B. H., Grumbach, M. M., and Kaplan, S. L. Effect of thyrotropin-releasing factor on serum thyroid-stimulating hormone: An approach to distinguishing hypothalamic from pituitary forms of idiopathic hypopituitary dwarfism. *J. Clin. Invest.* 50:2219–2225, 1971.
12. Cryer, P. E., Jacobs, L. S., and Daughaday, W. H. Regulation of growth hormone and prolactin secretion in patients with acromegaly and/or excessive prolactin secretion. *Mt. Sinai J. Med.* 40:402–413, 1973.
13. Demura, R., et al. The effect of hGH on hypothalamic-pituitary-thyroid function in patients with pituitary dwarfism. *Acta. Endocrinol.* 93:13–19, 1980.
14. Eastman, R. C., Gorden, P., and Roth, J. Conventional supervoltage irradiation is an effective treatment for acromegaly. *J. Clin. Endocrinol. Metab.* 48:931–940, 1979.
15. Eipper, B. A., and Mains, R. E. Structure and biosynthesis of proadrenocorticotropin/endorphin and related peptides. *Endocr. Rev.* 1:1–27, 1980.
16. Faglia, G., et al. Evaluation of the results of transsphenoidal surgery in acromegaly by assessment of the growth hormone response to thyrotropin-releasing hormone. *Clin. Endocrinol.* (Oxf.) 8:373–380, 1978.
17. Ferland, L., Labrie, F., and Tobin, M. Physiological role of somatostatin in the control of growth hormone and thyrotropin secretion. *Biochem. Biophys. Res. Commun.* 68:149–156, 1976.
18. Fine, S. A., and Frohman, L. A. Loss of central nervous system component of dopaminergic inhibition of prolactin secretion in patients with prolactin secreting pituitary tumors. *J. Clin. Invest.* 61:973–980, 1978.
19. Foley, T. P., Jr., et al. Serum thyrotropin responses to synthetic thyrotropin releasing hormone in normal children and hypopituitary patients: A new test to distinguish primary releasing hormone deficiency from primary pituitary hormone deficiency. *J. Clin. Invest.* 51:431–437, 1972.
20. Frantz, A. G. Prolactin. *N. Engl. J. Med.* 298:201–207, 1978.
21. Furlanetto, R. W., et al. Estimation of somatomedin-C levels in normals and patients with pituitary disease by radioimmunoassay. *J. Clin. Invest.* 60:648–657, 1977.
22. Giovanelli, M. A., Motti, E. D. F., and Paracchi, A. Treatment of acromegaly by transsphenoidal microsurgery. *J. Neurosurg.* 44:677–686, 1976.

23. Glass, M. R., et al. The control of gonadotropin release in women with hyperprolactinemic amenorrhea: Effect of estrogens and progesterone on the LH and FSH response to LHRH. *Clin. Endocrinol.* (Oxf.) 5:521–530, 1977.

24. Golde, D. W., Bersch, N., and Kaplan, S. A. Peripheral unresponsiveness to human growth hormone in Laron dwarfism. *N. Engl. J. Med.* 303:1156–1159, 1980.

25. Goodman, H. G., Grumbach, M. M., and Kaplan, S. L. Growth and growth hormone. A comparison of isolated growth hormone deficiency and multiple pituitary-hormone deficiencies in 35 patients with idiopathic hypopituitary dwarfism. *N. Engl. J. Med.* 278:57–68, 1968.

25a. Guillemin, R., et al. Growth hormone–releasing factor from a human pancreatic tumor that caused acromegaly. *Science* 218:585–587, 1982.

26. Herington, A. C., Jacobs, L. S., and Daughaday, W. H. Radioreceptor and radioimmunoassay quantitation of growth hormone in acromegalic serum: Overestimation by immunoassay and systematic differences between antisera. *J. Clin. Endocrinol. Metab.* 39:257–264, 1974.

27. Hunter, W. M., Gillingham, F. J., and Harris, P. Serial assays of plasma growth hormone in treated and untreated acromegaly. *J. Endocrinol.* 63:21–34, 1974.

28. Illig, R., et al. Elevated plasma TSH and hypothyrodism in children with hypothalamic hypopituitarism. *J. Clin. Endocrinol. Metab.* 41:722–728, 1975.

29. Jackson, I. M. D. Thyrotropin releasing hormone. *N. Engl. J. Med.* 306:145–155, 1982.

30. Jacobs, L. S., and Daughaday, W. H. Pathophysiology and Control of Prolactin Secretion in Patients with Pituitary and Hypothalamic Disease. In J. L. Pasteels and C. Robyn (Eds.), *Human Prolactin*. Amsterdam: Excerpta Medica, 1973. Pp. 189–205.

31. Jacobs, L. S., et al. Prolactin response to thyrotropin-releasing hormone in normal subjects. *J. Clin. Endocrinol. Metab.* 36:1069–1073, 1973.

32. Jordan, R. M., Kendall, J. W., and Kerber, C. W. The primary empty sella syndrome. Analysis of the clinical characteristics, radiographic features, pituitary function, and cerebrospinal fluid adenohypophyseal hormone concentrations. *Am. J. Med.* 62:569–580, 1977.

33. Kanis, J. A., Gillingham, F. J., and Harris, P. Clinical and laboratory study of acromegaly: Assessment before and one year after treatment. *Q. J. Med.* (N.S.) 43:409–431, 1974.

34. Kapten, E. M., et al. Thyroxine metabolism in the low thyroxine state of critical nonthyroidal illnesses. *J. Clin. Endocrinol. Metab.* 53:764–771, 1981.

35. Kleinberg, D. L., Noel, G. L., and Frantz, A. G. Galactorrhea: A study of 235 cases, including 48 with pituitary tumors. *N. Engl. J. Med.* 296:589–600, 1977.

36. Kowarski, A. A., et al. Growth failure with normal serum RIA-GH and low somatomedin activity: Somatomedin restoration and growth acceleration after exogenous GH. *J. Clin. Endocrinol. Metab.* 47:461–464, 1978.

37. Kourides, I. A., Weintraub, B. D., and Rosen, S. W. Secretion of alpha subunit of glycoprotein hormones by pituitary adenomas. *J. Clin. Endocrinol. Metab.* 43:97–106, 1976.

38. Lawrence, J. H., et al. Successful treatment of acromegaly: Metabolic and clinical studies in 145 patients. *J. Clin. Endocrinol. Metab.* 31:180–198, 1970.

39. Levin, S., et al. Cryohypophysectomy for acromegaly: Factors associated with altered endocrine function and carbohydrate metabolism. *Am. J. Med.* 57:526–535, 1974.

40. Neelon, F. A., Goree, J. A., and Lebovitz, H. E. The primary empty sella: Clinical and radiographic characteristics and endocrine function. *Medicine* 52:73–92, 1973.
41. Parks, J. S., et al. Growth hormone responses to propranolol-glucagon stimulation: A comparison with other tests of growth hormone reserve. *J. Clin. Endocrinol. Metab.* 37:85–92, 1973.
42. Patel, Y. C., and Burger, H. G. Serum thyrotropin (TSH) in pituitary and/ or hypothalamic hypothyroidism: Normal or elevated basal levels and paradoxical responses to thyrotropin releasing hormone. *J. Clin. Endocrinol. Metab.* 37:190–196, 1973.
43. Pederson, R. C., Brownie, A. C., and Ling, N. Pro-adrenocorticotropin/endorphin-derived peptides: Coordinate action on adrenal steroidogenesis. *Science* 208:1044–1046, 1980.
44. Penny, R., Blizzard, R. M., and Davis, W. T. Sequential arginine and insulin tolerance tests on the same day. *J. Clin. Endocrinol. Metab.* 29:1499–1501, 1969.
45. Peters, L. L., Hoefer, M. T., and Ben-Jonathan, N. The posterior pituitary: Regulation of anterior pituitary prolactin secretion. *Science* 213:659–661, 1981.
46. Phillips, L. S., and Vassilopoulou-Sellin, R. Somatomedins. *N. Engl. J. Med.* 302:371–380, 438–446, 1980.
47. Rabkin, M. T., and Frantz, A. G. Hypopituitarism: A study of growth hormone and other endocrine functions. *Ann. Intern. Med.* 64:1197–1207, 1966.
48. Richmond, I. L., Newton, T. H., and Wilson, C. B. Indications for angiography in the preoperative evaluation of patients with prolactin-secreting pituitary adenomas. *J. Neurosurg.* 52:378–380, 1980.
49. Ridgway, E. C., et al. Pure alpha-secreting pituitary adenomas. *N. Engl. J. Med.* 304:1254–1259, 1981.
50. Rudman, D., et al. Suprahypophyseal hypogonadism and hypothyroidism during prolonged coma after head trauma. *J. Clin. Endocrinol. Metab.* 45:747–754, 1977.
51. Rudman, D., et al. Children with normal-variant short stature: Treatment with human growth hormone for six months. *N. Engl. J. Med.* 305:123–131, 1981.
52. Salassa, R. M., et al. Transsphenoidal removal of pituitary microadenoma in Cushing's disease. *Mayo Clin. Proc.* 53:24–28, 1978.
53. Schlechte, J., et al. Prolactin-secreting pituitary tumors in amenorrheic women: A comprehensive study. *Endocr. Rev.* 1:295–308, 1980.
54. Schuster, L. D., et al. Acromegaly: Reassessment of the long-term therapeutic effectiveness of transsphenoidal surgery. *Ann. Intern. Med.* 95:172–174, 1981.
55. Snyder, P. J., Jacobs, L. S., and Rabello, M. M. Diagnostic value of thyrotropin-releasing hormone in pituitary and hypothalamic disease. *Ann. Intern. Med.* 81:751–757, 1974.
56. Snyder, P. J., Reitano, J. F., and Utiger, R. D. Serum LH and FSH responses to synthetic gonadotropin-releasing hormone in normal men. *J. Clin. Endocrinol. Metab.* 41:938–945, 1975.
57. Swanson, H. A., and du Boulay, G. Borderline variants of the normal pituitary fossa. *Br. J. Radiol.* 48:366–369, 1975.
58. Terry, L. C., and Martin, J. B. The effects of lateral hypothalamic-medial forebrain stimulation and somatostatin antiserum on pulsatile growth hormone secretion in freely behaving rats: Evidence for a dual regulatory mechanism. *Endocrinology* 109:622–627, 1981.
59. Tindall, G. T., and Hoffman, J. C. Evaluation of the abnormal sella turcica. *Arch. Intern. Med.* 140:1078–1083, 1980.

60. Tyrrell, J. B., et al. Cushing's disease. Selective trans-sphenoidal resection of pituitary microadenoma. *N. Engl. J. Med.* 298:753–758, 1978.
61. Vale, W., et al. Characterization of a 41-residue ovine hypothalamic peptide that stimulates secretion of corticotropin and β-endorphin. *Science* 213:1394–1397, 1981.
62. Van Wyk, J. J., and Grumbach, M. M. Syndrome of precocious menstruation and galactorrhea in juvenile hypothyroidism: An example of hormonal overlap in pituitary feedback. *J. Pediatr.* 57:416–435, 1960.
63. Vezina, J. L. Prolactin-secreting pituitary adenomas: Radiologic diagnosis. In C. Robyn and M. Harter (Eds.), *Progress in Prolactin Physiology and Pathology.* Amsterdam: Elsevier, 1978. Pp. 351–360.
64. Weldon, V. V., et al. Evaluation of growth hormone release in children using arginine and L-dopa in combination. *J. Pediatr.* 87:540–544, 1975.
65. Weisberg, L. A., Zimmerman, E. A., and Frantz, A. G. Diagnosis and evaluation of patients with an enlarged sella turcica. *Am. J. Med.* 61:590–596, 1976.
66. Woolf, P. D., et al. Secondary hypopituitarism: Evidence for continuing regulation of hormonal release. *J. Clin. Endocrinol. Metab.* 38:71–76, 1974.
67. Wright, A. D., et al. Mortality in acromegaly. *Q. J. Med.* (N.S.) 39:1–16, 1976.
68. Youlton, R., Kaplan, S. L., and Grumbach, M. M. Growth and growth hormone IV. Limitations of the growth hormone response to insulin and arginine and of the immunoreactive insulin response to arginine in the assessment of growth hormone deficiency in children. *Pediatrics* 43:989–1004, 1969.
69. Zervas, N. T., and Martin, J. B. Management of hormone-secreting pituitary adenomas. *N. Engl. J. Med.* 302:210–213, 1980.

Hyperthyroidism, Hypothyroidism, and Thyroiditis; Goiters and Thyroid Nodules

Paul D. Woolf

Under normal conditions, regulation of thyroid hormone secretion is mediated by release of thyrotropin (thyroid-stimulating hormone, TSH) from the pituitary gland. TSH, in turn, is controlled by the hypothalamic factor, thyrotropin releasing hormone (TRH). The interactions of thyroid hormones on TSH secretion exhibit classic negative feedback relationships, that is, changes in thyroid hormone levels cause reciprocal changes in TSH. Furthermore, the system is responsive to very slight changes in thyroid hormone. Small decreases in thyroxine (T_4) concentrations of as little as 1 μg/dl, which would still leave the T_4 well within the normal range, increase TSH levels and augment the response to TRH [16,24]. Derangement of the hypothalamic-pituitary-thyroid axis at the level of the thyroid gland itself is most commonly responsible for clinical thyroid disease.

Of all the diseases of the endocrine-metabolism system, maladies of the thyroid gland and its hormonal secretions are second in frequency only to abnormalities of carbohydrate metabolism. Evaluation is often initiated because of either suspected inappropriate thyroid hormone secretion or thyroidal masses due to goiters or nodules. In this discussion, disease states that alter thyroid hormone production will be considered in one section under the headings of hyperthyroidism, hypothyroidism and thyroiditis. Goiters and thyroid nodules are presented in the second section.

Hyperthyroidism, Hypothyroidism, and Thyroiditis

CLINICAL CONSIDERATIONS

Hyperthyroidism

Diffuse toxic goiter, commonly called *Graves' disease*, is the most common cause of thyrotoxicosis (Table 3-1). Exophthalmos, unilateral or more commonly bilateral, is present during some stage of the illness in two-thirds of the patients. Pretibial myxedema is present only rarely, usually in patients with exophthalmos. Exophthalmos may occur in the absence of hyperthyroidism, so called euthyroid Graves' disease [27], but must be differentiated from other causes. Graves' disease usually occurs in young to middle aged women and is less likely to be the cause of

Table 3-1. Etiology of Hyperthyroidism

Diffuse toxic goiter—Graves' disease
Toxic multinodular goiter
Solitary hot nodule
Thyroiditis
Metastatic thyroid carcinoma
TSH hypersecretion
Molar pregnancy
Factitious

hyperthyroidism in the elderly, a group in whom toxic multinodular goiter predominates [28]. Although an insidious onset is common, hyperthyroidism may also be precipitated by a major stress. In the United States, both biologically active thyroid hormones, thyroxine (T_4) and triiodothyronine (T_3), are elevated in over 95% of cases [19]. In the remainder, isolated T_3 elevation may occur (T_3 thyrotoxicosis), but this entity is more common in iodine-deficient areas of the world. T_3 elevation may also precede the T_4 rise [19].

Although the basic defect in Graves' disease is still a matter of investigation, early evidence suggested that long-acting thyroid stimulator (LATS), an immunoglobulin G (IgG), plays an important role. More recently an antibody directed against the TSH binding site on the thyroid cell membrane (thyroid-stimulating immunoglobin, TSI) [15] has received increasing attention. Nevertheless, the hallmark of Graves' disease is the failure of exogenous thyroid hormone to inhibit the ^{131}I uptake [27]. Lack of thyroid suppressibility may also be present in patients with euthyroid Graves' disease.

Toxic multinodular goiters are the most prevalent cause of thyrotoxicosis in the elderly [28]. The thyroid gland is always enlarged and on palpation contains multiple small to large nodules. Thyroidal scan usually reveals many hyperfunctioning areas surrounded by areas with suppressed function. Although it has been postulated that this condition arises over years from a diffuse nontoxic goiter, evidence to support this contention is sparse. Clinically, symptoms of hyperthyroidism may be subtle and limited to complaints of fatigue, irritability, weight loss, or such signs as atrial fibrillation.

Hyperthyroidism may also be caused by autonomously functioning solitary adenoma. The etiology of adenoma formation is obscure, and this lesion is encountered much less frequently than diffuse toxic goiter. Once the adenoma secretes thyroid hormone independently of TSH, it suppresses pituitary TSH release, resulting in diminished activity throughout the remainder of the gland. Thus, on thyroid scan it appears as a "hot" area surrounded by diminished or absent thyroid activity. The development of thyrotoxicosis is dependent upon the relative activity of the adenoma. Earlier studies suggested that hyperfunctioning nodules without hyperthyroidism rarely evolved to hyperthyroidism, although their size might change [11]. However, recently it has been estimated that about one patient in five with a nontoxic, autonomously functioning thyroid nodule 3 cm or larger will develop hyperthyroidism within 1 to 6 years [12].

Hyperthyroidism may also be caused by other less common conditions. Thyroiditis with or without thyroidal pain may present with transient hyperthyroidism because of the release of preformed thyroid hormone and may account for 4 to 23% of all cases of thyrotoxicosis [29]. Widespread metastatic follicular carcinoma of the thyroid may rarely lead to thyrotoxicosis, which is caused by a large mass of hormonally active tissue. There have been several recent reports of a small group of patients with hyperthyroidism secondary to TSH hypersecretion due to either a pituitary tumor or an altered set point in the negative feedback interactions of thyroid hormone and TSH. These patients have both elevated TSH and T_4, in contrast to other etiologies in which TSH levels are low [7,19b]. Hyperthyroidism has been reported in women with molar pregnancies [7]. The administration of radiologic dyes containing organic iodine has also been associated with hyperthyroidism, but this form of thyrotoxicosis may be transient [7,9a].

Surreptitious use of thyroid hormone must be considered. Because of TSH suppression by exogenous thyroid hormone, these patients will usually have small thyroid glands, unlike the previously described conditions, and will have no radioactive iodine uptake. Therefore, in the absence of thyroiditis, particularly if the thyrotoxicosis lasts for more than 6 months and if the gland is nonpalpable, abuse of thyroid hormone must be strongly considered.

Lastly, the T_4 and T_3 may be affected by changes in hormonal binding to thyroxine binding globulin (TBG). In pregnancy or after estrogen therapy, T_3 and T_4 levels are elevated but thyroid function remains normal. The free (unbound) thyroid hormone level, which is the biologically active fraction, remains normal and can be determined by measuring the free T_4 or some other index that correlates closely with the free T_4. Conversely, in rare cases T_4 and T_3 levels may be paradoxically low in hyperthyroid patients with critical nonthyroid illness [26a]. However, these patients usually have elevated free T_4 levels.

Hypothyroidism
Like other thyroid disorders, hypothyroidism is more prevalent in women than in men. The most common etiology is treatment of antecedent thyrotoxicosis. Idiopathic glandular atrophy is the next most commonly encountered condition (Table 3-2).

Biochemically, hypothyroid patients have low circulating levels of T_3 and T_4. If the thyroid gland itself is diseased, pituitary secretion of TSH

Table 3-2. Etiology of Hypothyroidism

Treatment of antecedent hyperthyroidism
Idiopathic "autoimmune" disease
Pituitary deficiency
   Intrinsic
   Hypothalamic failure
Organification defect
Iodine deficiency
Radiation therapy for head and neck malignancies

will be enhanced (primary hypothyroidism). If the gland itself is normal but is not being stimulated because of TSH deficiency, TSH levels will be low or inappropriately normal (secondary and tertiary hypothyroidism).

The treatment of hyperthyroidism with radioactive iodine leads to universal hypothyroidism if the duration of follow-up is sufficiently long [4]. The probability of developing permanent hypothyroidism within the first year of treatment, however, is dependent upon the dose of radioactive iodine administered. Thereafter, there is a 2 to 4% incidence of new hypothyroidism per year that is independent of the dose of ^{131}I used [4]. Although the commonly seen constellation of a mild elevation in TSH, a normal T_4 level, and clinical euthyroidism following ^{131}I therapy may indicate impending hypothyroidism, other studies have shown that only 1% of these patients develop frank thyroid deficiency per year [22].

The risk of hypothyroidism following a subtotal resection of the thyroid gland depends, in part, upon the aggressiveness of the surgeon, since there is a 20 to 30% incidence of either permanent hypothyroidism or a continuation of the hyperthyroid state [4] following surgery. The proportion of patients with postoperative hypothyroidism will obviously be increased if the surgeon is more concerned about controlling the original condition. Even if the patient is rendered euthyroid, there is still a small incidence of hyperthyroidism developing many years after surgery, although this phenomenon is not as well documented as after ^{131}I treatment.

So-called idiopathic hypothyroidism may well be the end stage of an autoimmune thyroiditis. On thyroid biopsy, lymphocytic infiltration of the gland is commonly seen and is indistinguishable from Hashimoto's thyroiditis. In addition, many patients have antithyroid antibodies, and may have antibodies to other endocrine tissues as well. The correlation of T_4 levels with clinical symptoms is poor, but patients with long-standing hypothyroidism will have elevated TSH values, often 10 to 20 times higher than normal.

Deficiency of TSH secretion is a less common cause of thyroid underactivity. TSH deficiency is rarely isolated and is more commonly associated with multiple hormonal deficits. The hypopituitarism may be due to a diseased pituitary such as hypophysitis, mass lesion (adenoma), or vascular catastrophe (Sheehan's syndrome). Alternatively, the pituitary gland may be intact, but it may not be receiving appropriate hypothalamic stimulation [16,30] (tertiary hypothyroidism, hypothalamic hypothyroidism, secondary hypopituitarism). The etiology of this form of hypopituitarism includes head trauma, surgical stalk section, metastatic tumors, irradiation, and idiopathic disease [30]. Both forms of hypopituitarism are characterized by low T_4 and T_3 levels with inappropriately normal or low TSH concentrations. With the availability of synthetic TSH-releasing hormone (TRH), it is possible to distinguish between hypothalamic insufficiency and pituitary insufficiency, since the TSH response is generally normal in the former and absent in the latter [14,20].

Because of the confusion between hypothyroidism and the "euthyroid sick syndrome," it is important that the latter be discussed in this section. (See [26a] for an extensive recent review.) In this entity, the T_4 and T_3 levels are markedly depressed to well within the hypothyroid range. Depending upon the methodology used, the free T_4 may be low, normal, or elevated, although only the latter two occur when the equilibrium dialysis method is used [14b]. When reverse T_3 (rT_3) has been measured, it is elevated. In contrast to primary hypothyroidism, TSH levels are normal. The TSH response to TRH may be mildly increased, but not to levels that are outside the normal range. Consequently, the finding of a frankly elevated TSH level in the setting of an acute illness suggests that primary hypothyroidism is present in addition to the patient's other medical problems.

The pathogenesis of the T_4 abnormalities appears to be enhanced T_4 metabolism with increased metabolic clearance [14a] due to altered T_4 binding to TBG by a circulating immunoglobulin [6a]. The changes in T_3 and rT_3 are caused by the effects of illness on the peripheral conversion of T_4 to T_3 due to a compensatory increase in rT_3 caused by decreased 5'-deiodination.

The euthyroid sick syndrome is quite prevalent in the intensive care unit. It has been observed following a wide variety of clinical disorders including surgery, myocardial infarction, renal insufficiency, anorexia nervosa, protein-calorie malnutrition, ketoacidosis, cirrhosis, thermal injury, and critical illnesses. It has also been seen following the administration of dopamine and corticosteroids, but it is unclear whether this is due to the drug or the underlying clinical condition [26a].

Since the euthyroid sick syndrome occurs in the severely ill patient, it must be differentiated from thyroid disease as clearly as possible. The finding of an elevated TSH is sufficient evidence to institute careful thyroid hormone replacement. However, based on laboratory test findings, it is not possible to differentiate between the euthyroid sick syndrome

Table 3-3. Etiology of Thyroiditis

Acute suppurative thyroiditis
Subacute (granulomatous) thyroiditis
Chronic thyroiditis (Hashimoto's lymphocytic)
Riedel's struma
Painless thyroiditis

and hypothyroidism due to a pituitary or hypothalamic etiology. This distinction can be made only on clinical grounds.

Thyroiditis
Inflammatory diseases of the thyroid gland are listed in Table 3-3. In most clinical circumstances either subacute or Hashimoto's thyroiditis will be encountered. The relative frequency of painless thyroiditis has only recently become apparent. Acute thyroiditis and Riedel's struma are very rare.

Subacute thyroiditis is probably caused by a viral infection or the reaction to such infections. It is a self-limited disease, although subject to recurrences. Classic symptoms include a very tender, firm, enlarged thyroid gland, often with pain referred to the ears or jaws. The erythrocyte sedimentation rate and white cell count are often high. Fever may be present. Histologically, giant cells and inflammatory cells are noted.

The illness typically evolves through four phases [26]. In the first, the sudden release of preformed hormone causes the patient to become biochemically and clinically hyperthyroid, with elevated T_3 and T_4 levels. The protein-bound iodine (PBI) may be disproportionately elevated due to the release of iodoproteins. Antithyroglobulin and antimicrosomal antibodies are not elevated either initially or later. Second is a transient euthyroid phase that may be a prelude to a hypothyroid third phase. Third, within 1 to 3 months of onset the patient may become hypothyroid, with low T_3 and T_4 levels, persistently low ^{131}I uptake, elevated TSH, and an exaggerated response to TRH. The uptake of ^{131}I may then become supranormal [26]. Finally, the thyroid hormone and TSH levels then return to normal. Long-term sequelae are rare.

Hashimoto's thyroiditis is a disease closely related to Graves' disease and is found most commonly in women. From 20 to 30% of patients are hypothyroid when first seen, but Hashimoto's thyroiditis is also a rare cause of hyperthyroidism (hashitoxicosis) [17]. The thyroid gland in this form of thyroiditis is usually diffusely enlarged and rubbery, with a cobblestone texture and a few discrete nodules. Biopsy reveals disrupted thyroid follicles and lymphocytic infiltration. Lymphoid germinal centers and fibrosis may be present. These features, plus the elevated titers of circulating antithyroglobulin and antimicrosmal antibodies, support an autoimmune etiology.

Painless thyroiditis was first described in detail in 1974. Subsequent studies suggest that it accounts for 4 to 23% of cases of hyperthyroidism [29]. There has been a great deal of confusion as to whether this entity is a form of lymphocytic thyroiditis or a painless form of subacute thyroiditis. Features compatible with subacute thyroiditis include the clinical course, depressed radioactive iodine uptake and negative to low titers of conventional antibody studies, whereas the biopsy findings and radioimmunoassayable antithyroglobulin antibodies suggest Hashimoto's disease [29].

Reidel's thyroiditis is very rare. The fibrotic process involving the thyroid may infiltrate into surrounding structures leading to tracheal compression. Fibrosis in other areas (retroperitoneum and mediastinum) may accompany the thyroidal disease.

Acute suppurative thyroiditis is a bacterial infection of the thyroid gland that usually develops from direct extension of an infection in the neck. This is a rare but potentially life-threatening illness. When full-blown, its presentation is similar to that of a furuncle or abscess elsewhere.

DIAGNOSTIC METHODS

Because of the multiplicity of thyroid tests, care must be exercised to choose those that provide the most data for each patient. Furthermore, because each laboratory may have a different normal range, it is as important to have the normal range as it is to have the value for the test ordered. The normal ranges that are given in the following sections, therefore, should be viewed as being only representative (Table 3-4).

Circulating Thyroxine Concentration

The most commonly used and appropriate initial tests of thyroid function are those that measure the circulating concentrations of the thyroid hormones, T_4 and T_3. Total T_4 measurement first became available in 1965 utilizing the competition of tracer quantities of radioactive T_4 for binding to TBG. This method, frequently called the *Murphy-Pattee method* (T_4 [D]), is rapid, reliable, and unaffected by organic iodides. A T_4 range of 4.6 to 11.2 μg/dl is typical. To a large extent, the availability of antibodies to T_4, which were raised against T_4 conjugated to large molecular weight proteins, such as albumin, has led to the replacement of the T_4 (D) by the radioimmunoassay methodology. In addition, this method has the advantages of being faster and more reproducible. The normal range is slightly broader (5.0–13.5 μg/dl). Since T_4 is 99.9% bound to the circulating proteins (TBG 75%, albumin 10%, and prealbumin 15%), T_4 levels will reflect both alterations in thyroid activity and changes in binding proteins. Thus, elevated T_4 levels are seen not only in patients with hyperthyroidism caused by excessive thyroid hormone pro-

Table 3-4. Thyroid Function Tests

Test	Normal Range	Factors Affecting Test
Circulating Hormone Concentrations		
Thyroxine (T$_4$)	5.0–13.5 µg/dl	Increased: Hyperthyroidism, thyroiditis (early), TBG increase (genetic, estrogens, infectious hepatitis–early, acute intermittent porphyria, perphenazine)
		Decreased: Hypothyroidism, thyroiditis (mid–late), TBG decrease (genetic, androgens, anabolic steroids, salicylate, growth hormone), nephrotic syndrome, cortico-steroids, goitrogens (sulfonamides, lithium), euthyroid sick syndrome, Dilantin
Triiodothyronine (T$_3$)	50–200 ng/ml	Increased: See T$_4$, T$_3$ toxicosis
		Decreased: See T$_4$, decreased T$_4$ to T$_3$ conversion (due to acute illness, starvation, propranolol, T$_4$ therapy, glucocorticoids, propylthiouracil, newborn)
Free T$_4$	0.8–2.3 ng/dl	Increased: Hyperthyroidism, heparin, acute febrile illness
		Decreased: Hypothyroidism, Dilantin (chronic)
Free T$_4$ index = T$_4 \times \dfrac{\text{patient's RT}_3\text{U}}{\text{control RT}_3\text{U}}$		Increased: See free T$_4$
(T$_7$) = T$_4 \times$ RT$_3$U		Decreased: See free T$_4$
Reverse T$_3$ (rT$_3$)	36–84 ng/dl	Increased: Hyperthyroidism, starvation, acute illness, newborn
		Decreased: Hypothyroidism
Protein-bound iodine (PBI)	4–8 µg/dl	Increased: See T$_4$, exogenous iodine, iodinated contrast dyes, thyroiditis
		Decreased: See T$_4$
Thyroid-stimulating hormone (TSH)	1–10 µU/ml	Increased: Primary hypothyroidism, after therapy for hyperthyroidism (with normal T$_4$), Hashimoto's thyroiditis, pituitary tumor (rare)
		Decreased: Hypopituitarism, secondary or tertiary hypothyroidism, glucocorticoid or dopamine therapy

Test	Value	Interpretation
TSH-releasing hormone (TRH)	TSH rises 5 μU/ml over basal level following TRH administration	Increased: Primary hypothyroidism Decreased: Hyperthyroidism, exogenous thyroid hormone, pituitary tumor, primary pituitary deficiency
Measurement of Thyroid Hormone Binding		
Thyroid-binding globulin	10–26 μg/dl of T_4 (binding capacity)	Increased: Estrogens (pregnancy, oral contraceptives, Premarin), newborn, infectious hepatitis, acute intermittent porphyria, genetic Decreased: Androgenic or anabolic steroids, acromegaly, large doses of glucocorticoids, nephrotic syndrome, genetic
T_3 resin uptake (RT_3U)	8–14%	Increased: Hyperthyroidism, dicumarol, heparin, salicylates, Butazolidin, prednisone, phenytoin, androgenic and anabolic steroids, nephrotic syndrome Decreased: Hypothyroidism, estrogens, pregnancy
Radioisotope Studies		
^{131}I uptake	8–30%	Increased: Hyperthyroidism, recovery from thyroid suppression, recovery from subacute thyroiditis, diuretics, iodine deficiency, dyshormonogenesis Decreased: Primary hypothyroidism, subacute thyroiditis, thyroid hormone administration, inorganic iodine, iodinated contrast dyes, cardiac and renal insufficiency, corticosteroids
T_3 suppression	50% decrease in pre-therapy value	Increased: (Failure to suppress): Graves' disease
TSH stimulation	100%	Decreased: (Failure to stimulate): primary hypothyroidism
Perchlorate washout	10% ^{131}I decrease in uptake	Increased: Dyshormonogenesis, goitrogens, Hashimoto's thyroiditis
Scan	See text	
Antibodies		
Long-acting thyroid stimulator (LATS), thyroid-stimulating antibody (TSAb), thyrotropin binding-inhibiting immunoglobulin (TSII)	Not detectable	Increased: Graves' disease
Antithyroglobulin antibody	1 : 100	Increased: Hashimoto's thyroiditis, Graves' disease
Antimicrosomal antibody	1 : 10	Increased: Hashimoto's thyroiditis, Graves' disease

duction or release but also in conditions that lead to increased binding. The most common causes of increased TBG levels are shown in Table 3-4. Anabolic steroids and androgens decrease TBG and hence T_4 levels. The nephrotic syndrome leads to excessive urinary loss of binding proteins, lowering the total T_4. Dilantin, in addition to displacing T_4 from TBG, enhances hepatic degradation. The euthyroid sick syndrome is an important cause of low T_4 levels that are not due to thyroid disease [26a].

Circulating Triiodothyroxine Concentration
Circulating T_3 levels are affected in many respects in a fashion parallel to T_4 and are increased in hyperthyroidism and by TBG elevations. In addition, elevated T_3 levels have been found in approximately 5% of hyperthyroid patients who have normal T_4 concentrations — so-called T_3 thyrotoxicosis [4].

Although T_3 levels are low in the same conditions as for T_4, there are several other causes of low T_3 levels. Since two-thirds of circulating T_3 is derived from peripheral deiodination of T_4, a decrease in peripheral formation leads to low T_3 levels [6]. Acute illnesses, starvation, poorly controlled diabetes mellitus, and therapy with propranolol, glucocorticoids, and propylthiouracil, but not methimazole, will all cause low T_3 levels [19]. Because of these considerations and because T_3 levels may be within the normal range in hypothyroid patients, T_3 measurements have little role in the diagnosis of hypothyroidism.

Free (Unbound) Thyroxine
The tests previously described measure the total, but not the biologically active, thyroid hormone concentration. Since the biologically active component represents much less than 1% of the total circulating concentration, it is important to know that these tests are accurately reflecting the state of thyroid hormone secretion and not alterations in hormonal binding. Therefore, in patients with suspected thyroid disorders in whom the binding proteins are altered (most commonly by estrogen), it is important to determine the amount of biologically active hormone present. This can be done with a "free" T_4 that assesses the amount of biologically active T_4 that is circulating and that correlates with the patient's clinical condition (normal range, 0.8–2.3 ng/dl). The only conditions in which the free T_4 does not accurately reflect thyroid function are following heparin therapy, which releases T_4 from tissue stores, and chronic phenytoin therapy, which accelerates thyroxine metabolism. Although equilibrium dialysis remains the "gold standard," several manufacturers have developed rapid kit methods. However, care must be exercised in choosing the appropriate manufacturer [14b].

Triiodothyronine Resin Uptake
The T_3 resin uptake test (RT_3U) is a measure of the available thyroid hormone-binding capacity of the serum. A known amount of radioac-

tively labeled T_3 is added to a sample containing the patient's serum and a T_3 binding resin. The amount of labeled T_3 bound to the resin will be the reciprocal of the amount bound to TBG. Thus, in hypothyroidism with low T_4 and decreased occupancy of TBG binding sites, RT_3U will be diminished. Because a similar unsaturation of TBG binding sites will also be present if TBG levels are increased (as with estrogen therapy), independent assessment of T_4 levels is necessary. Consequently, if the T_4 is normal, the RT_3U test provides useful data on the state of thyroid hormone binding, whereas if the TBG is normal, the RT_3U test can be used as a measure of thyroid hormone concentration. A useful rule of thumb is that the RT_3U changes in the same direction as primary thyroid disorders (increases in hyperthyroidism, decreases in hypothyroidism), whereas in conditions of altered TBG, the RT_3U changes in the opposite direction (estrogen-induced TBG increase will lower RT_3U). A typical normal range is 8 to 14%. Frequently, this test is expressed as a ratio of patients' results over control results, yielding values clustering about 1. Because of careless terminology, this test is frequently confused with a T_3 concentration, which it does not measure.

Free Thyroxine Index
The free T_4 index correlates closely with the free T_4 and has several synonyms. Basically all adjust for alterations in thyroid hormone binding, and in the T_4 index this is accomplished by comparing the patient's RT_3U to that of a control population and multiplying the ratio by the total T_4.

$$\text{Free } T_4 \text{ index} = \frac{RT_3U \text{ patient}}{RT_3U \text{ control}} \times T_4$$

Thyroxine Binding Globulin
TBG binds approximately 75% of the circulating thyroid hormones, with the remainder bound to albumin and thyroid binding prealbumin (except for about 0.04% of the T_4 fraction, which is free). T_3, unlike T_4, is not bound to prealbumin, and the free fraction is approximately 0.4%. The causes of alteration in TBG levels are shown in Table 3-4. Patients with any of the disorders that affect TBG will have abnormalities in their T_4 and T_3 concentrations, which are independent of, but frequently confused with, thyroid disease. Nevertheless, these patients can also have abnormal thyroid function, and the "artifactual" changes in T_4 and T_3 levels caused by abnormal TBG can be assessed by measuring the TBG binding capacity, expressed as micrograms of T_4 per deciliter (normal range, 10–26). Radioimmunoassays for TBG have recently been developed that correlate closely with the T_4 binding capacity. TBG levels of 2.4 mg/dl are typical. However, TBG determination under most circumstances offers no advantages over measurement of the fraction of T_4

that is unbound, that is, free T_4 or a free T_4 index, which are accurate reflections of thyroid gland function.

Thyroid-Stimulating Hormone

TSH measurements are performed using radioimmunoassay (normal range, 1–10 μU/ml). TSH determination is of great utility in four areas. First, it will differentiate between hypothyroidism due to lack of pituitary stimulation with decreased TSH release and hypothyroidism due to primary thyroid disease. In the former, not only will the T_3 and T_4 be low, but so will the TSH (or inappropriately normal), whereas in the latter, the TSH will be distinctly elevated. It is also extremely helpful in diagnosing hypothyroidism in the critically ill patient with the possible euthyroid sick syndrome [26a]. Second, by extension of these observations, measurement of TSH levels may be used to assess the adequacy of thyroid hormone replacement. Finally, mild elevation of TSH with normal T_3 and T_4 levels in patients with Hashimoto's thyroiditis or following treatment of thyrotoxicosis may indicate that these patients are at risk for the development of frank hypothyroidism. Because of significant overlap in most clinical assays between TSH levels from hyperthyroid and euthyroid patients, measurement of TSH in hyperthyroidism does not provide useful information.

Thyrotropin-Releasing Hormone

The availability of synthetic thyrotropin-releasing hormone (TRH, protirelin, Relefact, Thypinone) [14,18] has made it possible to do dynamic studies of TSH release. The administration of 500 μg of TRH as an intravenous bolus to euthyroid subjects causes a rise in TSH within 10 minutes, a peak response at 20 to 30 minutes, and a return to baseline by 120 minutes. A normal response is one in which TSH rises at least 5μU/ml but not more than 25 to 30 μU/ml. From 10 to 15% of normal subjects will not respond by these criteria to the first test [14]. For clinical purposes, samples should be obtained at 0, 20, and 60 minutes for TSH determination.

There are three main uses of TRH testing. In patients with pituitary disease who have hypothyroidism and inappropriately low TSH values, TRH administration will not cause a rise in TSH. In hypothalamic disease, the TSH response to exogenous TRH is quantitatively normal but frequently delayed [20]. Because clinically trivial increases in thyroid hormone levels abolish the TSH response [21], TRH testing, in patients who have symptoms suggestive of hyperthyroidism but whose thyroid tests are within the upper limits of normal, will be useful for establishing the diagnosis of hyperthyroidism. Since this clinical combination is frequently present in the elderly, the TRH test should replace the T_3 suppression test since T_3 administration is not without hazard in this population. Similarly, 40% of patients with exophthalmos and normal thyroid function tests will not have a TSH response to TRH, supporting the diagnosis of euthyroid Graves' disease and obviating the need for a T_3 suppression test [6]. Exaggerated TRH-mediated TSH release in patients with suspected primary hypothyroidism, but with equivocal abnormalities of their routine thyroid function tests, may be useful for the documentation of hypothyroidism.

Antibody Tests
Long-acting thyroid stimulation (LATS) is a 7 S antibody directed against thyroidal microsomes. It is present in the majority of patients with both euthyroid and typical Graves' disease, and it is measured with a bioassay based on the release of ^{131}I from pretreated mice. There are few current indications for its use. However, because LATS has been implicated as the cause of neonatal hyperthyroidism, its determination in the pregnant patient with active or treated Graves' disease may be useful.

Within the past few years, two types of assays have been developed for the investigation of the role of autoimmunity in Graves' disease. One is based on an increase in the generation of cyclic AMP in human thyroid tissue by the patient's serum and has been termed *thyroid-stimulating antibody (TSAb)* [30a] or *thyroid-stimulating immunoglobulin (TSI)*. The other is based on the inhibition of ^{125}I-thyrotropin binding to human thyroid membranes and has been called *thyroid binding inhibitory immunoglobulin (TBII)* [3a,19a]. Both procedures are more sensitive than the older LATS, with 70 to 100% of patients with Graves' disease having positive values [3a,19a,30a]. Like the LATS assay, these newer procedures can be used to identify pregnant women who are at high risk for having infants with neonatal hyperthyroidism. More important, however, is their use in the prediction of the percentage of patients who will remain in remission or who will relapse following treatment with antithyroid drugs [30a]. A positive TSAb result indicates that most patients will relapse within 3 months, whereas those with a negative result are likely to have a prolonged remission. Although both assays tend to give comparable results, the TSAb assay appears to be more specific and reliable than the TBII assay. However, the former remains a research tool, whereas the latter is only now becoming commercially available.

Antithyroglobulin and antimicrosomal antibody titers are important in establishing the diagnosis of autoimmune thyroid disease. They may be measured by immunofluorescence or by indirect hemagglutination. The agglutination of thyroglobulin-coated erythrocytes is the standard method for determination of antithyroglobulin antibodies. However, this test is less sensitive (50% positive) than the antimicrosomal antibody studies (70–80% positive) in the diagnosis of autoimmune thyroid disease. Normal titers for antithyroglobulin antibodies range up to 1 : 250. Titers greater than 1 : 1000 strongly suggest Graves' disease or

Hashimoto's thyroiditis. Antithyroid microsomal antibodies measured by immunofluorescence are normally not present (<1 : 10), and titers of 1 : 100 measured by hemagglutination techniques are abnormal. In Hashimoto's thyroiditis antibody titers may reach several thousand to several hundred thousand. Diagnostic accuracy may approach 80 to 90% if both tests are ordered.

Radioactive Iodine Uptake
The radioactive iodine uptake test (RAIU, ^{131}I uptake) provides an index of the avidity of the thyroid gland for iodine — the necessary constituent of thyroid hormone. Traditionally, approximately 5 μCi of ^{131}I is given in the morning before breakfast and the percentage of the administered dose present in the thyroid gland is determined at a standard time — always at 24 hours and usually at 2, 4, or 6 hours after the dose is given. Table 3-4 shows the conditions that increase or decrease the ^{131}I uptake. An elevated ^{131}I uptake is helpful in establishing the diagnosis of hyperthyroidism. When thyroiditis is present, the uptake will be low instead of high. However, recent iodine exposure by contrast dyes, iodine-containing soaps, and food supplements containing large amounts of iodine (i.e., kelp) will diminish ^{131}I trapping by a dilutional effect. The ^{131}I uptake is not useful in the diagnosis of hypothyroidism because of the great overlap of values between normal and hypothyroid patients.
    The ^{131}I uptake may be converted into a dynamic test of thyroid function. By repeating the uptake following the 10-day administration of 75 to 100 μg of synthetic T_3 (taking care that any residual radioactivity is subtracted), it is possible to determine the suppressibility of the thyroid gland — the T_3 suppression test. Failure to decrease the uptake to less than 50% of the pretreatment value is an abnormal response and indicative of autonomous thyroid function. When evaluating "hot" or "warm" thyroid nodules, repeating the uptake after the 3-day administration of bovine TSH (10 U per day IM) is useful for determining the presence of thyroid tissue that has been suppressed by the hyperfunctioning nodule.

Perchlorate Washout Test
Because the trapping of iodine against a concentration gradient is the rate-limiting step in thyroid hormone synthesis, very little inorganic iodide is present within the normal gland. Consequently, abolition of the trapping mechanism by the administration of perchlorate or thiocyanate prevents the continuation of iodide accumulation, and the uptake value remains relatively constant since all of the ^{131}I is organically bound. In a patient with an organification defect, free iodide is present within the gland, and blockade of the trapping mechanism results in its rapid discharge, so that the counts of ^{131}I within the gland diminish. Perchlorate is usually given 2 to 4 hours after the administration of ^{131}I, and the uptake

is calculated before and serially after the perchlorate is given. A decrease in the uptake by more than 10% from the peak value is a positive test and indicative of an organification defect.

Thyroid Scans
Thyroid scans provide information on the function of the thyroid gland, as well as supplemental information on the morphology of the gland. Isotopes of either iodine (^{123}I or ^{131}I) or technetium (99m pertechnetate) have been used for imaging; the latter isotope is preferred over ^{131}I because of its availability and low radiation exposure. Furthermore, the study can be performed 30 minutes after the intravenous administration of the isotope compared to 24 hours for ^{131}I. Because pertechnetate is only trapped and not organified and because of its circulation in blood, a very vascular tumor may appear to be warm using this isotope but cold with radioiodine.

When ^{123}I is available, its use has emerged as the isotope of choice for thyroid imaging and uptake studies. It provides the detail of iodine scanning with only slightly more radiation exposure than technetium and only about 3% that of ^{131}I. However, because of its short half-life, it is more difficult and costly to obtain.

Thyroid scans are of little value in hypothyroidism because of decreased trapping of iodine. They are important in the management of single or multiple thyroid nodules in determining activity of nodules (hot vs. cold), although they are of limited value in distinguishing benign from malignant disease. Scans are sometimes helpful in clarifying the etiology of hyperthyroidism (i.e., toxic adenoma vs. multinodular goiter) and in identifying ectopic or unsuspected lesions.

DISCUSSION
T_4 is preferred over T_3 as the initial screening test for thyroid disease because it is less commonly affected by nonthyroid factors. The many factors that decrease peripheral conversion of T_4 and T_3 independently of thyroid function make T_3 determinations in the hospitalized patient difficult to interpret. Furthermore, there is a great deal of overlap in the T_3 values between normal and hypothyroid patients. The principal drawback in obtaining a T_4 level as a first thyroid test is the possibility of missing the very rare patient with T_3 thyrotoxicosis. Because of this possibility, a T_3 level should be obtained in all patients with symptoms suggestive of hyperthyroidism who have a normal T_4 level (Fig. 3-1). In patients on propylthiouracil (PTU) therapy for hyperthyroidism, T_4 is preferred to T_3 determinations because PTU, unlike methimazole, decreases the peripheral formation of T_3 from T_4; thus, T_3 measurements may not provide an accurate reflection of thyroid function during treatment.

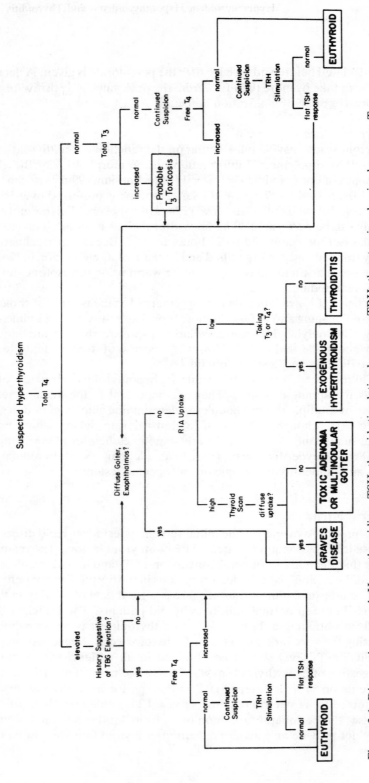

Figure 3-1. Diagnostic protocol: Hyperthyroidism. TSH, thyroid-stimulating hormone; TRH, thyrotropin releasing hormone; T_4, thyroxine; T_3, triiodothyronine; TBG, thyroxine binding globulin; RIA, radioimmunoassay.

In patients likely to have abnormalities in the thyroid binding proteins, such as those using oral contraceptives or most hospitalized patients, a measure of the free or active T_4 fraction should be obtained, as the free T_4 is a better index of thyroid function than total thyroid hormone.

Random TSH measurements have no place in the documentation of thyrotoxicosis. TRH stimulation tests are reserved for those patients with histories and physical examinations suggestive of hyper- or hypothyroidism but in whom the laboratory tests are equivocal. An absent response supports the diagnosis of hyperthyroidism and makes unnecessary the T_3 suppression test.

An elevated T_4 in the absence of TBG abnormalities establishes the diagnosis of hyperthyroidism. The next step is to determine its cause. Graves' disease is diagnosed by the presence of hyperthyroidism, diffuse goiter, and exophthalmos (Fig. 3-1). Painless thyroiditis is suggested by a low RAIU in the presence of hyperthyroidism and must be distinguished from factitious hyperthyroidism and ectopic thyroid hormone production. The decreased uptake distinguishes thyroiditis from unsuspected Graves' disease, toxic adenoma, or multinodular goiter conditions in which the iodine uptake is normal to elevated. Thyroid scanning with technetium 99 or ^{123}I will identify hot nodules or toxic multinodular goiter as the cause of hyperthyroidism.

The RAIU is also useful for differentiating the various forms of thyroiditis. In an acute suppurative thyroiditis the ^{123}I or ^{131}I uptake may be preserved (unless the thyroid has been replaced by pus), despite the extensive inflammatory processes. Thus, the persistence of RAIU differentiates acute suppurative from subacute thyroiditis, since the uptake is suppressed in the latter condition. In subacute thyroiditis, the inflammation may occur first in one lobe before migrating to the contralateral side. If this occurs, the depressed uptake will be limited to the involved side. Occasionally, the hyperthyroid phase is missed and the patient may be seen initially in the hypothyroid condition. If this occurs, the diagnosis may be difficult to establish.

If hypothyroidism is suspected, T_4 and TSH should be measured (Fig. 3-2). T_3 levels and the RAIU are less reliable because of the overlap of values between hypothyroid and euthyroid patients. The finding of an elevated TSH and a low T_4 establishes the diagnosis of primary hypothyroidism. Occasionally, the TSH may be slightly elevated with a low normal T_4, indicating compensated thyroid failure, and is suggestive of Hashimoto's thyroiditis (in the absence of prior radioactive iodine treatment for Graves' disease). A patchy thyroid scan also supports this diagnosis, which can be definitely established by the presence of high antithyroglobulin or antimicrosomal antibody titers. Very rarely, Hashimoto's thyroiditis may present with hyperthyroidism with an elevated RAIU [17].

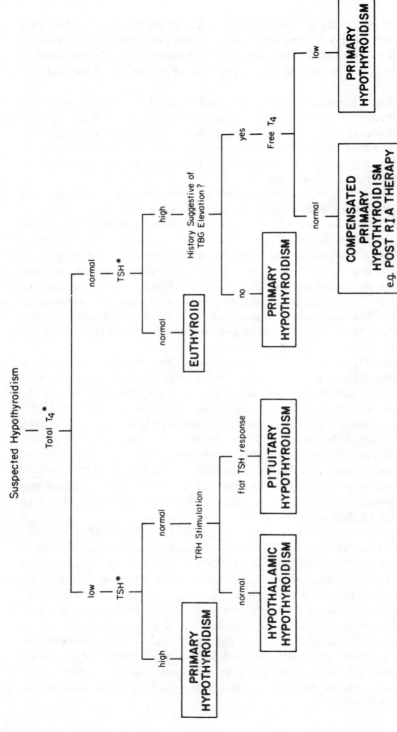

Figure 3-2. Diagnostic protocol: Hypothyroidism. TRH, thyrotropin releasing hormone; TSH, thyroid-stimulating hormone; TBG, thyroxine binding globulin; T_4, thyroxine; RIA, radioimmunoassay. *Obtain TSH with initial T_4 determination.

A low TSH in the presence of low T_4 values raises the question of hypothalamic or pituitary disease. It should be remembered that a decrease in binding proteins or in the affinity of T_4 for TBG (phenytoin) will lower T_4 values. Therefore, a free T_4 determination may be necessary before a TRH stimulation test is performed. If the pituitary is diseased, the TSH response is absent, whereas in hypothalamic disease the response may be delayed. However, these patterns are also seen in a small percentage of normal subjects [14,18]. More intensive evaluation of hypothalamic-pituitary function is usually indicated in these circumstances.

Measurement of TSH is also helpful in determining the adequacy of thyroid hormone replacement. When, because of inadequate evaluation, the diagnosis of hypothyroidism is in doubt, the medication must be discountinued for at least 1 month because of the slow return of TSH secretion to normal following prolonged thyroid hormone therapy [23].

Goiters and Thyroid Nodules

CLINICAL CONSIDERATIONS

Enlargement of the thyroid can be divided into (1) diffuse enlargement—either symmetrical and uniform or multinodular—and (2) solitary nodules. Such a division is convenient for both diagnosis and treatment, although there is some overlap.

Goiter formation may be a compensatory response of the thyroid to overcome deficient hormone synthesis. Hence, goiters are common in iodine-deficient areas of the world as well as those where goitrogens are present in the diet. Neither of these conditions is prevalent in the United States at the present time, but they may occur in food faddists. Lithium treatment of manic-depressive illness is accompanied by TSH elevation in 20 to 30% of the patients so treated, but goiters and hypothyroidism are much less common [9]. A family history of goiter with or without hypothyroidism suggests a partial organification defect. The presence of deafness, along with thyroid enlargement due to an organification defect, has been given the eponym *Pendred's syndrome*. Diffusely enlarged glands are very common in pregnancy and in adolescence. In both cases, the goiter usually resolves with time and no cause is found.

Multinodular goiters are much more common in middle-aged and elderly women. In some cases, they may have evolved from successive cycles of incomplete regression and stimulation of diffuse goiters. Frequently, only a single nodule is palpated, but several are found on thyroid scan or at surgery. Many of these patients are either mildly hyperthyroid or may become so in the future. Furthermore, the clinical signs and symptoms of thyrotoxicosis are not as dramatic in this population as they are in younger individuals, and the ^{131}I uptake may not be as elevated. Infrequently, these goiters may become so large as to cause compressive symptoms.

From a clinical perspective, goitrous enlargement of the thyroid is a common disorder, particularly in women. It is concern about thyroid malignancy that often prompts further evaluation, although the incidence of thyroid cancer among goitrous individuals is very small. As a general rule, a single nodule in an otherwise normal gland must be viewed with suspicion. The presence of more than one nodule lowers the probability of cancer and increases the probability of a benign multi-nodular goiter.

Solitary thyroid nodules require more attention than simple goiters [13]. Most solitary thyroid nodules are found on either a routine physical examination or by the patient, who notices a lump in the neck. These nodules rarely cause symptoms. Because of the markedly increased incidence of thyroid cancer in patients who have received head and neck irradiation in early childhood, it is imperative that this history be sought. Fixation of the nodule to the surrounding tissue, lymphadenopathy, hoarseness with vocal cord paralysis, or evidence of distant metastases strongly suggests a thyroid malignancy. Although the incidence of carcinoma is higher in solitary nodules, most solitary nodules are benign.

Estimates of cancer incidence in solitary cold nodules range from 10 to 30%. Cysts, adenomas, colloid nodules, thyroiditis, and other benign conditions account for most solitary nodules. Since goiters and noncarcinomatous nodules are common, the basic problem is the selective application of diagnostic procedures to direct appropriate medical or surgical therapy.

DIAGNOSTIC METHODS
In addition to the diagnostic methods discussed earlier, there are several tests that are particularly applicable to the evaluation of the nodular thyroid.

Thyroid Ultrasound
The superficial location of the thyroid gland allows the use of ultrasound to assess further the morphology of abnormal structures. Cold nodules identified by a scan may be further classified on the basis of density differences to ultrasound waves [13]. Cystic lesions are completely echo-free and usually benign. Mixed or solid lesions have echo recordings within the nodule. Carcinomas are mixed or solid lesions and are rarely echo-free. In addition to distinguishing between cystic and solid lesions, ultrasound is an excellent method for accurately determining and serially following nodule size. However, ultrasound cannot reliably distinguish between a benign and a malignant lesion [25].

Needle Biopsy of the Thyroid Gland

Percutaneous core needle biopsy of thyroid tissue may be accomplished using the large-bore Vim-Silverman or Tru-cut needle. Such specimens may be helpful in evaluation of the diffusely enlarged thyroid gland and are most helpful in establishing the diagnosis of thyroiditis. Large needle biopsy is less helpful in the diagnosis of thyroid nodules, particularly those less than 2 cm in diameter. For this reason, fine-needle aspiration (vs. "core" biopsy with large needles) has recently received emphasis [2,8,10,25]. It is important to realize that fine-needle biopsy yields cytologic specimens (vs. histologic samples using the core biopsy), and its success is critically dependent on the presence of a cytopathologist who is well trained in this technique. Fine-needle aspiration is currently the most accurate method for selecting patients with thyroid nodules for surgery [2,25]. Negative cytology after fine-needle aspiration does not exclude the presence of a malignancy when it is suspected on clinical grounds [5]. The reported accuracy of aspiration cytology varies from 50 to 97% [25]. In a recent analysis of various diagnostic tests used in evaluation of thyroid nodules, fine-needle aspiration was found to be the single best test currently available to differentiate benign from malignant nodules [2,25].

DISCUSSION

Goiter

The work-up of a diffuse nontoxic goiter should include a very careful family, dietary, and drug history. T_4 and TSH should be obtained to verify the clinical impression of euthyroidism. In the vast majority of patients, if these tests are normal, no further evaluation will be required. There is little need to obtain a thyroid scan unless there is a suggestion of nodularity or a rapid increase in gland size. A rapidly enlarging thyroid mass should be scanned and biopsied, particularly in an elderly patient, because of the high risk of anaplastic carcinoma. A ^{131}I uptake is necessary only when there is a clinical suspicion of painless thyroiditis or if the T_4 is suggestive of the more conventional forms of hyperthyroidism. Whenever the T_4 is normal and the TSH is mildly elevated, antithyroid antibody titers may be useful in establishing the diagnosis of Hashimoto's thyroiditis. In patients with a striking family history of goiter, particularly in association with hypothyroidism and deafness, an organification defect must be excluded by a perchlorate washout test.

The evaluation of multinodular goiter should include T_4 and T_3, since T_3 thyrotoxicosis is more common with multinodular goiters. A thyroid scan should be obtained to determine the presence of autonomously functioning nodules. This is particularly important when thyroid hormone levels are high normal or elevated. The absence of isotopic accumulation between the nodules is evidence of suppression of function of the remaining thyroid tissue, indicating escape of the hyperfunctioning areas from TSH regulation. The thyroid scan in patients whose disease has not progressed this far may show only an irregular distribution of uptake without distinct areas of accumulation. The TRH stimulation test may be very helpful in the documentation of mild hyperthyroidism in this group of patients because small increases in T_4 levels block the TSH response to TRH.

Solitary Nodule
Because the probability of a cancer within a solitary nodule varies considerably with the functional status of the nodule, the thyroid scan has traditionally been the initial screening test. If the scan shows discrete areas of increased uptake, thyroid function tests (T_4 and possibly T_3 as well) should be done to determine whether the patient is hyperthyroid.

For convenience and because of different management, solitary nodules may be divided, on the basis of scan findings, into (1) hyperfunctioning (hot), (2) functioning (warm), and (3) nonfunctioning (cold), nodules.

HYPERFUNCTIONING NODULE. Hyperfunctioning nodules demonstrate enhanced uptake of the radionuclide on a scan compared to the remainder of thyroid tissue. The scan image provides information only on the relative uptake of nuclide; it does not define the overall level of hormone production. Thus, although a nodule may be described as hyperfunctioning or hot based on its scan presentation, the patient may be euthyroid. In those instances in which the net thyroid hormone production is excessive, the hot nodule may be accompanied by hyperthyroidism. In either case, the remaining thyroid is hypofunctioning (because TSH secretion is diminished) and the scan shows a solitary area of isotope accumulation. In most instances, this is due to an adenoma that synthesizes hormone autonomously. The administration of exogenous thyroid will not result in a decrease in nodule size but will likely cause the patient to become hyperthyroid. The administration of bovine TSH will, however, stimulate the remaining thyroid tissue to accumulate tracer, distinguishing this group from patients with hemiagenesis of one thyroid lobe.

Hyperfunctioning nodules are rarely malignant, and no further evaluation for carcinoma is indicated unless there is evidence of extrathyroidal metastases. Evaluation should be directed toward determining the extent of thyroid hormone secretion.

FUNCTIONING NODULES. Functioning nodules are those that on thyroid scan cannot be differentiated from the remaining gland. There are currently no widely available tests that will indicate with acceptable accuracy the presence of malignancy, with the exception of a positive cytologic evaluation of thyroid aspirates [10]. The likelihood of finding

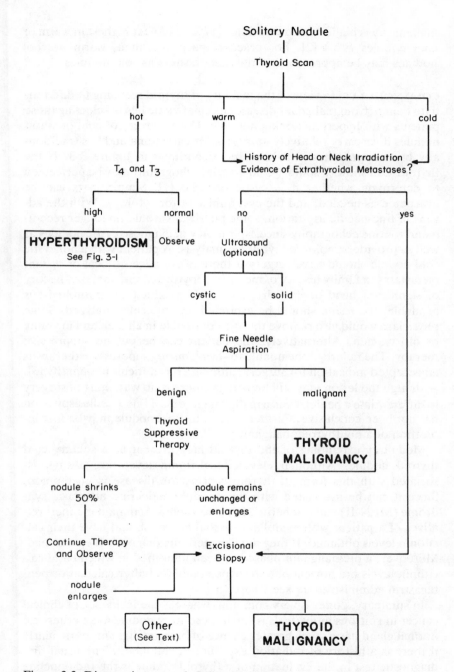

Figure 3-3. Diagnostic protocol: Solitary nodule. T_4, thyroxine; T_3, triiodothyronine.

malignancy is highest in cold nodules (17%) and next highest in warm or cool nodules (9%) [2]. For practical purposes, then, warm or cool nodules may be approached in the same fashion as cold nodules.

COLD NODULES. In view of the inability of thyroid scanning to differentiate benign from malignant disease, its chief value lies in selecting those patients with hyperfunctioning nodules. The discovery of cold or warm nodules does carry relatively more risk for carcinoma and has traditionally been approached with the studies outlined in Figure 3-3. If the thyroid scan shows a solitary cold nodule, echography may be performed to determine whether it is cystic or solid [1]. Simple cysts can be evacuated as needed, and the cyst fluid sent for cytology. With the advent of fine-needle aspiration, some physicians would no longer recommend routine echography since aspiration will diagnose cystic nodules as well as provide samples for cytologic analysis. A patient with a noncystic cold nodule should have surgery if there is evidence of local or distant metastases, a family history of medullary thyroid carcinoma, or a history of significant head or neck irradiation. If a skilled cytopathologist is available, the lesion should be aspirated and the cells analyzed. Some physicians would also remove this type of nodule in all men and in young or old women. Alternatively, the patient can be put on suppressive therapy. The failure of the nodule to shrink during suppressive therapy is an accepted indication for surgery, although it is difficult to quantify [3]. Although the lesion may still be benign, there is no way short of surgery to differentiate a benign from a malignant nodule if fine-needle aspiration has not been conclusive. Furthermore, a thyroid nodule may be first indication of a nonthyroid malignancy.

Medullary carcinoma of the thyroid may present as a solitary cold thyroid nodule. Although elevated calcitonin levels are always associated with this form of thyroid cancer, the disease is uncommon. Since it can be associated with the multiple endocrine neoplasia syndrome (MEN-II) and is inherited in an autosomal dominant manner, relatives of a patient with medullary thyroid cancer should have their calcitonin levels obtained. If they are elevated, the diagnosis is established. Moreover, a premalignant phase has been identified in which basal calcitonin levels are normal but are hyperstimulated after calcium or pentagastrin administration (see Chap. 15).

In summary, goiter is very common, whereas the incidence of clinical cancer in goitrous individuals is small. A solitary nodule in an otherwise normal gland has a much greater chance of being malignant, particularly if there is a history of radiation exposure in childhood. The usual first diagnostic test in the evaluation of a thyroid nodule is the radionuclide scan, which distinguishes hot from warm or cold nodules. [123]I or technetium pertechnetate scanning is currently preferred over radioiodine scanning with [131]I. Hot nodules on scan are rarely malignant. Evaluation of the hot nodule should be directed toward defining autonomy of function. With the exception of identifying hyperfunctioning nodules, scanning techniques offer little discrimination between benign and malignant nodules. Thyroid ultrasound provides supportive data for decisions regarding surgical or medical management since true cysts that are completely echo-free are rarely malignant. Fine-needle aspiration biopsy of solitary nodules is useful in skilled hands and has emerged as a sensitive and specific test in the evaluation of thyroid nodules. In groups not at high risk, a suppressive trial of thyroid therapy may be used as a diagnostic test, with failure of nodules to regress serving as an indication for surgery. In a multinodular gland, a dominant cold nodule that fails to suppress may be approached as a solitary nodule. The risk of malignancy, however, remains less than that of a solitary nodule.

REFERENCES

1. Ashcraft, M. W., and Van Herle, A. J. Management of thyroid nodules: I. History and physical examination, blood tests, x-ray tests, and ultrasonography. *Head Neck Surg.* 3:216–230, 1981.
2. Ashcraft, M. W., and Van Herle, A. J. Management of thyroid nodules: II. Scanning techniques, thyroid suppressive therapy, and fine needle aspiration. *Head Neck Surg.* 3:297–322, 1981.
3. Blum, M., and Rothschild, M. Improved nonoperative diagnosis of the solitary "cold" thyroid nodule: Surgical selection based on risk factors and three months of suppression. *J.A.M.A.* 243:242–245, 1980.
3a. Borges, M., et al. A new method for assessing the thyrotropin binding inhibitory activity in the immunoglobulins and whole serum of patients with Graves' disease. *J. Clin. Endocrinol. Metab.* 54:552–558, 1982.
4. Braverman, L. E. Therapeutic considerations (thyrotoxicosis). *Clin. Endocrinol. Metab.* 7:221-241, 1978.
5. Burrow, G. N. Aspiration needle biopsy of the thyroid. *Ann. Intern. Med.* 94:536–537, 1981.
6. Chopra, I. J., Chopra, U., and Orgiazzi, J. Abnormalities of hypothalamo-hypophyseal-thyroid axis in patients with Graves' ophthalmopathy. *J. Clin. Endocrinol. Metab.* 37:955–967, 1973.
6a. Chopra, I. J., et al. In search of an inhibitor of thyroid hormone binding to serum proteins in nonthyroid illnesses. *J. Clin. Endocrinol. Metab.* 49:63, 1979.
7. Cooper, D. S., Ridgway, E. C., and Maloof, F. Unusual types of hyperthyroidism. *Clin. Endocrinol. Metab.* 7:199–220, 1978.
8. Crile, G., Esselstyn, C. B., and Hawk, W. A. Needle biopsy in the diagnosis of thyroid nodules appearing after radiation. *N. Engl. J. Med.* 301:997–999, 1979.
9. Emerson, C. H., Dyson, W. L., and Utiger, R. D. Serum thyrotropin and thyroxine concentrations in patients receiving lithium carbonate. *J. Clin. Endocrinol. Metab.* 36:338–346, 1973.
9a. Fradkin, J. E., and Wolff, J. Iodide-induced thyrotoxicosis. *Medicine* 62:1–21, 1983.
10. Gershengorn, M. C., et al. Fine-needle aspiration cytology in the preoperative diagnosis of thyroid nodules. *Ann. Intern. Med.* 87:265–269, 1977.

11. Hamburger, J. I. Solitary autonomously functioning thyroid lesions. Diagnosis, clinical features and pathogenetic considerations. *Am. J. Med.* 58:740–748, 1975.

12. Hamburger, J. I. Evolution of toxicity in solitary nontoxic autonomously functioning thyroid nodules. *J. Clin. Endocrinol. Metab.* 50:1089–1093, 1980.

13. Hoffman, G. L., Thompson, N. W., and Heffron, C. The solitary thyroid nodule. *Arch. Surg.* 105:379–385, 1972.

14. Jackson, I. M. D. Thyrotropin-releasing hormone. *N. Engl. J. Med.* 306:145–155, 1982.

14a. Kaptein, E. M., et al. Thyroxine metabolism in the low thyroxine state of critical nonthyroidal illnesses. *J. Clin. Endocrinol. Metab.* 53:764–771, 1981.

14b. Kaptein, E. M., et al. Free thyroxine estimates in nonthyroidal illness: Comparison of eight methods. *J. Clin. Endocrinol. Metab.* 52:1073–1077, 1981.

15. Kidd, A., et al. Immunologic aspects of Graves' and Hashimoto's diseases. *Metabolism* 29:80–99, 1980.

16. Larsen, P. R. Thyroid-pituitary interaction: Feedback regulation of thyrotropin secretion by thyroid hormones. *N. Engl. J. Med.* 306:23–32, 1982.

17. McConahey, W. M. Hashimoto's thyroiditis. *Med. Clin. North Am.* 56:885–896, 1972.

18. Sawain, C. T., and Hershman, J. M. The TSH response to thyrotropin-releasing hormone (TRH) in young adult men: Intraindividual variation and relation to basal serum TSH and thyroid hormones. *J. Clin. Endocrinol. Metab.* 42:809–816, 1976.

19. Schimmel, M., and Utiger, R. D. Thyroidal and peripheral production of thyroid hormones. Review of recent findings and their clinical implications. *Ann. Intern. Med.* 87:760–768, 1977.

19a. Schleusener, H., et al. Relationship between thyroid status and Graves' disease-specific immunoglobulins. *J. Clin. Endocrinol. Metab.* 47:379–384, 1978.

19b. Smallridge, R. C., and Smith, C. E. Hyperthyroidism due to thyrotropin-secreting pituitary tumors. *Arch. Intern. Med.* 143:503–507, 1983.

20. Snyder, P. J., et al. Diagnostic value of thyrotropin-releasing hormone in pituitary and hypothalamic diseases: Assessment of thyrotropin and prolactin secretion in 100 patients. *Ann. Intern. Med.* 81:751–757, 1974.

21. Snyder, P. J., and Utiger, R. D. Inhibition of thyrotropin response to thyrotropin-releasing hormone by small quantities of thyroid hormones. *J. Clin. Invest.* 51:2077–2084, 1972.

22. Toft, A.D., et al. Thyroid function in the long-term follow-up of patients treated with iodine-131 for thyrotoxicosis. *Lancet* 2:576–578, 1975.

23. Vagenakis, A. G., et al. Recovery of pituitary thyrotropic function after withdrawal of prolonged thyroid-suppression therapy. *N. Engl. J. Med.* 293:681–684, 1975.

24. Vagenakis, A. G., et al. Hyperresponse to thyrotropin-releasing hormone accompanying small decreases in serum thyroid hormone concentrations. *J. Clin. Invest.* 54:913–918, 1974.

25. Van Herle, A. J. The thyroid nodule. *Ann. Intern. Med.* 96:221–232, 1982.

26. Volpe, R., Johnston, M. W., Huber, N. Thyroid function in subacute thyroiditis. *J. Clin. Endocrinol. Metab.* 18:65–78, 1958.

26a. Wartofsky, L., and Burman, K. D. Alterations in thyroid function in patients with systemic illness: "The euthyroid sick syndrome." *Endocr. Rev.* 3:164–217, 1982.

27. Werner, S. C. Euthyroid patients with early eye signs of Graves' disease. Their responses to L-triiodothyronine and thyrotropin. *Am. J. Med.* 18:608–612, 1955.
28. Werner, S. C. Hyperthyroidism. In S. C. Werner and S. H. Ingbar (Eds.), *The Thyroid.* Hagerstown, Md., Harper & Row, 1978. Pp. 591–603.
29. Woolf, P. D. Transient painless thyroiditis with hyperthyroidism: A variant of lymphocytic thyroiditis? *Endocr. Rev.* 1:411–430, 1980.
30. Woolf, P. D., et al. Secondary hypopituitarism: Evidence for continuing regulation of hormone release. *J. Clin. Endocrinol. Metab.* 38:71–76, 1974.
30a. Zakarija, M., McKenzie, J. M., and Banovac, K. Clinical significance of assay of thyroid-stimulating antibody in Graves' disease. *Ann. Intern. Med.* 93(Part 1):28–32, 1980.

4   Hypercalcemia

Angelo A. Licata
William F. Streck

Serum calcium is maintained within normal limits by the combined actions of parathyroid hormone (PTH) and vitamin D through their effects on bone, intestine, and kidney. Only 1% of total body calcium is normally present in the blood and extracellular space [31]. This circulating total serum calcium level is regulated within normal limits of 8.5 to 10.5 mg/dl and consists of the sum of ionized calcium, diffusible calcium complexes, and protein-bound calcium. Approximately 50% of the total serum calcium is in the ionized fraction. This form is the biologically active component that affects calcium-regulating hormones and a number of neuromuscular, metabolic, hormonal, and enzymatic processes.

Most calcium in the body (99%) is located in the skeleton, where it provides both structural support and a reservoir for the small but critical circulating pool of calcium. Total body calcium averages about 1 kg in a 70-kg man. A portion of this skeletal calcium is readily exchangeable with the extracellular calcium to allow ready modification of circulating levels. However, overall calcium balance is largely dependent on the intestinal absorption and renal handling of calcium.

In the adult, calcium intake averages 500 to 800 mg per day, with average absorption in the range of 30 to 35% [33]. Intestinal absorption of calcium is dependent on a vitamin D–mediated active transport process as well as on passive diffusion down a concentration gradient. As calcium intake increases in normal individuals, urinary calcium excretion increases, but to a much lesser extent [33]. This results from feedback mechanisms on the active transport process that protect the body from hyperabsorption of calcium and consequent hypercalciuria. In normal individuals, urinary excretion of calcium approximates 100 to 250 mg per day and maintains a normal overall calcium balance [33].

Parathyroid hormone and vitamin D and its metabolites are the major hormones affecting calcium metabolism. Calcitonin has demonstrable effects on calcium metabolism, primarily by inhibiting bone resorption, but the clinical role of calcitonin in calcium homeostasis has not been clearly defined. PTH affects calcium levels directly through mobilization of bone calcium and reduction of renal calcium excretion and increased loss of urinary phosphorous. Less directly, PTH affects intestinal calcium absorption, a process mediated largely by vitamin D.

Vitamin D undergoes hydroxylation in the liver to 25-hydroxyvitamin D (25-OHD). This agent serves as the substrate for the formation of 1,25-dihydroxyvitamin D [1,25-$(OH)_2$D] by the kidney. Formation of 1,25-$(OH)_2$D, in turn, is stimulated by PTH and low serum phosphate. Vitamin D metabolites elevate calcium levels by stimulating increased calcium absorption at the intestine and playing a permissive role for PTH-mediated bone resorption [22].

Calcium homeostasis is then focused on a small but critical circulating pool supported by a larger skeletal reserve, which is influenced by dietary intake and modified by the combined actions of PTH and vitamin D. Hypercalcemia may be a consequence of primary abnormalities in the controlling hormones or may be secondary to disease processes directly affecting bone resorption or intestinal absorption of calcium.

CLINICAL CONSIDERATIONS

In most clinical circumstances, hypercalcemia indicates the presence of either hyperparathyroidism or malignancy (Table 4-1). Hyperparathyroidism is more likely to be the cause of hypercalcemia noted in studies of the general population or unselected series of outpatients. In a general hospital population, malignancy accounts for most cases of hypercalcemia [16].

The duration of symptoms and the degree of hypercalcemia provide the initial clues to the diagnosis. Acute hypercalcemia, such as that developing over several days or weeks, produces anorexia, nausea and vomiting, azotemia, and marked neurologic manifestations ranging from lethargy to coma. Chronic hypercalcemia may be asymptomatic or may present with specific features such as band keratopathy. Renal, gastrointestinal, and skeletal features may be less apparent. Neurologic manifestations, in particular, may be less overt in chronic than in acute hypercal-

Table 4-1. Etiology of Hypercalcemia

Primary hyperparathyroidism
Neoplasia
    Bone metastases
    Ectopic PTH
    Prostaglandins
    Osteoclast-activating factor
    Other humoral mediators (cAMP-stimulating factor)
Drugs
    Thiazides
    Vitamins A and D
    Alkali antacids
    Lithium carbonate
Nonparathyroid endocrine disorders
    Hyperthyroidism
    Pheochromocytoma
    Adrenal insufficiency
    MEN syndromes
Granulomatous disease
Immobilization
    Paget's disease
    Fractures
Familial hypocalciuric hypercalcemia

cemic states. However, subtle neurologic abnormalities that improve with correction of chronic hypercalcemia have been noted in several studies. A picture of chronic hypercalcemia favors a diagnosis of non-malignant disease such as primary hyperparathyroidism, sarcoidosis, or vitamin D intoxication. Acute hypercalcemia or a serum calcium level greater than 13 mg/dl is more suggestive of malignant disease.

Primary hyperparathyroidism has been diagnosed with increasing frequency since the advent of routine multichannel analyzers. Studies have suggested a prevalence in the adult U.S. population of 0.12%, or 1 of every 834 adults [7]. The incidence of this disorder is higher in persons 40 or more years of age [23].

The ready availability of diagnostic tests has not only increased the recognition of primary hyperparathyroidism but has changed the characteristic presentation of this disorder [2,30,34]. Skeletal and renal manifestations are less often apparent. The size of parathyroid tumors at operation has decreased with earlier diagnosis. In the usual slowly progressive form of the disease, the development of hypercalcemia may be unaccompanied by overt symptoms in 50% of cases [23,30]. However, careful evaluation may reveal renal dysfunction (14%), hypercalciuria or stones (20–25%), ulcer disease or pancreatitis (8–15%), skeletal complaints (10–20%), and neurologic manifestations (20%). Hypertension also appears more frequently than in age-matched populations [23,30].

In the rapidly progressive form of hyperparathyroidism, which is usually due to parathyroid carcinoma or the rare fulminant parathyroid crisis, the symptoms described are intensified. Serum calcium levels tend to be higher than 13 mg/dl. Parathyroid carcinoma, however, is a rare cause of hyperparathyroidism; most cases are due to adenomas or hyperplasia [31]. The presence of parathyroid hyperplasia raises the possibility of an associated multiple endocrine neoplasia (MEN) syndrome.

Two aspects of hyperparathyroidism warrant brief comment. Radiation-induced hyperparathyroidism has been suggested in recent studies. In these cases, the interval between exposure and clinical presentation of hyperparathyroidism has been more than 30 years, and the development of hyperparathyroidism appeared to be dependent on the radiation dose [45,57]. Thus, the clinical history should include questions about prior radiation.

Normocalcemic hyperparathyroidism is defined as primary hyperparathyroidism with a normal serum calcium level. There is debate as to whether such an entity exists in the presumed early stages of hyperparathyroidism. Nephrogenous cyclic adenosine monophosphate (cAMP) may be consistently increased in spite of fluctuating values of total serum calcim [10]. In addition, ionized calcium levels have been shown to be elevated in some patients with symptoms of hypercalcemia but normal total calcium [58]. In suspected cases of hyperparathyroidism with borderline normal calcium levels, determination of ionized calcium and nephrogenous cAMP may prove helpful.

Neoplastic disease of nonparathyroid origin accounts for 70% of cases of hypercalcemia encountered in a hospital setting [29,31,38,47]. Tumors may cause hypercalcemia through direct metastatic involvement of bone or by other less well-characterized mechanisms. Carcinoma of the breast is a frequent cause of hypercalcemia usually secondary to bone metastases. It is important to note, however, that the extent of metastatic disease does not necessarily correlate with the degree of hypercalcemia. Lung carcinoma (epidermoid and large cell) [4], renal cell tumors, epidermoid tumors of the head, neck, and esophagus, and hepatobiliary and gastrointestinal tumors are the most frequent neoplasms causing hypercalcemia without apparent bone involvement. PTH-like substances [46,53,54] are suspected agents in these apparently humorally mediated hypercalcemic states. More specifically identified humoral factors are found in multiple myeloma, in which the hypercalcemia appears to be secondary to a specific osteoclast-activating factor [39], and in certain cases of tumor hypercalcemia apparently caused by prostaglandins [48].

Primary hyperparathyroidism may coexist with malignancy of nonparathyroid origin [15,26]. Such an association has been reported with breast, stomach, thyroid, and renal carcinomas. Although simultaneous presentations are obviously not common, they may be suspected when atypical clinical courses are found.

Drugs may cause hypercalcemia through several mechanisms. Excessive doses of vitamins A or D produce hypercalcemia through increased bone resorption (A and D) and increased intestinal calcium absorption (D) [18]. Thiazide diuretics will decrease urinary calcium excretion and transiently raise serum calcium in most patients [14]. A sustained increase in serum calcium levels suggests primary hyperparathyroidism. Chronic ingestion of calcium and absorbable alkali in the form of antacids is now an infrequent cause of hypercalcemia but may lead to significant hypercalcemia and renal impairment [40]. Lithium carbonate may also cause hypercalcemia [13]. This may be a result of an altered setpoint in the control of PTH secretion [12].

Endocrine disorders other than the MEN syndromes may be associated with hypercalcemia. In hyperthyroidism the excess of thyroid hormone directly increases bone resorption [43]. Overproduction of catecholamines by pheochromocytoma may stimulate parathormone release, leading to hypercalcemia [27]. The apparent hyperparathyroidism is corrected with removal of the adrenal tumor. This must be distinguished from the coexistence of primary hyperparathyroidism and pheochromocytoma in the MEN-II syndrome. Hypercalcemia may be present in adrenal insufficiency as a result of increased protein-bound calcium from hemoconcentration [25].

Other causes of hypercalcemia include immobilization and granulomatous diseases. Immobilization will not cause hypercalcemia unless the patient has a rapid bone turnover. Such states are present in growing children and in adults with preexisting diseases such as Paget's disease, hyperparathyroidism, neoplasia, and hyperthyroidism. Sarcoidosis is often associated with altered calcium metabolism due to an increased serum level of 1,25-$(OH)_2D$ [3,24,42]. In sarcoidosis, hypercalciuria is more frequent than hypercalcemia. Other granulomatous diseases, including tuberculosis, histoplasmosis, and coccidioidomycosis, have been found to cause hypercalcemia [32,49].

Familial hypocalciuric hypercalcemia (FHH) [37], also known as *familial benign hypercalcemia (FBH)* [17], is a newly recognized syndrome characterized by true hypercalcemia (ionized calcium is increased) without hypercalciuria (urinary calcium is usually less than 150 mg per day). This disorder is inherited in an autosomal dominant pattern and usually produces few symptoms [36]. PTH and urinary cAMP levels may be normal, whereas serum magnesium levels may be somewhat elevated. However, these findings are not invariably present. Clinically, this condition should be suspected when hypercalciuria does not accompany hypercalcemia or when hypercalcemia fails to improve with parathyroidectomy. Urinary calcium : creatinine clearance ratios are lower in this disorder compared to primary hyperparathyroidism or hypercalcemic disorders that suppress PTH activity [37].

Finally, it must be remembered that factitious hypercalcemia may result from laboratory error or prolonged use of a phlebotomy tourniquet. Volume depletion may cause minimal hypercalcemia.

DIAGNOSTIC METHODS
In most cases of hypercalcemia, the diagnosis can be made by an adequate history, physical examination, radiologic tests, and laboratory data obtained quickly and inexpensively from modern multichanneled analyzers. The major differential diagnosis is usually between hypercalcemia due to parathyroid disease and that due to neoplasia.

Serum Calcium and Phosphorus
Changes in serum albumin may alter the total calcium. A change in serum albumin of 1.0 g/dl will change the total calcium by approximately 0.8 mg/dl in the same direction. Measurements of total calcium are readily available by standard autoanalyzer techniques. Measurement of ionized calcium is not routinely indicated. *Ultrafilterable calcium* is a term encompassing nonprotein-bound calcium salts (i.e., calcium salts plus the ionized fraction).

Serum phosphorus levels are subject to much less regulation than calcium levels. The normal range in adults is 2.5 to 4.5 mg/dl, and higher levels may be found in children. Serum levels may also change with diurnal variation or dietary intake. For best interpretation, a fasting morning sample while the patient is on an adequate phosphorus diet is required.

Urinary Calcium
Normal urinary calcium levels are below 250 mg per day (males) and 200 mg per day (females) on a low-calcium diet. For practical purposes, such a diet may be considered to be one free of cheese and milk products. Calcium excretion parallels sodium excretion, so that urinary sodium measurements may be helpful in ensuring that calcium values are not altered by sodium intake or diuretics.

Serum Chloride and the Chloride/Phosphorus Ratio
In hyperparathyroidism, there is a tendency toward hyperchloremia and hypophosphatemia. A serum chloride level of 103 mEq/L or more was found in 97% of 76 patients with primary hyperparathyroidism in one study [30]; only 20% of other hypercalcemic subjects had values this high. The ratio of serum chloride and phosphorus may be diagnostically useful [41]. Patients with hyperparathyroidism characteristically have a Cl/PO_4 ratio above 33, whereas nonparathyroid hypercalcemic patients have a ratio below 30. Significant overlap has been noted in some studies, however.

Parathyroid Hormone Assay
Available radioimmunoassays for PTH have greatly simplified the diagnosis of hyperparathyroidism [1]. The diagnosis of primary hyperparathyroidism is supported by elevated PTH levels in 85 to 95% of cases, depending on the quality of the assay employed. However, problems do exist [52]. The assay is technically difficult, and measurement of the same serum in different laboratories may produce discrepant results [21,44]. This difficulty is partially related to the complex metabolism of the hormone that produces peptide fragments characterized by terminal amino or carboxy ends of the molecule. Carboxy terminal fragments represent the chronic secretory state and are measured in most available assays. Hormonal values should be interpreted in light of simultaneously measured serum calcium in the specimen since a normal PTH level may be abnormal for a given calcium value. PTH assays are time-consuming and thus are rarely useful in the immediate management of hypercalcemia.

Urinary Cyclic AMP
Since PTH dramatically increases the excretion of urinary cAMP (UcAMP), measurement of total UcAMP has emerged as a reliable and more available indirect assay of PTH action [50]. The measurement of total UcAMP includes the plasma cAMP (PcAMP) filtered and excreted by the kidney plus the cAMP produced primarily through PTH stimulation of the kidney, nephrogenous cAMP (NcAMP) [8,50]. Calculation of the NcAMP has been used to enhance interpretation of total UcAMP values. This calculation attempts to determine only that cAMP that is renally derived (NcAMP = UcAMP − PcAMP) [8,9]. However, since the plasma level and the filtered load of cAmp tend to remain fairly constant, studies have demonstrated that the use of UcAMP is almost equal

to the more time-consuming NcAMP determination in the assessment of hypercalcemic states [11].

Absolute measurements of UcAMP are not useful in diagnosis because the overlap of values between normals and hyperparathyroid patients is over 60%. However, when UcAMP is corrected for glomerular filtration rate (GFR), the resultant expression is comparable to the determination of NcAMP. Impaired renal function (GFR less than 20 ml per minute) may alter UcCAMP or NcAMP expressions.

Use of UcAMP expressed per deciliter/GF (glomerular filtrate) appears to be a simpler test and precludes the need for PcAMP measurement. A volume of urine is collected from a fasting recumbent patient for measurement of UcAMP and creatinine. A serum sample is obtained for creatinine. UcAMP, expressed as a function of GF (nanomoles per dl GF), may be conveniently computed by the product of the serum creatinine and UcAMP (in nanomoles per milligram creatinine) [9].

$$UcAMP/GF = \frac{\text{total UcAMP}}{\text{total urine creatinine}} \times \text{serum creatinine}$$

$$= \frac{\text{nmoles}}{\text{mg}} \times \text{mg/dl}$$

$$= \text{nmole/dl}$$

Elevated values have been found in 90% of patients with primary hyperparathyroidism [8,9]. Upper limits are relative, depending on the laboratory used; however, values greater than 3.5 nanomoles per dl are suggestive of hyperparathyroidism. Suppression of UcAMP or NcAMP by use of intravenous or oral calcium loads has also been advocated to aid in the diagnosis of subtle primary hyperparathyroidism [10,11]. Attempts to extend the use of cAMP to distinguish among the causes of hypercalcemia in association with malignant disease have shown inconsistent results [28,46,54].

Tubular Reabsorption of Phosphorus and the Renal Phosphorus Threshold

Since PTH enhances excretion of phosphorus, renal phosphate reabsorption is less than the normal 85% in about 70% of cases of primary hyperparathyroidism. Extraneous factors such as diminished renal function, decreased dietary phosphorus, and circadian rhythms can obscure the correct interpretation of this test. To avoid this problem, the test should be performed in a fasting, well-hydrated subject who has had an adequate dietary intake of phosphorus (1–2 gm) for at least 3 days. A timed fasting urine sample is collected. At the midpoint of the urine collection, a serum sample is drawn for phosphorus and creatinine. The percentage of tubular phosphorus reabsorption is then calculated:

$$TRP (\%) = 100 \times \left(1 - \frac{\text{urine phosphorus} \times \text{serum creatinine}}{\text{serum phosphorus} \times \text{urine creatinine}}\right)$$

The usefulness of this test is limited by the overlap between normal and hyperparathyroid patients.

Better discrimination between these groups may be obtained by determining the maximum tubular reabsorption of phosphate (TmP/GFR) [5]. The TmP/GFR is an index of phosphate clearance that expresses phosphate reabsorption as a function of both the serum phosphorus and the GFR. This determination gives an indication of the renal phosphorus threshold as it may be altered by PTH action. To determine TmP/GFR, the TRP is calculated and the TmP is derived from a nomogram [55]. Normal ranges are age and sex dependent but approximate 2.5 to 5.2 mg/dl. Patients with primary hyperparathyroidism have lower TmP/GFR (< 2.5) reflecting the lower setpoint for phosphorus reabsorption. This test has the advantages of being available and easily performed in most clinical settings.

Other Tests

Steroid suppression tests using high-dose glucocorticoids to suppress hypercalcemia have been employed in attempts to distinguish parathyroid from nonparathyroid disease [19,56]. The assumption in such tests is that suppression does not occur in patients with hyperparathyroidism but does occur in patients with nonparathyroid malignant disease. Cortisone (120 mg per day) or prednisone (30 mg per day) given for 5 to 10 days may lower calcium in nonparathyroid hypercalcemia. In a recent study, 30 of 42 patients with malignant disease had a fall in corrected serum calcium of at least 1 mg/dl during 8 days of therapy with 40 mg of hydrocortisone given three times a day. In the same study, only 2 of 84 patients with primary hyperparathyroidism and no bone disease had such falls in calcium, although 6 of 14 patients with radiologic evidence of parathyroid bone disease did show suppression of calcium [56].

The serum alkaline phosphatase may be increased in hyperparathyroidism but offers little discriminatory information. Serum bicarbonate is usually normal to low in parathyroid-dependent hypercalcemia and normal to high in other hypercalcemic states such as malignancy. Urinary calcium is usually elevated in nonparathyroid hypercalcemia but may be normal or high in hyperparathyroidism.

Skeletal radiographs or scans may aid in the evaluation of hypercalcemia. Resorptive changes in the distal and middle phalanges of the hands or the presence of cysts in long bones suggest hyperparathyroidism. Such changes usually occur late in the course of the disease.

Parathyroid angiography and venography may be used in selected cases, including those in which prior neck surgery failed to correct hypercalcemia [6,35].

Arterial and venous neck catheterization may aid in the localization of a parathyroid adenoma but should be limited to patients who have undergone previously unsuccessful neck surgery or those with other special considerations [35]. The arterial phase of the study may localize an adenoma if a characteristic "blush" becomes apparent. During the venous phase of the study, measurement of the PTH concentration in samples of thyroid effluent may localize parathyroid disease. Unilateral increases in PTH suggest adenoma; bilateral increases suggest hyperplasia.

DISCUSSION

Hypercalcemia should be confirmed with more than one calcium determination. The serum protein status and the corrected calcium values made should be noted. When hypercalcemia is clearly present, the severity of the calcium elevation dictates the pace of diagnostic efforts. Moderate hypercalcemia (less than 13 mg/dl) that is well tolerated clinically may be approached in a systematic manner. The history and physical examination are critical elements of the evaluation. If no evidence of malignancy is apparent on examination, drug-induced hypercalcemia becomes the first consideration. If drugs that may cause hypercalcemia have been used, it is reasonable to discontinue them and observe the patient. If hypercalcemia persists, further evaluation is necessary. Since thiazides reduce urinary calcium excretion, it may be helpful to measure 24-hour urine calcium in a case of presumed thiazide-induced hypercalcemia. Urinary calcium values should also be low in FBH. High values suggest additional causes for hypercalcemia. Vitamin D intoxication may cause persistent hypercalcemia for months following discontinuation of the drug.

In the absence of evidence of malignant disease or use of drugs, primary hyperparathyroidism emerges as the major diagnostic consideration (Fig. 4-1). Efforts must then be directed toward confirming this diagnosis and excluding other causes of nonmalignant hypercalcemia. The most readily available tests are the least specific. A low serum phosphorus or a high Cl/PO_4 ratio in a well-nourished, ambulatory patient supports the diagnosis of hyperparathyroidism. TmP/GFR determinations provide further supportive data when values are less than 2.5 mg/dl. The relative ease and reliability of the measurement of UcAMP/dl GF allows an early assessment of parathyroid function. High values suggest primary hyperparathyroidism. PTH assay will confirm the diagnosis in most instances.

It may be reasonably argued that a high suspicion of primary hyperparathyroidism should lead to determination of PTH levels, bypassing the other studies. However, when clinical presentations are equivocal, the use of these other tests may prove helpful and in some instances necessary [30]. For instance, a high TRP is found in the phosphorus depletion syndrome. Normal UcAMP values are expected in sarcoidosis or occult drug ingestion. Since the results of the PTH assay may not be immediately available, the careful use of these other tests may provide as-

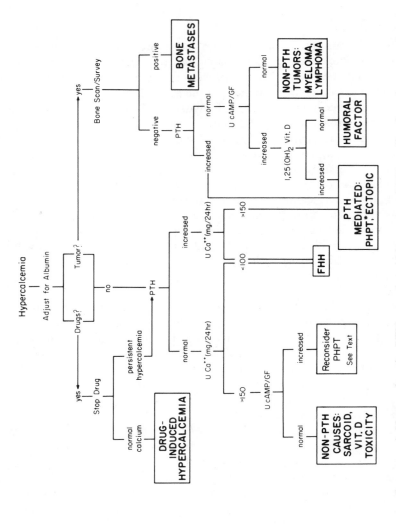

Figure 4-1. Diagnostic protocol: Hypercalcemia. PTH, parathyroid hormone; cAMP, cyclic adenosine monophosphate; PHPT, primary hyperparathyroidism; FHH, familial hypocalciuric hypercalcemia.

surance that other diseases are unlikely or, conversely, that other causes of hypercalcemia should be sought.

Primary hyperparathyroidism is confirmed by surgical exploration of the neck. Failure to correct hypercalcemia with surgery is an indication to localize parathyroid disease by neck catheterization studies or to re-evaluate for possible FBH.

Other forms of PTH excess leading to hypercalcemia include the hypercalcemia of chronic renal failure, so-called tertiary hyper-parathyroidism, and the hypercalcemia that may follow successful renal transplantation. Both of these disorders are characterized by increased parathyroid mass and high circulating PTH levels. In the case of successful transplantation, enhanced conversion of $1,25\text{-}(OH)_2D$ also is presumed to play a role. As with primary hyperparathyroidism, surgery may be required.

The other causes of nonneoplastic hypercalcemia listed in Table 4-1 may be confirmed by specific diagnostic tests. Commercial assays are now available to measure 25-OHD. The recent availability of the more potent $1,25 (OH)_2D$ makes this agent a possible source of intoxication. Assays for this compound are also now commercially available. Intoxication with this drug, however, should be briefer in duration than that noted with other vitamin D preparations.

Sarcoidosis, particularly in patients presenting without classic signs of hilar adenopathy or erythema nodosum, may be difficult to distinguish from the hypercalcemia of parathyroid or malignant origin. As noted in Figure 4-1, low UcAMP/dl GF may prove very useful in these cases, reflecting the low level of PTH. Diagnosis depends on appropriate biopsy confirmation. The response to a steroid suppression test may be dramatic in both sarcoidosis and vitamin D intoxication.

Hypercalcemia due to malignancy should be suspected when the serum calcium level is above 13 mg/dl, when no evidence of chronic hypercalcemia is present (neophrolithiasis, nephrocalcinosis, band keratopathy, or osteitis fibrosa), or when evidence of malignancy is found. Clinically, these patients tend to be more ill than others; therefore, the diagnostic evaluation must often be abbreviated in order to begin therapy for the elevated calcium. In such circumstances, it is critical that necessary studies be obtained prior to therapy that may obscure subsequent results.

Although hypercalcemia is often found in association with malignant disease, the mechanisms accounting for such elevations of calcium have been unclear. Two general pathophysiologic models have been proposed. The first mechanism, represented by carcinoma of the breast, attributes calcium elevation to local bone destruction by tumor that has metastasized to bone. Hence, a bone scan is a reasonable first step in evaluating hypercalcemia. A second proposed mechanism involves humoral substances, secreted by tumor, that mobilize calcium from bone. Occult malignancies (of the ovary or kidney) or those without metastases to bone are more likely to cause hypercalcemia through humoral mechanisms. PTH-like substances, prostaglandins, and the os-teoclast-activating factor of myeloma and some lymphomas have been implicated in cases of such humoral hypercalcemia.

The terms *pseudohyperparathyroidism* and *ectopic PTH syndrome* have been used to describe the hypercalcemic state resulting from pre-sumed PTH-like substances that cause hypercalcemia. However, several recent observations have complicated this concept. First, malignant dis-ease and primary hyperparathyroidism occur together with a frequency greater than that expected by chance [15,26]. Hence, the cause of an in-creased PTH level may be unclear. Second, PTH elevations in primary hyperparathyroidism and the hypercalcemia of malignancy overlap to some extent in many assays [21], reflecting some of the limitations of the current PTH assays. Third, the correlation between cAMP values and PTH levels, although high in primary hyperparathyroidism, has been in-consistent in cases of hypercalcemia in malignancy [28,46,54].

Recent studies have provided several important concepts that are quite helpful in explaining some of these inconsistencies and in further defining humoral mechanisms of hypercalcemia. Ectopic production of PTH does not appear to be a frequent cause of hypercalcemia in malig-nancy [53]. Elevated PTH levels have not been shown to account for hypercalcemia in recent studies [46,53,54]. Complementary data have emerged from studies suggesting that a humoral substance that is chemi-cally uncharacterized mimics certain aspects of PTH activity and may ac-count for hypercalcemia in many cases of malignancy. This humoral fac-tor, like PTH, is capable of stimulating production of nephrogenous cAMP and is associated with renal phosphate wasting and hypophos-phatemia, but unlike PTH, it does not decrease fasting calcium excretion or stimulate the conversion of 25-OHD to 1,25-$(OH)_2$D at the kidney [54]. The identification of the humoral cAMP-stimulating factor serves as a major conceptual advance in explaining the difficulty of characteriz-ing the mechanism of calcium elevation in malignancy. Studies using a cytochemical bioassay have demonstrated that this factor differs from PTH in patients with malignancy, hypercalcemia, and elevated NcAmp [20]. Further definition of this factor and more information on actual mechanisms of the humoral hypercalcemia of malignancy await studies of tumor cells themselves.

Since this humoral agent can increase nephrogenous cAMP, it has caused many problems in the use of UcAMP or NcAMP to investigate causes of hypercalcemia with cancer. Elevation of UcAMP or NcAMP appears to be common in malignancy, even in the absence of hypercal-cemia. In one study [46], UcAMP and NcAMP values were elevated in cancer patients with hypercalcemia from bone metastases and "pseudohyperparathyroidism" as well as in those without hypercal-cemia. Similar observations have been reported in patients with lung cancer [28]. Therefore, in the differential diagnosis of hypercalcemia, low UcAMP or NcAMP values suggest non-PTH–mediated causes of hypercalcemia. However, the presence of normal or high levels of UcAMP or NcAMP does not appear useful in distinguishing primary hyperparathyroidism from a humoral cAMP-stimulating factor or from the apparently rare case of true ectopic PTH secretion. Elevated PTH levels in the hypercalcemia of malignancy may be more suggestive of concurrent primary hyperparathyroidism than production of ectopic PTH by the malignancy. Very low PTH levels in the presence of increased UcAMP or NcAMP suggest the presence of the humoral cAMP-stimulatory factor. In the future, the use of fasting calcium excretion or the measurement of $1,25\text{-}(OH)_2D$ levels may prove helpful in distinguishing the causes of hypercalcemia in malignancy [54].

Therapy must often be initiated promptly in cases of malignant hypercalcemia. Samples for PTH determinations and cAMP levels should be obtained promptly. Phosphorus studies (Cl/PO_4 ratio and TRP) are less helpful in the acutely ill anorectic patient. In unusual instances in which studies eventually suggest PTH excess, particularly when PTH values are very elevated, neck catheterization studies [34] or surgery may be required to distinguish primary hyperparathyroidism from the uncommon ectopic-PTH syndrome. Alternatively, therapy directed at the neoplasm may be selected. Amelioration of the hypercalcemia should roughly parallel the tumor response.

REFERENCES
1. Arnaud, C. D., Tsao, H. S., and Littledike, T. Radioimmunoassay of parathyroid hormone in serum. *J. Clin. Invest.* 50:21–34, 1971.
2. Aurbach, G. D., et al. Hyperparathyroidism: Recent studies. *Ann. Intern. Med.* 79:566–581, 1973.
3. Bell, N. H., et al. Evidence that increased circulating 1,25-dihydroxy vitamin D is the probable cause for abnormal calcium metabolism in sarcoidosis. *J. Clin. Invest.* 64:218–225, 1979.
4. Bender, R. H., and Hansen, H. Hypercalcemia in bronchogenic carcinoma. A prospective study of 200 patients. *Ann. Intern. Med.* 80:205–208, 1974.
5. Bijvoet, O. L. M. Kidney Function in Calcium and Phosphate Metabolism. In L. V. Avioli and S. M. Krane (Eds.), *Metabolic Bone Disease.* New York: Academic Press, 1977. Pp. 50–140.
6. Bilezikian, J. P., et al. Preoperative localization of abnormal parathyroid tissue, cumulative experience with venous sampling and arteriography. *Am. J. Med.* 55:505–514, 1977.
7. Boonstra, C. E., and Jackson, C. E. Hyperparathyroidism detected by routine serum calcium analysis—prevalence in a clinic population. *Ann. Intern. Med.* 6:468–474, 1965.
8. Broadus, A. E. Nephrogenous cyclic AMP as a parathyroid function test. *Nephron* 23:136–41, 1979.
9. Broadus, A. E., et al. Nephrogenous cyclic adenosine monophosphate as a parathyroid function test. *J. Clin. Invest.* 60:771–783, 1977.

10. Broadus, A. E., et al. Primary hyperparathyroidism with intermittent hypercalcemia: Serial observations and simple diagnosis by means of an oral calcium tolerance test. *Clin. Endocrinol.* 12:225–235, 1980.
11. Broadus, A. E., and Rasmussen, H. Clinical evaluation of parathyroid function. *Am. J. Med.* 70:457–458, 1981.
12. Brown, E. M. Lithium induces abnormal calcium-regulated PTH release in dispersed bovine parathyroid cells. *J. Clin. Endocrinol. Metab.* 52:961–968, 1981.
13. Christiansen, C., Boastrup, P. C., and Transbol, I. Lithium induced "primary" hyperparathyroidism. *Calcif. Tissue Res.* 22 (suppl):341–343, 1977.
14. Duarte, C. G., et al. Thiazide induced hypercalcemia. *N. Engl. J. Med.* 284:828–830, 1971.
15. Farr, H. W., et al. Primary hyperparathyroidism and cancer. *Am. J. Surg.* 126:539–543, 1973.
16. Fisken, R. A., Heath, D. A., and Bold, A. M. Hypercalcemia: A hospital survey. *Q. J. Med.* 196:405–418, 1980.
17. Foley, T. P., et al. Familial benign hypercalcemia. *J. Pediatr.* 81:1060–1067, 1972.
18. Frame, B., et al. Hypercalcemia and skeletal effects in chronic hypervitaminosis. *Ann. Intern. Med.* 80:44–48, 1978.
19. Fucik, R. T., et al. Effect of glucocorticoids on function of the parathyroid glands in man. *J. Clin. Endocrinol. Metab.* 40:152–155, 1975.
20. Goltzman, D., Stewart, A. F., and Broadus, A. E. Malignancy-associated hypercalcemia: Evaluation with a cytochemical bioassay for parathyroid hormone. *J. Clin. Endocrinol. Metab.* 53:899–904, 1981.
21. Habener, J. F., and Segre, G. V. Parathyroid hormone radioimmunoassay. *Ann. Intern. Med.* 91:782–784, 1979.
22. Haussler, M. R., and McCain, T. A. Vitamin D metabolism and action. *N. Engl. J. Med.* 297:1041–1051, 1977.
23. Heath, H. H., Hodgson, S. F., and Kennedy, M. A. Primary hyperparathyroidism: Incidence, morbidity, and potential economic impact in a community. *N. Engl. J. Med.* 302:189–193, 1980.
24. Hornum, I., and Transbol, I. Observations on the different calcium metabolic patterns in sarcoidosis. A metabolic and kinetic study. *Acta Med. Scand.* 200:341–349, 1976.
25. Jorgensen, H. Hypercalcemia in adrenocortical insufficiency. *Acta Med. Scand.* 193:175–179, 1973.
26. Kaplan, L., et al. Malignant neoplasms and parathyroid adenoma. *Cancer* 28:401–407, 1971.
27. Kukreja, S. C., et al. Pheochromocytoma causing excessive parathyroid hormone production and hypercalcemia. *Ann. Intern. Med.* 79:838–840, 1970.
28. Kukreja, S. C., et al. Elevated nephrogenous cyclic AMP with normal serum parathyroid hormone levels in patients with lung cancer. *J. Clin. Endocrinol. Metab.* 51:167–169, 1980.
29. Lafferty, F. W. Pseudohyperparathyroidism. *Medicine* 45:247–259, 1966.
30. Lafferty, F. W. Primary hyperparathyroidism: Changing clinical spectrum, prevalence of hypertension, and discriminant analysis of laboratory tests. *Arch. Intern. Med.* 141:1761–1766, 1981.
31. Lee, D. B., Quawadu, E. T., and Kleeman, C. R. The pathophysiology and clinical aspects of hypercalcemic disorders. *West. J. Med.* 129:278–320, 1978.
32. Lee, J. C., et al. Hypercalcemia in disseminated coccidiomycosis. *N. Engl. J. Med.* 297:431–433, 1977.

33. Lemann, J., Adams, N. D., and Gray, R. Urinary calcium excretion in human beings. *N. Engl. J. Med.* 301:535–541, 1979.
34. Mallette, L. E., et al. Primary hyperparathyroidism: Clinical and biochemical features. *Medicine* 53:127–146, 1974.
35. Mallette, L. E., Gomez, L., and Fisher, R. G. Parathyroid angiography: A review of current knowledge and guidelines for clinical application. *Endocr. Rev.* 2:124–135, 1981.
36. Marx, S. J., et al. The hypocalciuric or benign variant of familial hypercalcemia: Clinical and biochemical features in fifteen kindreds. *Medicine* 60:397–412, 1981.
37. Marx, S. J., et al. Familial hypocalciuric hypercalcemia: Recognition among patients referred after unsuccessful parathyroid exploration. *Ann. Intern. Med.* 92:351–356, 1980.
38. Mundy, G. R., and Martin, T. J. The hypercalcemia of malignancy: Pathogenesis and management. *Metabolism* 31:1247–1277, 1982.
39. Mundy, G. R., and Raisz, L. G. Big and little forms of osteoclast activating factor. *J. Clin. Invest.* 60:122–128, 1977.
40. Orwoll, E. S. The milk-alkali syndrome: Current concepts. *Ann. Intern. Med.* 97:242–248, 1982.
41. Pak, C. Y. C., and Townsend, J. Chloride/phosphate ratio in primary hyperparathyroidism. *Ann. Intern. Med.* 85:830, 1976.
42. Papapoulos, S., et al. 1,25 dihydroxycholecalciferol in the pathogenesis of the hypercalcemia of sarcoidosis. *Lancet* 1:627–630, 1979.
43. Parfitt, A. M., and Dent, C. E. Hyperthyroidism and hypercalcemia. *Q. J. Med.* 39:171–187, 1970.
44. Raisz, L. G., et al. Comparison of commercially available parathyroid hormone immunoassays in the differential diagnosis of hypercalcemia due to primary hyperparathyroidism or malignancy. *Ann. Intern. Med.* 91:739–740, 1979.
45. Rao, S. D., et al. Hyperparathyroidism following head and neck irradiation. *Arch. Intern. Med.* 140:205–207, 1980.
46. Rude, R. K., et al. Urinary and nephrogenous cyclic adenosine 3'5'-monophosphate in the hypercalcemia of malignancy. *J. Clin. Endocrinol. Metab.* 52:765–771, 1981.
47. Rudman, J. S., and Sherwood, L. M. Disorders of Mineral Metabolism in Malignancy, in L. V. Avioli and S. M. Krane (Eds.), *Metabolic Bone Disease,* New York: Academic Press, 1978. Pp. 577–631.
48. Seyberth, H. W., Raisz, L. G., and Oates, J. A. Prostaglandins and hypercalcemic states. *Ann. Rev. Med.* 29:23–29, 1978.
49. Shai, F., et al. Hypercalcemia in mycobacterial infection. *J. Clin. Endocrinol. Metab.* 34:251–256, 1972.
50. Shaw, J. W., et al. Urinary cyclic AMP analyzed as a function of the serum calcium and parathyroid hormone in the differential diagnosis of hypercalcemia. *J. Clin. Invest.* 59:14–21, 1971.
51. Sherwood, L. M. The multiple causes of hypercalcemia in malignant disease. *N. Engl. J. Med.* 303:1412–1413, 1980.
52. Silverman, R., and Yalow, R. S. Heterogeneity of parathyroid hormone. Clinical and physiological implications. *J. Clin. Invest.* 52:1958–1971, 1973.
53. Skrabanek, P., McPartkin, J., and Powel, D. Tumor hypercalcemia and ectopic hyperparathyroidism. *Medicine* 59:262–282, 1980.
54. Stewart, A. F., et al. Biochemical evaluation of patients with cancer-associated hypercalcemia: Evidence for humoral and nonhumoral groups. *N. Engl. J. Med.* 303:1377–1383, 1980.

55. Walton, R. J., and Bijvoet, O. L. M. Normogram for derivation of renal threshold phosphate concentration. *Lancet* 2:309–310, 1975.
56. Watson, L., Moxham, J., and Fraser, P. Hydrocortisone suppression test and discriminant analysis in differential diagnosis of hypercalcemia. *Lancet* 2:1320–1325, 1980.
57. Tissell, L. E., et al. Hyperparathyroidism in persons treated with x-rays for tuberculosis cervical adenitis. *Cancer* 40:846–854, 1977.
58. Transbol, I. On the diagnosis of so-called normocalcemic hyperparathyroidism. *Acta Med. Scand.* 202:481–487, 1977.

5 Hypocalcemia

Angelo A. Licata
William F. Streck

Whereas hypercalcemia is a pathologic process for which the body has few compensatory mechanisms, hypocalcemia elicits a series of complex hormonal responses that serve to protect the body from the potentially serious effects of low calcium levels. Parathyroid hormone (PTH) and vitamin D, acting both independently and in concert, correct hypocalcemia and maintain the serum calcium level in the normal range [3]. Deficiencies of either of these hormones or ineffective action of either may lead to symptomatic hypocalcemia [14].

Hypocalcemia normally elicits an increased release of PTH. PTH, in turn, stimulates the renal conversion of 25-hydroxyvitamin D (25-OHD) to the more active form, 1,25-dihydroxyvitamin D [1,25-$(OH)_2$D]. PTH and the 1,25-$(OH)_2$D, acting synergistically, stimulate mobilization of calcium from bone [25]. In addition, the vitamin D metabolite enhances calcium and phosphorus absorption at the intestine, thus providing the complementary influx of calcium necessary to ensure that correction of hypocalcemia is not accomplished by depletion of bone calcium reserves. Calcium is then conserved through a PTH-mediated renal conservation of calcium [3,4,10]. Thus, in the normal compensatory state, the body is able both to mobilize more calcium and to conserve this calcium in order to correct hypocalcemia (Fig. 5-1).

Disorders of vitamin D may not be characterized by very low serum calcium levels. This reflects the fact that in these states PTH is still capable of mobilizing calcium from bone to maintain normal calcium levels. Such calcium elevations are achieved at the price of hypophosphatemia and metabolic bone disease. Conversely, in states of PTH deficiency, hypocalcemia is expected but metabolic bone disease is less common. The absence of PTH depresses tubular resorption of calcium and decreases clearance of phosphate; both hypocalcemia and hyperphosphatemia then ensue. The combination of low PTH and increased phosphate leads to decreased levels of 1,25-$(OH)_2$D [12]. Since both bone resorption and calcium absorption are reduced, hypocalcemia may result but metabolic bone disease may not occur.

CLINICAL CONSIDERATIONS

Hypocalcemia is present if the total serum calcium is less than 8.5 mg/dl in a patient with normal serum albumin levels. The ionized serum calcium may be lowered in the presence of a normal total calcium in such conditions as hyperventilation or acute severe vomiting because these lead to alkalosis, which enhances the binding of calcium to protein. In the absence of obvious acid-base disorders, the total calcium value is a useful but imprecise indication of ionized calcium levels [18]. In most

A.

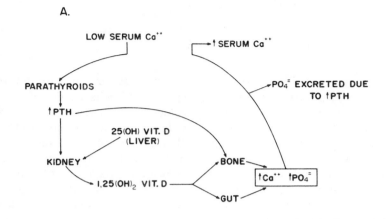

B.

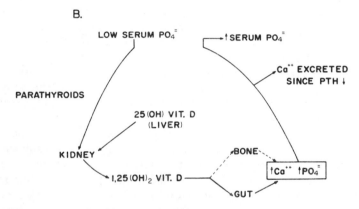

Figure 5-1. Parathyroid hormone (PTH)/vitamin D interactions in mineral homeostasis. **A.** Hypocalcemia elicits a PTH response with consequent conversion of 25-OHD to 1,25-(OH)₂D at the kidney. Calcium absorption is increased due to the effect of 1,25-(OH)₂D at the intestine. Increased bone mobilization of calcium occurs via the effects of both 1,25-(OH)₂D and PTH. The net result of these processes is an increase of calcium and phosphorus in the blood. The excess phosphorus is excreted by the kidney due to the phosphaturic effect of PTH. **B.** Hypophosphatemia does not stimulate secretion of PTH but leads directly to increased formation of 1,25-(OH)₂D with consequent increased gut absorption of calcium and phosphorus. In the absence of PTH, calcium is excreted and phosphorus retained. 25(OH) vit. D = 25-hydroxyvitamin D; 1,25(OH)₂ vit. D = 1,25-dihydroxyvitamin D.

Table 5-1. Causes of Hypocalcemia

Parathormone failure or ineffectiveness
  Hypoparathyroidism
    Postsurgical
    Idiopathic
  Pseudohypoparathyroidism
Vitamin D disorders
  Renal failure [↓ production of $1,25\text{-}(OH)_2D$]
  Malabsorption of vitamin D
  Hepatic disease (↓ formation of 25-OHD)
  Dietary vitamin D deficiency
  Vitamin D–dependent rickets
    Type I [defective production of $1,25\text{-}(OH)_2D$]
    Type II [end-organ resistance to $1,25\text{-}(OH)_2D$]
Magnesium deficiency

Drugs
  Phosphate
  Anticonvulsants
  Mithramycin
  Calcitonin

Other
  Neonatal tetany
  Acute pancreatitis
  Increased skeletal uptake
  Multiple transfusions

---

clinical circumstances, hypocalcemia reflects a chronic process (Table 5-1). Exceptions include the hypocalcemia of acute pancreatitis and drug ingestion (phosphate loads).

The rapidity of development of hypocalcemia determines symptoms more directly than the absolute calcium level (Table 5-2). Acute hypocalcemia may lead to tetany, which is first manifested by carpopedal spasm. During a tetanic episode, tonic contraction of separate muscle groups may progress to involve the hands, arms, legs, and face. Convulsions, laryngeal stridor, and gastrointestinal symptoms may be present.

Latent tetany is a state in which tetanic symptoms may be elicited by diagnostic measures such as Chvostek's or Trousseau's signs. Chvostek's sign is elicited by tapping the facial nerve in front of the ear. A positive test consists of contraction of the mouth, the nostril, and the orbicularis oculi. Trousseau's sign consists of carpopedal spasm after blood flow to the hand is impeded by inflating a blood pressure cuff to systolic levels for 3 minutes. Trousseau's sign is the more reliable indicator of hypocalcemia. Ten percent of normal persons may have a positive Chvostek's sign.

Chronic hypocalcemia causes subtle and less specific symptoms. Mental symptoms may dominate. Depression, irritability, memory loss, and emotional disturbances are common. Other associated findings are listed

Table 5-2. Manifestations of Hypocalcemia

Acute
  Paresthesias (acral and circumoral)
  Carpopedal spasm
  Tetany
  Seizures
Chronic
  Mental changes
  Neurologic changes
    Headache
    Extrapyramidal symptoms
  Basal ganglia calcification
  Cataracts
  Dystrophic changes
    Alopecia
    Abnormal nails
  Moniliasis
  Abnormal dentition
  Hyperostosis

---

in Table 5-2. Chronic hypocalcemia may be clinically inapparent until the calcium balance is stressed, for example, with a calciuric diuretic such as furosemide or in situations of increased demand such as pregnancy [17].

Parathyroid Hormone Disorders
PTH disorders that result in hypocalcemia include deficient production of PTH and end-organ unresponsiveness to biologically active hormone [24].

Postsurgical hypoparathyroidism is the most common cause of hypocalcemia due to PTH deficiency. Consequent abnormalities in vitamin D metabolism also occur [20]. PTH deficiency may be transient after the removal of hyperplastic or adenomatous glands. This is due to suppression of the remaining parathyroid tissue in combination with "hungry bones" of the previously hyperstimulated state. Surgical injury to the glands may cause hypoparathyroidism immediately after surgery or much later.

Idiopathic hypoparathyroidism is a rare disorder that may present in several forms. Di George's syndrome is recognized during the neonatal period. Developmental abnormalities of the pharyngeal pouches and branchial arches result in absent or rudimentary parathyroid glands, hypoparathyroidism, and thymic aplasia. Such infants present with hypocalcemia, recurrent fungal and viral infections, and failure to thrive. Death often occurs by 6 years of age.

A familial form of hypoparathyroidism and an isolated form occurring in the fifth and sixth decades are also known. Idiopathic hypoparathyroidism is frequently associated with cutaneous moniliasis and multiple endocrine deficiencies, particularly hypoadrenalism, thyroiditis, and pernicious anemia [5,24]. Dental abnormalities are often prominent. Seizures or behavioral problems may provide clues in childhood. Calcium levels may be 5 to 7 mg/dl, phosphorus levels are increased, and both PTH and 1,25-$(OH)_2$D levels are low.

Pseudohypoparathyroidism (PHP) represents a state of end-organ resistance to PTH, characterized by hyperplasia of the parathyroid glands and excessive secretion of hormone. Hypocalcemia develops from relative resistance to the action of the hormone at kidney and bone. In the classic state, this condition is associated with specific skeletal and developmental abnormalities, including short stature, dental aplasia, extraosseus calcifications, shortened metacarpals, and mental retardation. Recent studies have demonstrated that various end-organ deficiencies may characterize this condition, including selective skeletal and/or renal resistance to PTH and cyclic AMP (cAMP) abnormalities [5]. Since bone resistance may be incomplete, very high PTH levels may lead to evidence of metabolic bone disease [16].

Pseudo-pseudohypoparathyroidism (PPHP) describes a condition characterized by normal calcium levels but skeletal and developmental features suggestive of pseudohypoparathyroidism [5]. This disorder may be part of a continuum of incompletely expressed forms of the PTH-resistant state.

Vitamin D Disorders

Relative or absolute deficiencies of vitamin D or its metabolites may cause hypocalcemia. Decreased production of 25-hydroxyvitamin D (25-OHD) appears to be present in some cases of severe liver disease, including alcoholic and biliary cirrhosis [19,22]. In patients on chronic anticonvulsant therapy, decreased levels of 25-OHD have also been noted, due either to increased catabolism by the induction of hepatic microsomal mixed-oxidase activity or to disordered formation of the metabolite [13]. Steatorrhea may lead to malabsorption of both calcium and vitamin D. Nutritional vitamin D deficiency is relatively rare in young adults but may be more common in elderly persons who have unusual degrees of sun deprivation [9].

Chronic renal failure remains the most common cause of hypocalcemia due to altered metabolism of vitamin D. Damage to the kidney prevents conversion of the 25-hydroxy form to the active 1,25-$(OH)_2$D [8,21]. Even in the presence of elevated PTH, decreased calcium absorption ensues, since PTH elicits a subnormal calcemic response at bone. Vitamin D–dependent rickets (type I) also results from defective 1,25-hydroxylation. However, it is not renal damage but a metabolic block of the 1,25-hydroxylation process that causes this disorder [11]. Vitamin D–dependent rickets (type II) is caused by target-organ resistance to normal or elevated levels of this metabolite [6]. Hypophosphatemic vitamin

D–resistant rickets, usually a sex-linked dominantly inherited disorder, is characterized by diminished renal tubular phosphorus absorption. Hypocalcemia is not a usual feature. In contrast to the vitamin D–dependent disorders, phosphorus supplementation is required for normal growth and maturation.

Other Disorders

Hypomagnesemia is an increasingly recognized cause of hypocalcemia in such conditions as malabsorption, chronic alcoholism, and malnutrition. Magnesium deficiency leads to decreased synthesis and secretion of PTH and probable impairment of its activity at target organs [28].

Selected drugs that may cause hypocalcemia are listed in Table 5-1. Phosphate infusion may lead to calcium-phosphate complexes and acutely lower serum calcium. Such therapy is rarely indicated. Mithramycin inhibits bone resorption [15]. Dilantin alters hepatic microsomal metabolism of 25-OHD [13]. Calcitonin may lower serum calcium in hypercalcemic states; however, clinical states of hypercalcitonemia (i.e., medullary thyroid tumors) do not result in hypocalcemia [2].

Other causes of hypocalcemia include neonatal hypocalcemia, a multifactorial disorder that may occur in up to 50% of premature infants. Functional hypoparathyroidism may play a role, particularly in cases of maternal hypercalcemia. Increased phosphate loads and abnormalities of vitamin D have also been implicated [27]. The transient hypocalcemia of acute pancreatitis is not well understood but may be associated with concurrent magnesium deficiency [29]. The infusion of multiple units of citrated blood may lead to calcium-citrate complexes and hypocalcemia. In rare situations, hypocalcemia has resulted from the osteoblastic activity of metastatic tumor [26].

DIAGNOSTIC METHODS

Serum Calcium and Phosphorus ⎫
Parathormone Measurement   ⎬ (See Chap. 4).
Urinary Cyclic AMP   ⎭

Vitamin D Metabolites

Assays for 25-OHD are commercially available. Normal ranges in the United States are 15 to 80 ng/ml. Diet and exposure to sunlight affect the level in a given patient. Low levels may be found in malabsorption, biliary cirrhosis, and vitamin D deficiency. Assays for $1,25-(OH)_2D$ have recently become commercially available.

Parathyroid Hormone Infusion

In the hypocalcemic patient, the response to infused PTH will differentiate PTH deficiency from the end-organ insensitivity of pseudohypoparathyroidism [7,23].

Following 5 days of a low-phosphate diet, a fasting patient collects three consecutive 1-hour urine samples for measurement of creatinine, calcium, phosphorus, and cAMP. At the end of the third hour, 200 to 400 units of bovine PTH is administered intravenously over 10 minutes.

Urine is collected in periods of 0 to 30, 30 to 60, 60 to 120, and 120 to 180 minutes and analyzed as noted. A normal response shows about a 10-fold increase in cAMP and a 4- to 6-fold rise in phosphorus. A rise in serum calcium may also occur.

Two additional points require mention. First, a control subject should undergo the protocol to ensure biologic potency of the PTH preparation. Second, intradermal skin tests with 0.1 mg of a 1 : 10 dilution of the hormone with normal saline may be used before testing to avoid allergic reactions.

Alternatively, to avoid dependence on a single test, repeated PTH injections may be given every 6 hours for 2 or 3 days. Intramuscular or subcutaneous injection of 600 to 800 units a day will double phosphorus excretion and elevate serum calcium levels in PTH-deficient individuals, usually within 3 days. Because the commercial source of PTH may be limited in the future, this testing may be available only in referral centers.

Serum and Urinary Magnesium
The normal range for serum magnesium is 1.8 to 2.7 mEq/L. Serum levels may remain normal despite depletion of 10 to 20% of body stores. Symptomatic hypomagnesemia is usually accompanied by serum levels below 1.0 mEq/L, although hypocalcemia may be associated with normal levels. Urinary magnesium depends directly on dietary intake and body stores. In patients with suspected hypomagnesemia, daily urinary losses should be small (1 mEq per day) even if serum levels are in the normal range.

DISCUSSION
The more common causes of hypocalcemia are chronic renal disease, hypoparathyroidism, and magnesium deficiency [14,24]. As in the evaluation of hypercalcemia, total serum calcium must be adjusted for changes in serum proteins (Fig. 5-2). Use of calcium-lowering drugs or the presence of acute pancreatitis is usually revealed by history and physical examination. Similarly, a surgical scar on the neck indicates possible postsurgical hypoparathyroidism. A history of prior neck irradiation with radioactive iodine may also be sought since there is a report that parathyroid function may be impaired after ^{131}I therapy in hyperthyroidism [1].

In the patient who has not had prior neck surgery, an elevated serum phosphorus should initiate evaluation of renal function. If renal function is abnormal and the phosphorus is above 4.5 mg/dl, acute or chronic

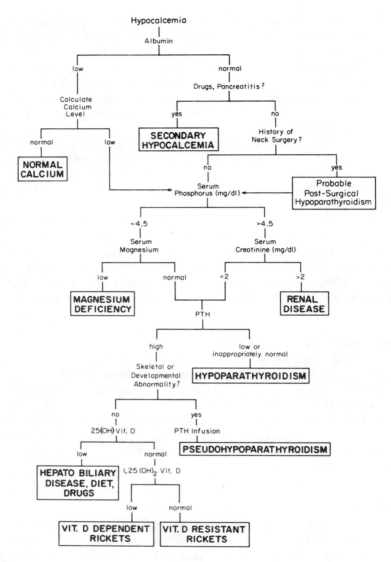

Figure 5-2. Diagnostic protocol: Hypocalcemia. PTH, parathyroid hormone; 25(OH) vit. D = 25-hydroxyvitamin D; 1,25(OH)$_2$ = 1,25-dihydroxyvitamin D.

renal insufficiency is suggested. Hypocalcemia in renal failure rarely presents as tetany due to the increased ionized calcium fraction associated with metabolic acidosis.

Hypocalcemia in the presence of hypophosphatemia should lead to measurement of serum magnesium. Hypomagnesemia occurs in alcoholics or subjects with steatorrhea or other malabsorptive problems. Magnesium replacement is necessary before PTH determinations are of value. If hypocalcemia is not corrected with magnesium replacement, additional abnormalities of PTH or vitamin D systems should be sought. In this setting, a high PTH value suggests vitamin D disorders. A low PTH value suggests hypoparathyroidism as a contributing factor but does not fully explain the hypophosphatemia.

Hypoparathyroidism is indicated by a low PTH in the presence of hypocalcemia, hyperphosphatemia, and normal renal function. Magnesium levels are normal. In contrast, PTH levels are elevated in pseudohypoparathyroidism, although the biochemical markers are similar. Pseudohypoparathyroidism usually has associated skeletal and developmental defects, or a family history of skeletal disorders is noted. However, the definitive diagnosis of such disorders must be made through the PTH stimulation test. Since the basic problem is end-organ resistance to biologically normal PTH [23], there is a minimal increase in urinary cAmp excretion after PTH infusion compared to a normal increase of 4- to 10-fold.

As outlined in Figure 5-2, the selective measurement of vitamin D metabolites may be used to identify other causes of hypocalcemia in the presence of increased PTH levels. Low 25-OHD levels suggest hepatobiliary or malabsorptive disorders. Normal levels of 25-OHD may indicate more selective problems of $1,25-(OH)_2D$ deficiency or resistance.

REFERENCES

1. Adams, P. A., and Chalmers, T. M. Parathyroid function after I-131 therapy in hyperthyroidism. *Clin. Sci.* 29:392–395, 1965.
2. Austin, L. A., and Heath, H. H., III. Calcitonin: Physiology and pathophysiology. *N. Engl. J. Med.* 304:269–279, 1981.
3. Avioli, L. V. Hormonal aspects of vitamin D metabolism and its clinical implications. *Clin. Endocrinol. Metab.* 8:547–577, 1979.
4. Bilezikian, J. P., et al. Response of 1,25-dihydroxyvitamin D_3 to hypocalcemia in human subjects. *N. Engl. J. Med.* 299:437–441, 1978.
5. Breslau, N. A., and Pak, C. Y. Hypoparathyroidism. *Metabolism* 28:1261–1275, 1979.
6. Brooks, M. H., et al. Vitamin D dependent rickets Type II, resistance of target organs to 1,25-dihydroxyvitamin D. *N. Engl. J. Med.* 298:996–999, 1978.
7. Chase, L. R., Nelson, G. C., and Aurbach, G. D. Pseudohypoparathyroidism: Defective excretion of 3′,5′-AMP in response to parathyroid hormone. *J. Clin. Invest.* 48:1832–1844, 1969.

8. Coburn, J. W., Hartenbower, D. L., and Massry, S. G. Intestinal absorption of calcium and the effect of renal insufficiency. *Kidney Int.* 4:96–101, 1973.
9. Corless, D., et al. Response of plasma 25-hydroxyvitamin D to ultraviolet irradiation in long stay geriatric patients. *Lancet* 2:649–652, 1978.
10. DeLuca, H. F. Vitamin D metabolism and function. *Arch. Intern. Med.* 138:836–847, 1978.
11. Fraser, D., et al. Pathogenesis of hereditary vitamin D dependent rickets. *N. Engl. J. Med.* 289:817–822, 1973.
12. Gray, R. W., et al. The importance of phosphate in regulating plasma 1,25-(OH)$_2$-vitamin D levels in humans: Studies in healthy subjects, in calcium stone formers and patients with hyperparathyroidism. *J. Clin. Endocrinol. Metab.* 45:299–306, 1977.
13. Hahn, T. J., et al. Serum 25 hydroxycholecalciferol levels and bone mass in children on anticonvulsant therapy. *N. Engl. J. Med.* 292:550–554, 1975.
14. Juan, D. Hypocalcemia, differential diagnosis and mechanisms. *Arch. Intern. Med.* 139:1166–1171, 1979.
15. Kiarn, D. T., Lokan, M. K., and Kennedy, B. J. Mechanism of the hypocalcemic effect of mithramycin. *J. Clin. Endocrinol. Metab.* 48:341–344, 1979.
16. Kidd, G. S., et al. Skeletal responsiveness in pseudohypoparathyroidism. *Am. J. Med.* 68:772–781, 1980.
17. Kumar, R., et al. Elevated 1,25 dihydroxyvitamin D plasma levels in normal human pregnancy and lactation. *J. Clin. Invest.* 63:342–344, 1979.
18. Landenson, J. H., Lewis, J. W., and Boyd, J. C. Failure of total calcium corrected for protein, albumin, and pH to correctly assess free calcium states. *J. Clin. Endocrinol. Metab.* 46:986–992, 1978.
19. Long, R. G., et al. Serum 25 hydroxyvitamin D in untreated parenchymal and cholestatic liver disease. *Lancet* 2:650–652, 1976.
20. Lund, B., et al. Vitamin D metabolism in hypoparathyroidism. *J. Clin. Endocrinol. Metab.* 51:606–610, 1980.
21. Massry, S. G., et al. Divalent ion metabolism in patients with acute renal failure. *Kidney Int.* 5:437–445, 1974.
22. Meyer, M., et al. Malabsorption of vitamin D in man and rat with liver cirrhosis. *J. Lab. Clin. Med.* 74:472–479, 1978.
23. Neer, R. M., Tregear, G. W., and Potts, J. J., Jr. Renal effects of native parathyroid hormone and synthetic biologically active fragments in pseudohypoparathyroidism and hypoparathyroidism. *J. Clin. Endocrinol. Metab.* 38:420–423, 1977.
24. Nusynowitz, M. L., Frame, B. L., and Kolb, S. O. The spectrum of the hypoparathyroid states: A classification based on physiologic principles. *Medicine* 55:105–119, 1976.
25. Parfitt, A. M. The actions of parathyroid hormone on bone: Relation to bone remodeling and turnover, calcium homeostasis and metabolic bone disease. Part II. PTH and bone cells. Bone turnover and plasma calcium regulation. *Metabolism* 25:909–955, 1976.
26. Smallridge, R. C., Wray, H. L., and Schaaf, M. Hypocalcemia with osteoblastic metastases in a patient with prostate carcinoma. *Am. J. Med.* 71:184–188, 1981.
27. Tsang, R. C., Steichen, J. J., and Chan, G. M. Neonatal hypocalcemia: Mechanism of occurrence and management. *Crit. Care Med.* 5:56–61, 1977.
28. Weigmann, T., and Kaye, M. Hypomagnesemic hypocalcemia. *Arch. Intern. Med.* 137:953–955, 1977.
29. Weir, G. C., et al. The hypocalcemia of acute pancreatitis. *Ann. Intern. Med.* 83:185–189, 1975.

6 Diabetes Insipidus and SIADH

S. Zane Burday
William F. Streck

The movement of our remote ancestors from a fluid to a terrestrial environment necessitated the development of a means of maintaining water balance. The homeostatic regulation provided by the secretion of arginine vasopressin (AVP) and the induction of thirst and drinking behavior are evolutionary solutions to this problem [22]. In a classic series of experiments performed more than 30 years ago, Verney [26] demonstrated that the secretion of AVP is largely regulated by the osmolality of body water. The recent development of sensitive and specific methods for measuring AVP has facilitated more detailed understanding of the control system for this hormone [19,20]. Despite its name, AVP serves primarily as an antidiuretic hormone (ADH). Its role in blood pressure control is not clearly defined [4,18], and the terms *AVP* and *ADH* are often used interchangeably.

AVP is synthesized in the neurons of the supraoptic and paraventricular nuclei and transported down axons in secretory vesicles to the posterior pituitary, where it is stored. It is released into the circulation in response to a wide variety of stimuli (Table 6-1). Under physiologic conditions, plasma osmolality is the major determinant of AVP release. Osmoreceptor neurons, functionally separate from the secretory neurons, are able to detect small changes in plasma osmolality and translate these into appropriate signals to the neurohypophyseal system, which modifies AVP secretion [22]. As the plasma osmolality increases to about 292 mOsm/kg, plasma levels of AVP rise rapidly in proportion to changes in plasma osmolality [21]. According to Robertson et al., a plasma osmolality of 295 mOsm/kg produces AVP levels of 5 pg/ml, a concentration able to induce maximal antidiuresis. At plasma levels below 280 mOsm/kg, plasma AVP is usually suppressed and a maximal water diuresis may occur. Within the range of 280 to 295 mOsm/kg, small changes in plasma osmolality effect large changes in urine osmolality and volume by altering AVP. The significant "gain" in the osmoregulatory system is illustrated by the fact that a 1% increase in plasma osmolality (2.8–2.9 mOsm/kg) will raise plasma AVP by approximately 1 pg/ml, which in turn may effect an increase in urine osmolality of 250 mOsm/kg [19,21]. The full range of renal concentration and dilution is found in AVP levels of 0.5–5.0 pg/ml and has been expressed in a series of formuli derived from the work of Robertson et al. [19].

The threshold and sensitivity of AVP release may vary considerably from person to person but are reproducible in an individual. Sensitivity, the slope of the line describing effects of osmolar changes on plasma AVP, varies by a factor of five- to sixfold (0.14–0.98) in normal adults [21]. Furthermore, the sensitivity of the osmoreceptor to osmolar changes induced by sodium and its anions is not paralleled by other sol-

Table 6-1. Known Stimuli and Inhibitors of Vasopressin Release and Action

Stimuli

Osmotic

   Increased osmolality of ECF leading to contracted intracellular volume of hypothalamic osmoreceptors

Nonosmotic

   Decreased pressure in carotid and aortic baroreceptors

   Decreased left atrial and large pulmonary vein tension resulting from reduced intrathoracic blood volume (blood loss, upright position, positive-pressure breathing)

   Stimulation of the renin-angiotensin system

   Emesis, pain, emotional stress

   Drugs

      Stimulate release: acetylcholine, nicotine, beta agonists, morphine, bradykinin, vincristine

      Potentiate effect: chlorpropamide, carbamazepine, clofibrate

   Glucopenia

Inhibitors

Osmotic

   Decreased osmolality of ECF leading to expanded intracellular volume of hypothalamic osmoreceptors

Nonosmotic

   Increased pressure in carotid and aortic baroreceptors

   Increased left atrial and large pulmonary vein tension resulting from increased intrathoracic blood volume (hypervolemia, reclining position, negative-pressure breathing, exposure to cold)

   Drugs

      Inhibit release: ethanol, diphenylhydantoin, atropine, alpha agonists

      Block action: lithium, demethylchlortetracycline, methoxyflurane, amphotericin B

utes such as urea, which distributes throughout body water, and glucose, which may actually suppress AVP release, presumably by extracellular fluid (ECF) volume expansion.

Physiologic alterations in intravascular volume affect AVP release and are important to recognize in assessing the clinical disorders of water metabolism. Volume depletion lowers the threshold for AVP release and increases the rate of secretion. Conversely, hypervolemia elevates the osmolar threshold for AVP release. In addition to these osmotic and volume-mediated influences, a number of other variables may affect the release and action of AVP (Table 6-1).

Regulation of water metabolism is effected through two major organ systems. First, the supraoptic neurohypophyseal tract synthesizes, stores, and releases ADH as needed [19]. Second, the kidney must respond in an appropriate fashion to the presence of AVP [14]. The dilution of urine involves active transport of chloride out of the ascending limb of the loop of Henle, with subsequent sodium transport. Simultaneously, the transport of sodium, chloride, and urea into the medullary interstitial area generates a hyperosmolar gradient in the interstitium. The dilute urine in the collecting duct then passes through this hyperosmolar environment. In the presence of AVP, the collecting duct is permeable to water that is osmotically attracted into the hypertonic medullary interstitium, with subsequent water conservation. In this manner, the kidney serves as the end organ for AVP action and water conservation.

CLINICAL CONSIDERATIONS

Disorders of water metabolism are best understood by reference not to body water but rather to solute concentrations [5,13,27]. Water is permeable between the ECF and the intracellular fluid (ICF) compartments. Solutes, in contrast, reside largely on one side or the other of the cell membrane, a process regulated by various physiologic mechanisms. Solute concentrations (osmolality) affect the flow of water between the two basic fluid compartments and thus determine the distribution of water throughout the body [8]. Disorders of water metabolism are reflected by changes in the solute concentration, primarily as seen in the ECF, which is most easily assessed [23].

As sodium is the primary ECF solute, changes in serum sodium levels are most commonly encountered in problems of water metabolism. Hyponatremia indicates an absolute or relative excess of water over sodium due to either water retention or sodium loss. Hypernatremia, in contrast, reflects an absolute or relative water deficit and is only rarely related to excessive sodium retention. The serum sodium concentration gives little information about total body sodium stores. Sodium balance can be assessed by clinical means, such as skin turgor, orthostatic blood pressure changes, and neck vein distention. The combination of serum sodium or serum osmolality determinations in conjunction with assessment of volume status provides the basis for clinical estimate of the activity of AVP in the body.

Deficiencies of Arginine Vasopressin

The presence of polyuria, with or without hypernatremia and hyperosmolality, raises the question of a possible defect in water conservation. Such defects fall into four major categories (Table 6-2). First, there may be damage to the posterior pituitary or hypothalamic region with failure to secrete AVP. Second, there may be damage to the kidney such that it is unresponsive to AVP. Nephrogenic diabetes insipidus of the congenital and acquired types falls into this category. Third, there is the possibility of primary polydipsia, that is, excessive drinking of water. Finally, osmotic diuresis such as may occur in diabetes mellitus must be considered. The majority of causes of polyuria, unrelated to AVP deficiency, are easily distinguished clinically and present little problem in differential diagnosis.

Table 6-2. Etiology of Major Polyuric Syndromes

Inadequate secretion of AVP—diabetes insipidus
Inability to reabsorb adequate amounts of filtered water despite adequate AVP
  secretion
  Nephrogenic diabetes insipidus—congenital
  Nephrogenic diabetes insipidus—acquired
    Drug-induced—lithium, demethylchlortetracycline, methoxyflurane, etc.
    Chronic renal disease
    Obstructive uropathy
    Multiple myeloma
    Amyloid
    Hypokalemia
    Renal effects of hypercalcemia
    Sickle cell anemia
    Polyuric phase of acute tubular necrosis
Primary polydipsia—psychogenic, postencephalitic (rare)
Osmotic diuresis

Table 6-3. Etiology of Diabetes Insipidus

Primary
  Idiopathic
  Hereditary, dominant or recessive
Secondary
  Posttraumatic—head injury, neurosurgery
  Tumor
    Primary pituitary or suprasellar
    Secondary breast or lung carcinoma
Miscellaneous
  Sarcoidosis
  Histiocytosis
  Tuberculosis
  Syphilis
  Encephalitis

In states of AVP deficiency (neurogenic diabetes insipidus), the clinical presentation of the patient is determined by the normality of the thirst mechanism and the availability of water for ingestion. If these do not present a problem, the manifestations of the disease are polyuria and polydipsia. Patients often note an acute onset of the polydipsia, and there is a preference for cold water. If, however, thirst is not appropriate or water is not available, then rapid dehydration, hypotension, hyperosmolarity, and hypernatremia with confusion, coma, and vascular collapse may ensue. The history provides clues to the etiology in the evaluation of a patient with possible diabetes insipidus, with secondary causes far more commonly encountered [16] (Table 6-3).

Individuals with nephrogenic diabetes insipidus, whether congenital or acquired, have minimal responsiveness to endogenous AVP and to standardized tests of AVP action. Acquired causes of nephrogenic diabetes insipidus include renal disease, starvation with decreased urea in the medullary interstitium, electrolyte disorders including hypokalemia and hypercalcemia, and drug-induced disease.

In the last category, two drugs warrant particular attention. Lithium, because of its frequent use in psychiatric disorders, is a common cause of nephrogenic diabetes insipidus. The clinical manifestations are unpredictable, and there is no definite dose-response relationship. Demethylchlortetracycline (Demeclocycline), in contrast, has been shown to produce a dose-dependent nephrogenic diabetes insipidus [10]. This characteristic has been utilized in clinical trials to induce a controlled state of diabetes insipidus as a countermeasure in states of inappropriate ADH secretion.

The compulsive water drinker may be difficult to distinguish from someone with true diabetes insipidus of a central or nephrogenic origin because he or she may have an abnormal concentrating mechanism. The compulsive water drinking and high urinary flow result in some "washout" of urea in the medullary interstitium, with a consequent loss of the hyperosmolar gradient in this area. Thus, even in the presence of AVP, they may have diminished ability to concentrate the urine. Patients with primary polydipsia tend to be volume overloaded and generally have plasma osmolalities that are lower than normal. With water restriction, some time may be required for a reconstitution of the medullary interstitium before responsiveness is normal.

Arginine Vasopressin Excess
The syndrome of inappropriate secretion of antidiuretic hormone (SIADH) is a constellation of symptoms and signs resulting from continued AVP secretion that is inappropriate in the presence of a low plasma osmolality. The hallmark of the syndrome is the finding of dilutional hyponatremia. Patients are unable to excrete an appropriately dilute urine and hence expand their ECF volume. The diagnosis is generally suspected by the laboratory finding of hyponatremia and its clinical concomitants (Table 6-4), which are largely related to nervous system dysfunction. The severity of the signs and symptoms is related not only to the absolute level of serum sodium but to the rapidity of development of the hyponatremia [1,2].

Table 6-4. Signs and Symptoms of Hyponatremia

Symptoms	Signs
Headache	Abnormal or depressed reflexes
Confusion	Altered levels of consciousness
Muscle cramps, weakness	Cheyne-Stokes respiration
Lethargy, apathy, agitation	Hypothermia
Nausea, emesis, anorexia	Seizures, coma

Table 6-5. Clinical Conditions Associated with Hyponatremia

ECF volume depletion
Renal losses
    Diuretic excess
    Salt-losing nephritis
    Adrenal insufficiency with mineralocorticoid deficiency
    Panhypopituitarism with stress
    Renal tubular acidosis
  Extrarenal losses
    Vomiting
    Diarrhea
    "Third space"
    Pancreatitis
    Burns
    Muscle trauma
ECF volume excess
  Marked, with edema
    Nephrotic syndrome
    Cirrhosis
    Congestive heart failure
    Acute and chronic renal failure
  Modest, without edema
    Hypothyroidism
    Glucocorticoid deficiency
    Excess water intake
    Drug-induced—chlorpropamide, carbamazepine, clofibrate
    SIADH
  Pseudohyponatremia
    Hyperlipidemia
    Hyperglycemia
    Hyperproteinemia

As hyponatremia may exist in many pathologic states, the diagnosis of SIADH [3] can be considered only when other etiologies have been eliminated [5] (Table 6-5). A review of these entities indicates that the majority can be easily recognized on the basis of clinical symptoms and signs, along with routine laboratory data such as urinalysis, serum and urine electrolytes and osmolalities, and renal function tests. Others, that is, glucocorticoid deficiency, may be diagnosed only after more extensive evaluation.

The finding of an elevated AVP level with hyponatremia does not establish the diagnosis of SIADH. In many instances, appropriate physiologic stimuli to AVP secretion may be present, as for example the low cardiac output states associated with congestive heart failure [25] or the nephrotic syndrome. Criteria for the diagnosis of SIADH are listed in Table 6-6.

Many causes of SIADH not produced by recognized osmotic or volume stimuli have been described. These include ectopic production of AVP by neoplastic tissue, pulmonary disease, CNS disorders, and the

Table 6-6. Diagnostic Criteria for SIADH

Hypo-osmolality and hyponatremia of ECF
Absence of ECF volume depletion
Production of nonmaximally dilute urine, usually hypertonic relative to plasma
Continued excretion of ingested sodium despite hyponatremia; initial mild urinary salt wasting followed by a steady state
Normal renal, adrenal, pituitary, cardiac, and hepatic function
Inappropriately elevated AVP level

Table 6-7. Etiology of SIADH

Aberrant production of AVP
   Oat cell carcinoma of the lung
   Thymoma
   Pancreatic carcinoma
Endogenous AVP production
   Hemorrhage, trauma, stress, positive-pressure breathing
   Pulmonary disease: pneumonia, tuberculosis, aspergillosis
   CNS disease: head injury, meningitis, abscess, encephalitis, Guillain-Barré
      syndrome, acute intermittent porphyria, subarachnoid hemorrhage, tumor
Idiopathic
Drug-induced AVP release and/or increased renal sensitivity; chlorpropamide,
      carbamazepine, clofibrate, nicotine, vincristine
AVP and oxytocin administration

---

use of drugs that may stimulate the release of AVP or potentiate its renal effect (Table 6-7).

Acute or chronic water intoxication will cause hyponatremia and is more frequent in an individual who has limitation of renal function. It is possible, however, by drinking approximately 1 liter per hour, to overcome the normal kidney's ability to excrete water. Patients with primary polydipsia may present with hyponatremia [11], as may those with a "reset osmostat" in which AVP response occurs at inappropriately low osmolalities [6].

Patients with diuretic-induced hyponatremia may have an abnormality in water excretion. This is more likely to result from decreased delivery of sodium to the distal diluting segment than from AVP excess [2,9]. In some instances, rapidly developing hyponatremia may occur following the use of thiazide diuretics [2].

Factitious or pseudohyponatremia must be considered in the evaluation of any patient reported to have a low serum sodium level [7]. Hyperlipidemia and hyperproteinemia have both been demonstrated to give spurious results in serum sodium determinations. This is due to displacement of water from the standardized volume of serum measured to determine the sodium concentration. Thus, a standard serum aliquot with a high lipid content would have a significant amount of water displaced. The volume of water containing sodium would be smaller, and the amount of sodium per total volume (lipid plus water) would be lower. Hyperglycemia may also lower the measured sodium, without sodium loss or water retention, by osmotically attracting fluid from the ICF compartment, thus diluting the serum sodium.

DIAGNOSTIC METHODS

In investigating patients with abnormalities of water metabolism, individual variations in threshold and sensitivity of the osmoreceptors, the enormous gain of the AVP system, the effects of different osmotic stimuli, and differing states of hydration, as well as difficulties in osmotic measurements, make data interpretation difficult.

Serum Osmolality

Serum osmolality is normally maintained in a relatively narrow range of 280 to 295 mOsm/kg. Sodium is the dominant contributor to osmolality and may be used in its determination in the following formula:

$$\text{Serum osmolality} = 2 \times \text{serum sodium} + \frac{\text{glucose mg/dl}}{18} + \frac{\text{BUN mg/dl}}{2.8}$$

This and other formulas give a rough estimate of serum osmolality values (Table 6-8). It should be noted that both glucose and blood urea nitrogen (BUN) may significantly change osmolality. This clinical calculation is a readily available tool and correlates well with the measurement of osmolality. It is important to remember that blood must be drawn without the use of a tourniquet and promptly studied for accurate determinations of osmolality.

Urine Osmolality

A normal individual can dilute the urine to approximately 50 to 90 mOsm/kg and concentrate it to 800 to 1500 mOsm/kg. Determination of urine osmolality provides important information regarding AVP effect and renal integrity. However, an isolated observation is often not helpful if plasma osmolality or volume status is not defined.

Correlation of Serum and Urinary Osmolality

Superimposition of serum and urinary osmolality measurements on a plot of normal relationships between these two variables has been suggested as a rapid and reliable method to support a diagnosis of suspected diabetes insipidus [16]. This requires only random simultaneous blood and urine samples from dehydrated patients and may be further enhanced by administering AVP (Pitressin, 5 units subcutaneously) to investigate nephrogenic versus neurogenic causes [16,24].

Table 6-8. Useful Calculations

1. Osmolality (mOsm) = 2(Na mEq/L) + $\dfrac{\text{glucose mg/dl}}{18}$

   + $\dfrac{\text{BUN mg/dl}}{2.8}$

2. Total body water (TBW) = weight (kg) × 0.6
   Intracellular fluid (ICF) = weight (kg) × 0.4
   Extracellular fluid (ECF) = weight (kg) × 0.2

3. Estimated reductions in measured serum sodium
   a. Every 100 mg/dl of glucose lowers the serum sodium (SNa) by
      1.6 mEq/L, e.g.,

      Glucose $\dfrac{1000 \text{ mg/dl}}{100 \text{ mg/dl}}$ × 1.6 = 16 mEq/L decrease in SNa

   b. For lipids, lipid mg/dl × 0.002 = Change in SNa (mEq/L)
      For protein, (protein gm/dl − 8) × 0.25 = Change in SNa (mEq/L)

Dehydration Test
The standard method of diagnosing neurogenic diabetes insipidus is fluid deprivation followed by the administration of exogenous AVP [15,17,24]. This procedure usually allows the identification of patients with complete diabetes insipidus and their differentiation from patients with primary polydipsia and nephrogenic diabetes insipidus.

The test is performed by restricting fluid intake until the osmolality of hourly voided urines reaches a plateau. This usually occurs after 8 to 10 hours of fluid deprivation and may result in a 3 to 5% decrease in body weight. It must be emphasized that the initiation of water deprivation is a considered decision. Patients with severe polyuria subjected to overnight fluid deprivation may risk volume loss and vascular collapse. In addition, patients with severe diabetes insipidus have been known to go to extraordinary lengths to obtain fluids. For these reasons, it may be better to begin the test in the morning so that more careful observation of the patient can occur.

The protocol for the water deprivation study is as follows:
1. The patient is weighed before and then after completion of a predetermined period of water deprivation
2. Serum and urine osmolalities are determined
3. Urine osmolalities are determined on an hourly basis until the urine osmolality plateaus with a change of less than 30 mOsm/kg in two consecutive hourly samples
4. When this has been achieved, blood is drawn without the use of a tourniquet for determination of plasma osmolality to confirm adequate dehydration (Posm = 292 mOsm/kg)

5. Five units of aqueous Pitressin is then given subcutaneously
6. Urine and plasma osmolalities are measured 1 hour after this injection

In normal subjects the urine osmolality is higher than the serum osmolality after dehydration, and since AVP release is already maximal, there is no change after the administration of exogenous AVP. Thus, the post-AVP urine osmolality shows a change of 9% or less compared to the maximally stimulated pre-AVP level. In partial diabetes insipidus, although urine osmolality may be somewhat above plasma osmolality after dehydration, it is not possible for a maximal AVP effect to occur. As the responsiveness of the kidney is intact, the addition of exogenous AVP may be expected to increase urine osmolality further by 9 to 50%. In contrast, patients with neurogenic diabetes insipidus and severe AVP deficiency demonstrate a urine osmolality before AVP administration that is much less than plasma osmolality. After AVP injection, it is expected that urine osmolality will increase by 50% or more. Finally, patients with nephrogenic diabetes insipidus will not concentrate the urine appropriately before or after water deprivation and have little or no rise in osmolality after AVP is given [16].

Patients with primary polydipsia provide a diagnostic dilemma and may be difficult to distinguish from those with partial neurogenic diabetes insipidus. As they are often in an overhydrated state, prolonged water deprivation may be needed to reach a plateau in urine osmolality. Once this is achieved, little if any urine response to AVP is expected to result from endogenous AVP secretion. Recent studies using AVP measurements have demonstrated that some patients diagnosed as having primary polydipsia by the dehydration test may have partial diabetes insipidus [28,29].

Hypertonic Saline Infusion
For the diagnosis of diabetes insipidus, the water deprivation study has largely supplanted the saline infusion test, which is still useful for the assessment of osmoreceptor function and determination of the threshold for AVP release [6,13,17]. The infusion of hypertonic saline (5% NaCl) to increase plasma osmolality will cause an antidiuresis in normal subjects but not in patients with diabetes insipidus. This test requires measurements of plasma osmolality to document an increase to above the upper limit of the normal osmotic threshold (292 mOsm/kg). It is also necessary to measure free water clearance, as urine output may fail to fall significantly because of the saline diuresis that may ensue. Obviously, this study is contraindicated in any patient who cannot tolerate acute volume expansion.

To perform the study, the following protocol is used [16]:
1. Patients are given an oral water load (20 ml/kg) by mouth over 10

to 15 minutes; at the same time a slow infusion (0.5 ml per minute) of 5% NaCl is started
2. When a sustained diuresis has been present for six to eight successive urine collections of 15 minutes each, the rate of infusion of 5% NaCl is increased to 0.05 ml/kg per minute until a definite fall in three or more subsequent 15-minute urinary volumes has been recorded or until severe headache or thirst supervenes
3. If rapid determinations of plasma osmolality are not available to document the fact that the upper limits of the normal osmotic threshold have been reached, the infusion should be continued for at least 2 hours unless the urinary volumes have fallen or symptoms have supervened
4. Plasma and urine samples are measured for osmolality at 15-minute intervals until the study is terminated so that calculations of free water clearance may be made
5. Free water clearance should show a fall to zero or a negative value in normal individuals but no fall in subjects with diabetes insipidus

A modified version of this approach has been used by Zerbe and Robertson [28]. Hypertonic saline at 0.05 to 0.06 ml/kg per minute is infused for 2 hours. Plasma samples for AVP and osmolality measurements are obtained every 20 minutes. AVP as a function of osmolality is plotted on a nomogram [28]. This approach offers the advantage of being less cumbersome than urine collections and calculation of free water clearance values; however, reliable AVP assays are not widely available.

Arginine Vasopressin Levels
The studies outlined represent attempts to look at hormonal effects rather than circulating AVP levels. Basal levels of plasma AVP depend upon the state of hydration. There is an overlap in AVP levels in normals, patients with primary polydipsia, and patients with diabetes insipidus. It is only through the measurement of AVP and concomitant plasma and urine osmolalities that one is able to separate these groups. AVP has been shown to be elevated in patients with congestive heart failure [25] as well as in the majority of patients who satisfy the criteria for SIADH, but a subgroup has been identified with normal AVP levels [28]. Isolated plasma AVP values do not provide adequate differentiation of disease states. Plasma measurements of AVP are increasingly available but remain difficult assays and vary considerably in sensitivity and specificity [28]. In the assessment of clinical disorders, AVP levels are best used in the context of concurrent plasma and urinary osmolalities and basal urinary flows.

Diluting Capacity Assessment
Whereas many studies assess the ability of the kidney to conserve water, the use of the water load helps define the ability of the kidney to excrete water. The test is performed as follows:

1. A water load of 20 mg/kg is administered orally over 15 to 30 minutes. Hourly urine samples are then collected for volume and osmolality determinations.
2. To ensure adequate hydration, urine volumes are replaced with an NaCl infusion.
3. Normal subjects excrete more than 65% of the water load within 4 hours [16]. Urine osmolality should fall to below 100 mOsm/kg. The inability to excrete this water load demonstrates an excessive AVP effect. Intrinsic renal disease or decreased renal blood flow may also limit excretion of the water load.

This test must be used with caution in persons with an impaired ability to excrete a water load, such as those with hypothyroidism, adrenal insufficiency, heart disease, or drug-induced alterations in AVP function.

Free Water Clearance
The kidney's ability to excrete water is determined in large part by the maintenance of the interstitial hyperosmolality that allows the diluting segment to function. Thus, the chloride pump and the high medullary osmolality allow the generation of a dilute urine, which enters the distal tubule and collecting duct. In the absence of AVP, this dilute urine is excreted and "free water" is lost from the body. The urine may be considered as composed of two volumes: one that is excreted because it is bound to osmolar solutes such as urea and sodium, and another that is essentially free water, not bound to any solutes. It is the ability to excrete solute free water that indicates the effect of AVP on the kidney. High AVP levels decrease free water clearance; low AVP levels allow it.

Free water clearance (CH_2O) is determined by the following equations:

$$CH_2O = V - Cosm$$
$$Cosm = Uosm \times \frac{V}{Posm}$$

where Cosm = osmolar clearance, Uosm = urine osmolality, Posm = plasma osmolality, and V = urine volume in cubic centimeters per minute. As the equations indicate, the total urinary volume (V) minus the volume that is associated with urinary osmolality (Cosm) indicates the urine volume excreted as free water (CH_2O).

DISCUSSION
Polyuria and Hypernatremia
Evaluation of a patient for diabetes insipidus is often initiated by the finding of polyuria with or without hypernatremia. The symptom of

polyuria requires explanation but does not necessarily indicate disordered water metabolism. The clinical sign of hypernatremia is firm evidence of a disordered osmolar state.

Polyuria without hypernatremia is commonly found with disorders such as diuretic use, osmotic diuresis, and renal disease (Table 6-2) in which adequate water consumption allows high urine flow rates. Investigation of the polyuric state begins with determination of electrolytes, calcium, renal function, and a careful urinalysis (Fig. 6-1). The last needs emphasis, as it may be a clue to osmotic diuresis (glucose) or disorders of dilution and concentration (specific gravity).

Hypernatremia without polyuria is best approached by assessment of the ECF. Hypovolemia without polyuria suggests extrarenal volume loss such as may occur with vomiting or diarrhea. Polyuria would not be expected under these circumstances, with renal conservation of water (Uosm > Posm) and sodium (UNa < 10 mEq/L) expected as a normal response. Hypovolemia with polyuria raises the question of AVP deficiency or renal disease. Finally, nonosmotic polyuria may be due to AVP deficiency, yet it may not be characterized by volume depletion or hypernatremia if the deficiency is not severe and fluid intake is adequate.

As outlined in Figure 6-1, the patient with unexplained polyuria may be studied using the standard dehydration test. The patient who demonstrates an ability to concentrate urine has evidence of some ADH effect. Calculation of the Uosm/Posm ratio immediately separates the normal (or polydipsic) individual from the patient with severe diabetes insipidus. The Uosm response to Pitressin allows further discrimination of disorders within the two groups defined by Uosm/Posm ratios following dehydration. The normal individual or the patient with primary polydipsia if dehydrated shows little response to exogenous AVP since endogenous AVP secretion is already maximal. Conversely, the response to exogenous AVP is dramatic in the patient with severe diabetes insipidus.

The patient with nephrogenic diabetes insipidus may have little or no response to exogenous AVP. This finding, in conjunction with both increased plasma osmolality and hypotonic urine, confirms the renal origin of the disorder. In many instances of nephrogenic diabetes insipidus, some response to exogenous AVP will be noted. The response may be similar to that noted in partial diabetes insipidus of neurogenic origin. In such instances, the use of plasma AVP levels will distinguish between neurogenic (low AVP) and renal (high AVP) disorders.

Partial neurogenic diabetes insipidus may also share certain features with primary polydipsia. These include a Uosm/Posm ratio above 1 after dehydration and a small rise in Uosm after exogenous AVP administration. To distinguish between these two disorders, measurement of AVP levels after hypertonic saline infusion may be used [28]. However, in most instances, review of plasma osmolality before and after dehydration will usually suffice since the patient with partial diabetes insipidus

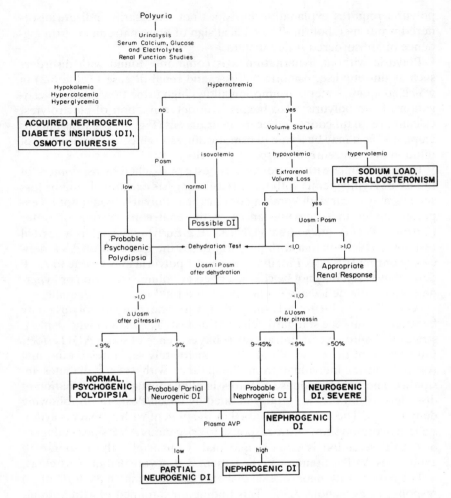

Figure 6-1. Diagnostic protocol: Polyuria. Posm, plasma osmolality; Uosm, urine osmolality; AVP, arginine vasopressin.

will characteristically have higher plasma osmolalities (>290 mOsm/kg) in both states. In contrast, the polydipsic patient often demonstrates plasma hypotonicity in the basal state and may require prolonged dehydration to attain a Posm adequate for assessment of AVP effect.

In practical terms, it is advisable to obtain a sample for AVP assay at the end of the dehydration test. This sample must be carefully and correctly obtained and frozen. In those instances in which the dehydration test proves equivocal, the sample will be available for assay and may preclude the need to repeat the entire dehydration test.

Hyponatremia

Hyponatremia usually indicates impairment of free water excretion. Assessment of the patient's volume status using skin turgor and orthostatic blood pressure and pulse changes remains basic to the evaluation of the hyponatremic state (Fig. 6-2). Volume expansion, with dilution of the serum sodium, such as may occur in congestive heart failure, the nephrotic syndrome, and cirrhosis, is the most common cause of hyponatremia.

The presence of hyponatremia and evidence of hypovolemia are indicative of a sodium deficit in excess of a water deficit. This may occur following the use of diuretics or after episodes of diarrhea or vomiting with volume loss that is replaced largely by consumption of solute free liquids. The presence of orthostatic blood pressure changes confirms the presence of intravascular volume depletion.

Diuretic-induced hyponatremia may be difficult to diagnose. The presence of hypokalemia, hyponatremia, and volume depletion should immediately raise the question of diuretic use. Urinary sodium is usually low in volume-depleted states; however, in cases of diuretic use, the urinary sodium may be elevated secondary to the diuretic effect. Diuretic-induced hyponatremia may simulate the syndrome of inappropriate ADH secretion if the patient consumes amounts of water adequate to maintain an isovolemic state. The serum potassium level is, however, usually low in diuretic-induced disorders.

The diagnosis of SIADH is made on the basis of certain defined criteria after other causes of AVP excess have been ruled out [2]. Careful clinical evaluation of the hyponatremic patient will rapidly narrow the number of diagnostic possibilities, with particular attention being paid to the volume status. Evidence for ECF volume depletion such as orthostatic hypotension, hemoconcentration, or an elevated BUN makes SIADH unlikely. The measurement of urinary sodium is helpful in that excess AVP is associated with continued urinary sodium excretion despite the hyponatremia. The simultaneous measurement of plasma and urinary osmolality will readily distinguish between the psychogenic water drinker (low Posm and Uosm) and the true SIADH (low Posm, increased Uosm). Thus, the combination of the absence of volume depletion, normal renal function, and urinary sodium over 20 mEq/L should

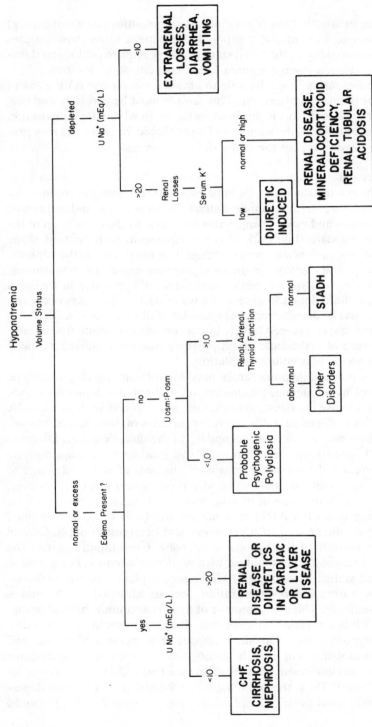

Figure 6-2. Diagnostic protocol: Hyponatremia. CHF, congestive heart failure; Uosm, urine osmolality; Posm, plasma osmolality.

raise the question of SIADH. If the patient is not on drugs, which may influence AVP secretion or action, and is not hypothyroid, the differential diagnosis is between glucocorticoid deficiency and SIADH. Measurement of plasma cortisol before and after stimulation with synthetic 1-24 ACTH will generally allow this distinction to be made.

There is no definitive test for the diagnosis of SIADH. In general, AVP levels are inappropriately high for the serum osmolality; however, as has been noted, a group of patients who satisfy all of the accepted criteria for SIADH but have normal AVP levels have been identified. The standard method for confirming the diagnosis, water deprivation, is also the standard mode of therapy. When the diagnosis is suspected, water restriction of 500 to 1000 ml per day will, over the course of 7 to 10 days, eliminate the body water excess and return the serum sodium and plasma osmolality to or toward normal.

Occasionally, patients are seen in whom SIADH is suspected but the osmolality and serum sodium are not definitive. In such cases, the response to water loading is a useful means of establishing the diagnosis. It must be recognized that water loading in such patients is not without risk and should not be done on patients who have symptomatic hyponatremia or a serum sodium below 130 mEq/L. Patients with AVP excess will fail to dilute the urine maximally, with the urine osmolality generally remaining greater than the plasma osmolality, and will excrete less than 40% of the water load. Patients with reset osmostats [6] are able to excrete a water load while maintaining persistently low sodium levels.

REFERENCES

1. Arieff, A. I., and Guisado, R. Effects on the central nervous system of hypernatremic and hyponatremic states. *Kidney Int.* 10:104–116, 1976.
2. Ashraf, N., Locksley, R., and Arieff, A. Thiazide induced hypoatremia associated with death or neurologic damage in outpatients. *Am. J. Med.* 70:77–88, 1981.
3. Bartter, F. C. The syndrome of inappropriate secretion of antidiuretic hormone. *Am. J. Med.* 42:790–806, 1967.
4. Bartter, F. C. Vasopressin and blood pressure. *N. Engl. J. Med.* 304:1097–1098, 1981.
5. Berl, T., et al. Clinical disorders of water metabolism. *Kidney Int.* 10:117–132, 1976.
6. DeFronzo, R. A., Goldberg, M., and Agus, Z. S. Normal diluting capacity in hyponatremic patients. *Ann. Intern. Med.* 84:538–542, 1976.
7. DeFronzo, R. A., and Thier, S. O. Pathophysiologic approach to hyponatremia. *Arch. Intern. Med.* 140:897–902, 1980.
8. Feig, P. V., and McCurdy, D. R. The hypertonic state. *N. Engl. J. Med.* 297:1444–1454, 1977.
9. Fichman, M. P., et al. Diuretic induced hyponatremia. *Ann. Intern. Med.* 75:853–863, 1971.
10. Forrest, J. N., Jr., et al. Superiority of demeclocycline over lithium in the treatment of chronic syndrome of inappropriate secretion of antidiuretic hormone. *N. Engl. J. Med.* 298:173–177, 1978.

11. Hariprasad, M. K., et al. Hyponatremia in psychogenic polydipsia. *Arch. Intern. Med.* 140:1639–1642, 1980.
12. Hickey, R., and Hare, K. Renal excretion of chloride and water in diabetes insipidus. *J. Clin. Invest.* 23:768–775, 1944.
13. Humes, H. D., Narins, R. C., and Brenner, B. M. Disorders of water balance. *Hosp. Prac.* 14:133–145, 1979.
14. Kokko, J. D. The role of renal concentrating mechanisms in the regulation of serum sodium concentration. *Am. J. Med.* 62:165–169, 1977.
15. Miller, M., et al. Recognition of partial defects in antidiuretic hormone secretion. *Ann. Intern. Med.* 73:721–729, 1970.
16. Moses, A. M., and Notman, D. Diabetes insipidus and syndrome of inappropriate antidiuretic hormone secretion (SIADH). *Adv. Intern. Med.* 27:73–100, 1982.
17. Moses, A. M., and Streeten, D. H. P. Differentiation of polyuric states by measurement of responses to changes in plasma osmolality induced by hypertonic saline infusions. *Am. J. Med.* 42:368–375, 1967.
18. Padfield, P. L., et al. Blood pressure in acute and chronic vasopressin excess: Studies of malignant hypertension and the syndrome of inappropriate antidiuretic hormone secretion. *N. Engl. J. Med.* 304:1067–1071, 1981.
19. Robertson, G. L., Aycinena, P., and Zerbe, R. L. Neurogenic disorders of osmoregulation. *Am. J. Med.* 72:339–353, 1982.
20. Robertson, G. L., et al. The development and clinical application of a new method for the radioimmunoassay of arginine vasopressin in human plasma. *J. Clin. Invest.* 52:2340–2352, 1979.
21. Robertson, G. L., Shelton, R. L., and Atnar, S. The osmoregulation of vasopressin. *Kidney Int.* 10:25–37, 1976.
22. Sawyer, W. H. Vertebrate neurohypophyseal principles. *Endocrinology* 79:981, 1964.
23. Skorecki, K., and Brenner, B. Body fluid homeostasis in man. *Am. J. Med.* 70:77–88, 1981.
24. Streeten, D. H. P., Moses, A. M., and Miller, M. Disorders of the Neurohypophysis. In K. J. Isselbacher et al. (Eds.), *Harrison's Principles of Internal Medicine.* (9th ed.). New York: McGraw-Hill, 1980. P. 1684.
25. Szatalowicz, V. L., et al. Radioimmuonassay of plasma arginine vasopressin in hyponatremic patients with congestive heart failure. *N. Engl. J. Med.* 305:263–266, 1981.
26. Verney, E. B. The antidiuretic hormone and the factors which determine its release. *Proc. R. Soc. Lond.* 135:25–106, 1947.
27. Weitzman, R. E., and Kleeman, C. R. The clinical physiology of water metabolism, Part III: The water depletion (hyperosmolar) and water excess (hypoosmolar) syndromes. *West. J. Med.* 132:16–38, 1980.
28. Zerbe, R. L., and Robertson, G. L. A comparison of plasma vasopressin measurements with a standard indirect test in the differential diagnosis of polyuria. *N. Engl. J. Med.* 305:1539–1546, 1981.
29. Zerbe, R. L., Stropes, L., and Robertson, G. L. Vasopressin function in the syndrome of inappropriate antidiuresis. *Annu. Rev. Med.* 31:315–327, 1980.

7   Adrenocortical Insufficiency

William F. Streck

CLINICAL CONSIDERATIONS

Adrenocortical insufficiency may be a result of primary adrenal gland failure (Addison's disease) or may be secondary to disordered regulation of adrenocorticotropic hormone (ACTH), with subsequent adrenal gland hypofunction. Causes of secondary failure include hypothalamic or pituitary disease and the use of exogenous glucocorticoids. By far the most common form of adrenocortical insufficiency is that occurring secondary to suppression of the hypothalamic-pituitary-adrenal (HPA) axis following prolonged use of pharmacologic doses of exogenous glucocorticoids.

The nonspecificity of presenting symptoms of adrenal insufficiency makes adrenal hypofunction a frequent clinical postulate in the patient who is seriously ill without apparent cause. The importance of correct diagnosis is emphasized by the fact that treatment initiated without adequate documentation of hypoadrenalism may induce the very disorder for which the therapy was initiated. Replacement doses of glucocorticoids may not cause total suppression of the HPA axis; however, even those doses used for prolonged periods with supplements for stress or illness may lead to axis suppression [4]. Thus, for the patient who is suspected of having either primary or secondary adrenal insufficiency, careful and complete definition of adrenocortical function is required since prolonged therapy with glucocorticoids may follow the incorrect as well as the correct diagnosis.

Adrenal insufficiency may present in an acute or chronic fashion. Acute adrenal insufficiency or adrenal "crisis" does not usually present as a de novo disorder. Rather, it is usually a result of superimposition of a new stress on a chronic deficiency. Acute presentations are more likely in cases of primary adrenal failure in which both glucocorticoid and mineralocorticoid deficiencies are present. The signs and symptoms of acute adrenocortical deficiency are nonspecific: fever, hypotension, nausea, vomiting, occasional diarrhea and abdominal pain, confusion, and weakness. The classic laboratory findings of hyponatremia, hyperkalemia, acidosis, and hypotension may not be present [15,25], especially in cases of secondary failure.

Chronic adrenal insufficiency is the more common presentation of primary adrenal failure and the expected outcome in most cases of secondary insufficiency. However, some clues as to the primary or secondary nature of the hypoadrenalism are provided by characteristic features at presentation. In chronic primary adrenal insufficiency, increased pigmentation of the skin, mucous membranes, palmar creases, and scars is often the first distinguishing clinical sign. This hyperpigmentation is a consequence of the absence of feedback inhibition of ACTH by cortisol.

Table 7-1. Signs and Symptoms in Confirmed Addison's Disease

Sign or Symptom	Incidence (%)	
	Irvine and Barnes, 1972 [15] (N = 84)	Nerup, 1974 [25] (N = 108)
Weakness	100	100
Weight loss	100	100
Hyperpigmentation	94	92
Hypotension	94	88
Orthostatic		12
Anorexia		100
Gastrointestinal symptoms	92	56
Electrolyte disturbances		92
Vitiligo	17	4

This deficiency of cortisol allows sustained elevation of ACTH and melanotropic peptides. Features of mineralocorticoid deficiency are also more frequent in primary failure since aldosterone deficiency reduces sodium conservation and potassium excretion at the distal tubule. In contrast, chronic secondary failure is not characterized by hyperpigmentation since ACTH is suppressed or deficient. Salt wasting and hyperkalemia are less common in secondary failure since the renin-aldosterone system remains intact. However, in secondary failure, dilutional hyponatremia may result because cortisol is required for optimal excretion of a water load.

Primary Adrenal Insufficiency

Adrenal failure due to destruction or loss of the adrenal glands is known as *Addison's disease* (Table 7-1). Idiopathic adrenal atrophy accounts for most (75%) cases of primary adrenal failure [15,25]. Fungal diseases and tuberculosis have consistently been described as the second most common causes in recent reviews. Surgical removal of adrenal glands for treatment of Cushing's syndrome is no longer common. However, adrenalectomy remains an occasional approach to the management of breast cancer. The remaining rare causes of primary adrenal insufficiency include adrenal infarction, tumor, amyloid, hemorrhage, and infection.

Idiopathic adrenal failure is characterized by adrenal antibodies in 50 to 70% of cases. Several clinical disorders, similarly characterized by organ-specific antibodies, are associated with the antibody-positive form of adrenal failure. Thyroid disease (Graves' disease, Hashimoto's disease, hypothyroidism), abnormal gonadal function, atrophic gastritis and pernicious anemia, hypoparathyroidism, diabetes mellitus, and vitiligo may be encountered in association with primary adrenal failure in up to 50% of cases. Such associations of adrenal and other disease are more common in women, show no correlation to adrenal antibody titer, and are not characterized by evidence of generalized autoimmune phenomena such as antinuclear antibodies. Antibodies to adrenal glands are rare in the normal population (1%) and in patients who have other autoimmune diseases without adrenal disease (4%) [5].

Secondary Adrenal Insufficiency
Adrenocortical failure secondary to hypothalamic-pituitary disorders and consequent decreased ACTH secretion characteristically presents in a clinical context of multiple hormone deficiencies [8]. Pituitary tumors and hypothalamic tumors (chromophobe adenomas and craniopharyngiomas) and postpartum pituitary hemorrhage account for most cases of secondary failure. The classic, although not invariable, sequence of deficiencies due to tumor consists of gonadotropins followed by growth hormone (apparent in the adult only after testing). ACTH and thyroid-stimulating hormone (TSH) deficiences may then follow.

Secondary adrenal insufficiency may, at least in theory, resemble idiopathic primary adrenal failure with associated thyroidal and/or gonadal failure due to a presumed autoimmune process. The suggestion of intracranial disease and the absence of pigmentation point toward secondary failure. In addition, the patient with pale, finely wrinkled skin and absent pubic and axillary hair provides a ready contrast to the thin, asthenic, hyperpigmented Addisonian. Since the renin-aldosterone system remains intact in secondary failure, evidence of mineralocorticoid deficiency is characteristically lacking. The measurement of aldosterone levels following ACTH stimulation has been used to improve diagnostic discrimination between primary and secondary failure [10]. Secondary hypoadrenalism may be difficult to recognize when combined hypothyroidism and ACTH deficiency are present. The reduced cortisol output is masked by a reduced metabolic clearance rate. This may obscure the relative hypoadrenalism until thyroid replacement is instituted.

Adrenal Insufficiency Secondary to Exogenous Glucocorticoids
The isolated lack of ACTH as a consequence of a pituitary or hypothalamic lesion is rare [30]. Yet, selective ACTH suppression from exogenous glucocorticoids represents the most frequently encountered form of adrenocortical insufficiency. Pharmacologic doses of glucocorticoids administered over several months may suppress the HPA axis for up to a year after discontinuation of therapy [23]. Short courses of glucocorticoids have also been shown to cause significant suppression of HPA function for up to a week or more after abrupt discontinuation of therapy [29,31].

Suppression of the HPA axis depends on a number of variables. Doses of 7.5 mg of prednisone or equivalent daily doses have generally been considered to be nonsuppressive, whereas doses of 20 to 30 mg for more than a week have been considered to be suppressive [4]. However, even the lower dose in a given individual or administered for a long enough period of time may lead to decreased adrenal responsiveness to ACTH. Shorter-acting compounds (cortisone, prednisone) are less suppressive than compounds with longer biologic half-lives (dexamethasone) [9,24]. Comparable doses of a given steroid are less suppressive when administered as a single daily morning dose than when given as divided doses [13,26]. Alternate-day therapy with short-acting compounds effects less HPA suppression than daily therapy [1]. In sum, HPA suppression is likely if more than 20 to 30 mg of prednisone or equivalent doses are administered on a daily basis in divided doses for a period of more than 1 month [4,11].

Clinically, the possibility of adrenocortical insufficiency secondary to exogenous glucocorticoids will be suggested by the history or by the paradoxical combination of a cushingoid patient with features of hypoadrenalism. Glucocorticoid-induced secondary adrenocortical failure has some of the features of secondary adrenal failure of hypothalamic-pituitary origin, that is, lack of pigmentation and an intact renin-aldosterone system. The lack of associated hormonal deficiencies emphasizes the selective ACTH suppression in the steroid-induced disorder.

Evaluation may be complicated by the fact that a steroid withdrawal syndrome may occur despite normal levels of plasma glucocorticoids and normal responsiveness of the HPA system. Anorexia, nausea, lethargy, arthralgia, weakness, desquamation, and weight loss characterize this still unexplained syndrome; all the symptoms are quite consistent with hypoadrenalism. A history of prior steroid therapy, usually with high doses, or a recent rapid taper to near physiologic doses may be obtained in this syndrome [2].

DIAGNOSTIC METHODS
Laboratory documentation remains the essential confirmation of adrenocortical insufficiency. In suspected hypoadrenalism, plasma steroid measurements have advantages as estimates of function compared to urinary metabolites such as 17-hydroxycorticoids (17-OHCS), 17-ketosteroids (17-KS), or free cortisol. Isolated single observations of plasma or urinary compounds provide less information than comparative values after testing of various parts of the HPA axis.

Plasma Cortisol
Currently, there are four major methods for the measurement of serum or plasma cortisol. These include fluorometric, colorimetric, competitive protein binding (CPB), and radioimmunoassay (RIA) procedures. Most current assay systems utilize RIA to measure total (bound and

free) cortisol. These assays in fact measure steroids other than cortisol to some extent (11-deoxycorticol, corticosterone). However, this is quantitatively unimportant except in instances of impaired cortisol synthesis such as congenital adrenal hyperplasia or after metyrapone administration.

The highest plasma cortisol levels are found from 6 to 10 AM and the lowest around midnight. Normal morning values range from 8 to 25 μg/dl in most assays, with evening values being 5 to 15 μg/dl. Whatever the particular normal range, a morning value of less than 5 μg/dl in a clinical situation suggesting hypoadrenalism is suspicious. However, such a single determination could be a result of an undocumented earlier peak or an alteration in the diurnal rhythm secondary to disease, drugs, or altered sleep patterns. Efforts to document a normal circadian rhythm are subject to the same variables. Further, normal basal plasma cortisols and an intact circadian rhythm do not preclude an absent stress reserve. In sum, single observations of low plasma cortisol levels, unless they occur in an acute setting or are consistently very low on retesting, are of little help in making a definitive diagnosis. Dynamic tests of adrenal function are usually required.

Adrenocorticotropic Hormone Stimulation
Direct stimulation of the adrenal gland should be the first step in the evaluation of adrenal insufficiency. This may be easily accomplished with the intravenous or intramuscular administration of synthetic ACTH (cosyntropin, Cortrosyn). The standard ampule of this drug contains 0.25 mg of synthetic ACTH, comparable in activity to 25 units of natural ACTH. Since 20 to 50 units of ACTH infused over 8 hours (3–6 units per hour) effect maximal adrenal stimulation in normals [19], use of 0.25 mg of synthetic ACTH in bolus fashion represents a pharmacologic stimulus to the adrenal gland that provides an index of adrenal responsiveness. Cosyntropin may be used as a single-dose screening test. In contrast, more sustained administration serves as a more definitive test of adrenal gland function.

Single-Dose Cosyntropin Stimulation Test
When administered intramuscularly or intravenously, cosyntropin effects a peak cortisol response within 1 hour and a return to basal values within 4 hours [28,32]. Sampling has been recommended at various times after drug administration: 30 minutes, 1 hour, both, and 2 hours in infants. As a general screen, the following brief protocol seems most reliable:

1. Basal plasma cortisol measurement
2. Cosyntropin, 0.25 mg intramuscularly or intravenously, over 2 to 3 minutes
3. Repeat cortisol measurements at 30 and 60 minutes

The definition of a normal response becomes a critical issue. Used as a screening test, the desirable error would be one that selected for further testing some proportion of individuals subsequently proven normal. Various criteria have been proposed in the literature. For a normal response, the best-established criteria appear to be:

1. Basal plasma cortisol, >5 µg/dl
2. Incremental cortisol (peak-basal) at 30 or 60 minutes, >7 µg/dl
3. Peak plasma cortisol at 30 or 60 minutes, >18 µg/dl

Since the basal plasma cortisol is subject to diurnal variation whereas the peak response tends to remain the same, the incremental response will vary with the basal level. This is important in evaluating patients who are taking spironolactone or estrogens, who will have elevated basal levels but normal incremental responses. The listed criteria are best applied to testing in the morning fasting state. At other times, the peak value becomes the primary criterion. A peak value of 20 µg/dl is strong presumptive evidence against adrenal insufficiency. Correct performance and interpretation of the single-dose test will resolve the bulk of clinical questions. If on single-dose testing or repeat testing the above criteria are not met, sustained ACTH stimulation should be considered.

Sustained Adrenocorticotropic Hormone Stimulation

More prolonged stimulation of the adrenal gland may be necessary to clarify adrenal gland status after an abnormal cosyntropin screening test. Various protocols with different normal response patterns have been proposed. Fundamental to all these protocols is the observation that secondarily atrophied or suppressed adrenal glands will show some response to persistent ACTH stimulation. Primary failure is characterized by a minimal or absent adrenal response to any level of ACTH. Of the protocols suggested for sustained stimulation, the 3-day protocols appear more reliable, particularly since adrenal gland responsiveness may be delayed in long-term secondary failure. It should be noted that glucocorticoid supplementation with a high-potency, minimally cross-reactive steroid such as dexamethasone may be provided if necessary during the study period.

Both 4-hour and 8-hour infusions, 1-day and 3-day protocols, and intramuscular and intravenous delivery routes have been suggested. A 3-day protocol using constant intravenous infusion of synthetic ACTH at 250 µg over 8 hours follows:

Days 1, 2   Baseline 24-hour urine collections for 17-OHCS and creatinine

Days 3, 4, 5   1. 250 μg of cosyntropin, constant infusion over 8 hours (8 AM–4 PM) in 5% dextrose and saline
2. Daily 24-hour urine collection for 17-OHCS and creatinine
3. Plasma cortisol level determination at 8 AM and 4 PM daily

Different criteria for a normal response to sustained ACTH infusion have been suggested. The critical observation, however, is that a substantial increase in adrenal steroids must occur to document intact adrenal tissue. Normal response criteria include:

Plasma cortisol
Days 1, 2   Baseline 10–25 μg/dl [21]
Day 3   Increase of 15–40 μg/dl by the eighth hour [21]
Days 4, 5   Plasma levels of 30–60 μg/dl [3]
17-OHCS (urine)
Days 1,2   Baseline 5–12 mg/24 hr; 3–7 mg/gm creatinine
Day 3   Total 15–40 mg/24 hr [3]
    12–25 mg/gm creatinine [21]
Days 4,5   30–40 mg/24 hr

Complete primary adrenal insufficiency is characterized by absent responses to ACTH (cortisol < 10 μg/dl, no increase in 17-OHCS). Secondary adrenal insufficiency may be characterized by responses less than normal, but with increasing levels of response through day 5.

Insulin Tolerance Test
When ACTH stimulation suggests secondary adrenal insufficiency, the hypothalamic pituitary response to the stress of hypoglycemia may be assessed [14,20]. The corticosteroid response to insulin-induced hypoglycemia is probably the most sensitive of the currently available tests for assessing HPA function [16]. A rise in plasma cortisol of 7 μg/dl after adequate hypoglycemia constitutes a normal response [14].

ACTH-responsive adrenal tissue is necessary in the insulin tolerance test (ITT) since the end result of testing is adrenal cortisol output. Thus, when secondary insufficiency is clinically suspected, prior ACTH stimulation may be necessary. If the presence of a demonstrated capacity of the adrenal gland to respond to ACTH, the absence of a cortisol increase after hypoglycemia indicates ACTH deficiency.

Clinical situations may arise when an ITT is considered prior to any formal testing of the adrenal gland. This occurs in suspected pituitary tumors or in the empty sella syndrome when adrenocortical failure is not the first consideration. However, when adrenocortical insufficiency is suspected on clinical grounds, prior ACTH stimulation is necessary to ensure interpretable test results.

The ITT is an effective tool for HPA evaluation, with advantages over metyrapone testing. Among these advantages is the ability to assess concurrently secretion of growth hormone and prolactin. If desired, gonadal and thyroidal function may be assessed since gonadotropin-releasing hormone (GnRH) and thyrotropin-releasing hormone (TRH) may be simultaneously administered (see Chap. 2). In the ITT the initial insulin dose should be 0.1 to 0.15 unit/kg initially. When hypopituitarism is suspected, 0.05 unit/kg should be used. Ampules of glucose and glucocorticoid preparations should be readily available for administration during the performance of the ITT. For details of testing see Chapter 2.

Metyrapone Test
Metyrapone blocks the enzymatic conversion of 11-deoxycortisol (compound S) to cortisol (compound F). The lowered cortisol prompts compensatory ACTH release from the pituitary. A normal ACTH response causes adrenal stimulation, with increased compound S as the major product due to the enzymatic blockade. Confirmation of adequate blockade should be obtained by measuring plasma cortisol, which should be low [27]. A post-metyrapone increase in 11-deoxycortisol thus becomes the indicator of normal pituitary adrenal reserve, and the post-metyrapone cortisol confirms the adequacy of 11-hydroxylation blockade.

An overnight (30 mg/kg of metyrapone) and a 3-day test (750 mg of metyrapone every 4 hours for 24 hours) have been utilized. The 3-day test appears more discriminating:

Day 1   Basal 24-hour urine for 17-OHCS
Day 2   750 mg of metyrapone every 4 hours (8 AM–4 AM)
             24-hour urine for 17-OHCS
Day 3   Plasma 11-deoxycortisol and cortisol levels at 8 AM
             Repeat 24-hour urine for 17-OHCS

Using both plasma steroids and urinary metabolites as response criteria, reasonable normal values would be:

1. Post-metyrapone 11-deoxycortisol, >10 μg/dl
   Post-metyrapone cortisol, <7 μg/dl
2. 17-OHCS of twice the basal level on day 3
   17-OHCS increment of 10 to 40 mg per 24 hours on day 3

The metyrapone test, like the ITT, is not useful if the presence of ACTH-responsive adrenal tissue has not been confirmed. Several points warrant consideration when metyrapone is used to evaluate a case of suspected secondary adrenal insufficiency:

1. Metyrapone may induce adrenal insufficiency in the borderline case. It should not be used when a strong suspicion of adrenocortical failure is present.
2. Since reduction of plasma cortisol is critical for ACTH stimulation, administration of glucocorticoids to "cover" the patient will suppress any ACTH response and negate the test.
3. Inadequate blockade may occur due to inadequate absorption or single-dose omission.
4. Normal metyrapone responsiveness does not necessarily indicate an intact hypothalamic-pituitary stress response.
5. The range of normal urinary metabolite responses is wide.

Measurement of plasma 11-deoxycortisol and cortisol may reduce the dependence on urine collections. Nonetheless, the metyrapone test appears most valuable when it is clearly normal, as in evaluating suspected asymptomatic pituitary tumors. Equivocal or abnormal results are often difficult to interpret.

Adrenocorticotropic Hormone Measurement
Studies to date indicate clear distinctions between primary and secondary adrenocortical failure by ACTH measurement. Using current methods, ACTH values for 8 to 10 AM are in the 10 to 80 pg/ml range. Addisonian patients have values in the 200 to 300 pg/ml range. Between these extreme values, ACTH levels in basal and stimulated states are not well defined. In current practice, more traditional assays of HPA function remain necessary, with ACTH measurement providing supplementary data.

Urinary Steroid Metabolites
Although direct measurement of plasma steroids is often more helpful in the investigation of hypoadrenalism, many data on urinary metabolites in response to testing are available. These determinations also supplement plasma data after ACTH infusion or metyrapone administration. Confusion over terminology and normal ranges have hindered interpretation. In general, accurate measurement of urinary steroids and metabolites provides an integrated assessment of episodic adrenocortical hormone secretion and metabolism over 24 hours.

URINARY FREE CORTISOL. Since cortisol-binding globulin is saturated at plasma cortisol levels of 20 to 25 µg/dl, further cortisol elevation causes a disproportionate elevation in the free fraction. Urinary quantitation of this free fraction thus provides a sensitive measure of changes in adrenocortical activity. Competitive protein-binding methods were initially developed, with normal values for adults up to 150 µg per 24 hours. More recently, RIA techniques have provided normal range values of up to 100 µg per 24 hours. This test is obviously of more value when plasma cortisol values are elevated. Urinary free cortisol determination is help-

ful in evaluation of adrenocortical insufficiency when used compara-
tively following ACTH stimulation.

17-HYDROXYCORTICOIDS AND 17-KETOSTEROIDS. Confusion among
17-ketosteroids (17-KS), 17-ketogenic steroids (17-KGS), and 17-hy-
droxycorticoids (17-OHCS) may hinder interpretation of the literature
on evaluation of adrenocortical insufficiency. The 17-KS are metabolites
of the androgenic steroids of adrenal and, to a lesser extent, gonadal origin, characterized by a keto group at C-17. As primarily androgen
metabolites, they have limited use in evaluation of adrenal insufficiency.
However, they are useful in evaluation of hirsutism and certain causes of
Cushing's syndrome (Chaps. 9 and 12).

The 17-KGS are steroids that may be oxidized to 17-KS and measured
as such, less baseline 17-KS, to approximate cortisol production. The 17-
KGS include cortisol, cortisone, 11-deoxycortisol, and their tetrahydro
derivatives as well as cortol, cortolone, and pregnanetriol. These
"genic" steroids obviously provide a less specific assessment of cortisol
production and are not preferred when 17-OHCS or free cortisol measurements are available.

Most commonly used now are the 17-hydroxycorticosteroids. These
are colorimetrically determined products (Porter-Silber chromogens).
They represent 30 to 40% of the total cortisol metabolites and include
primarily tetrahydrocortisol glucuronide and tetrahydrocortisone
glucuronide, but not the later degradation products of cortol and cortolone. Thus, the Porter-Silber chromogens assess less of the total output of cortisol metabolites than 17-KGS but are somewhat more specific.

Normal values for urinary metabolites are as follows:

17-KS	7-20 mg/24 hr (5–10 mg/gm creatinine)
17-KGS	5–20 mg/24 hr (5–10 mg/gm creatinine)
17-OHCS	4–12 mg/24 hr (2–7 mg/gm creatinine)

Measurement of creatinine in 24-hour urine collections provides an
idea of the completeness of a urine collection. Since creatinine excretion
is relatively constant day to day in a given patient, expressing urinary
metabolites per gram of creatinine allows comparison of results and recognition of collection errors. Creatinine excretion is approximately 15 to
20 mg/kg in men and 10 to 15 mg/kg in women.

DISCUSSION
Evaluation of the Patient with No Prior Steroid History
The single-dose 1-hour ACTH stimulation test has evolved as the first
diagnostic tool in the investigation of adrenocortical insufficiency. Basal
cortisol levels or the determination of diurnal rhythm do not provide the

quantitative assay of adrenocortical reserve afforded by the single-dose test.

In the emergent situation of suspected adrenal crisis, single-dose stimulation should be accomplished while glucocorticoid coverage is provided by a nonmeasured compound such as dexamethasone. In fact, basal and stimulated cortisol determinations under stress may prove very valuable in later evaluation of a patient's steroid requirement.

Beginning at the first step of the protocol (Fig. 7-1), a patient with a normal cosyntropin response by all three criteria is usually not adrenally insufficient. An exception to this general statement may be found in cases of acute pituitary infarction when the adrenal gland is tested before atrophy occurs. If some variables do not meet the accepted criteria (and this is more likely if testing is not done between 8 and 10 AM), a repeat test (single dose) under more standard conditions may be completed prior to the more sustained stimulation. If the repeat single dose does not meet all criteria, further testing is warranted. If all cortisol values are below normal and no response criteria have been met, this is very suggestive of adrenal insufficiency. Finally, in the critically ill individual, very high cortisol levels ($\geq$40 μg/dl) without large incremental responses may be found. This represents an appropriate and presumably a maximal response to the stress. The critically ill patient with basal cortisol (pre-ACTH) of less than 15 μg/dl and a peak cortisol response after ACTH of <20 μg/dl warrants further investigation.

Evaluation should proceed to the 3-day ACTH stimulation test when single-dose or repeated cosyntropin screening tests are abnormal. The 3-day protocol is a demanding evaluation. However, an unambiguous study will preclude multiple questions about future therapy and will limit the need for further evaluations. A normal response is easily distinguished from the absent response of primary adrenal insufficiency. ACTH tests are helpful in the confirmation of primary insufficiency, with levels often in excess of 200 pg/ml. Low or normal-range ACTH levels in combination with an absent or partial adrenal gland response to exogenous ACTH suggest secondary insufficiency. Studies suggest that even the most severely atrophied glands will show some response by the third day of ACTH stimulation.

In the absence of a history of steroid ingestion, evidence of secondary insufficiency should lead to an evaluation for intracranial disease. Skull films with tomography of the sella turcica, visual fields, computed tomography scan, and other radiologic procedures as indicated should be obtained (see Chap. 2). As discussed earlier, however, secondary adrenal insufficiency (in the absence of exogenous steroids) is often identified by the company it keeps. Thus, other secondary hormonal deficiencies would be expected.

Final confirmation of secondary ACTH deficiency as well as documentation of other deficiencies is afforded by the ITT in combination with TRH/GnRH administration and growth hormone determination.

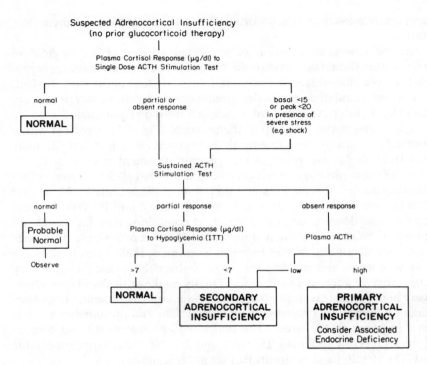

Figure 7-1. Diagnostic protocol: Adrenocortical insufficiency (no prior glucocorticoids). ACTH, adrenocorticotropic hormone; ITT, insulin tolerance test.

These may be done in a single combined procedure, as outlined in the section on hypopituitarism in Chapter 2.

Metyrapone remains an option in the assessment of secondary failure. However, less overall information is provided since normal feedback responses do not necessarily correlate with normal stress responses. Whatever the final tool of evaluation, it must be remembered that a responsive adrenal gland is necessary to provide evidence of ACTH action using metyrapone or the ITT.

Evaluation of the Patient with a Prior Steroid History

The patient who is receiving glucocorticoids or has recently completed glucocorticoid therapy presents a somewhat more complex diagnostic problem (Fig. 7-2). It has been well established that high doses of glucocorticoids given for long enough courses of therapy will lead to hypothalamic-pituitary suppression and secondary adrenal atrophy. The pattern of return of the HPA axis after long-term suppression has been characterized by a staged partial return of various parts of the axis. After suppression occurs, both ACTH and corticosteroid levels are low (1–2 months). Then (2–5 months) ACTH levels increase to the supranormal range, but adrenal responsiveness to exogenous ACTH remains subnormal. During the next phase (6–9 months), plasma and urine steroids return to normal but in the face of elevated ACTH levels. The recovery phase (9 months) is complete when ACTH levels are normal and the adrenal gland response to exogenous ACTH is normal [12].

The key concept in this observation is that adrenal gland responsiveness (to exogenous ACTH) lags behind hypothalamic-pituitary return. Thus, in evaluating a patient who has a history of steroid therapy, the single-dose cosyntropin test remains a reasonable first step. Since the adrenal gland is presumably the last component of the HPA axis to recover from suppression [12], a normal test suggests return of the entire axis to normal. Supportive data for this approach are found in studies showing that the short ACTH test accurately reflects the function of the HPA system as assessed by the insulin hypoglycemia test [18,22]. However, exceptions to this approach have been reported in which discordant cortisol responses to exogenous ACTH and the ITT were found in some patients with pituitary disease [6] or in patients withdrawn from long-term therapy with glucocorticoids [17]. At this time, it seems reasonable to consider a clearly normal short ACTH test as presumptive evidence of adrenal recovery. However, the ITT appears to be the more sensitive test and should be utilized if definitive characterization of the HPA axis is necessary.

Less information on HPA return after short-term, high-dose therapy is available. However, evidence exists that, as in long-term suppression, recovery of hypothalamic-pituitary function is apparent before normal adrenal gland responsiveness following short-term therapy. A normal

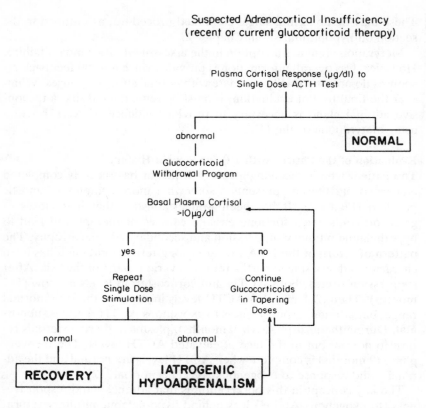

Figure 7-2. Diagnostic protocol: Adrenocortical insufficiency (prior or current steroid therapy). ACTH, adrenocorticotropic hormone.

response to synthetic ACTH appears to be a reliable measure of HPA axis integrity after short-term glucocorticoid suppression [31].

If the single-dose cosyntropin test is not normal, further evaluation may follow one of two courses: First, if there is an unresolved question of possible primary adrenal insufficiency in the past for which the patient is on steroids, the sustained ACTH test is a reasonable next step. A lack of response to sustained ACTH confirms a correct prior diagnosis of primary adrenal insufficiency and subsequent appropriate steroid therapy. A stepwise increase in 17-OHCS is consistent with glucocorticoid-induced suppression of the HPA axis. Second, if exogenous steroid therapy was begun to treat another disease (temporal arteritis, nephritis, etc.), it may reasonably be presumed that the adrenal insufficiency is secondary and the sustained ACTH infusion test is not required. In contrast to the evaluation of the patient with no prior steroid history, there is little point in pursuing further evaluation of the secondarily suppressed individual until evidence of HPA recovery is evident. Documentation of full HPA recovery becomes the goal.

Various protocols have been advocated to withdraw patients from glucocorticoids [7]. From these, several guidelines emerge:

1. Gradual tapering of glucocorticoids until maintenance of 40 mg of hydrocortisone or an equivalent single morning dose is attained.
2. Continued gradual tapering (supplementing for stress) to 10 to 20 mg of hydrocortisone per day.
3. Basal fasting morning cortisol testing as an initial measure of recovery. When the morning basal cortisol is >10 μg/dl, single-dose cosyntropin stimulation may be used at monthly intervals to assess adrenal gland responsiveness.
4. When the single-dose cosyntropin is normal, recovery may be assumed.

It follows from these considerations that more elaborate hypothalamic-pituitary testing in the steroid-suppressed patient is not required unless clinical considerations dictate the need for definitive study using the ITT.

REFERENCES

1. Ackerman, G., and Nolan, C. Adrenocortical responsiveness after alternate day corticosteroid therapy. *N. Engl. J. Med.* 278:405–409, 1968.
2. Amatruda, T., Hurst, M., and D'Esopo, N. Certain endocrine and metabolic facets of the steroid withdrawal syndrome. *J. Clin. Endocrinol. Metab.* 25:1207–1217, 1965.
3. Alsever, R. N., and Gottin, R. W. *Handbook of Endocrine Tests in Adults and Children* (2nd ed.). Chicago: Year Book, 1978. P. 130.
4. Axelrod, L. Glucocorticoid therapy. *Medicine* 55:39–67, 1976.
5. Blizzard, R. M., Chee, D., and Davie, W. The incidence of adrenal and other antibodies in the sera of patients with idiopathic adrenal insufficiency (Addison's disease). *Clin. Exp. Immunol.* 2:19–30, 1967.

6. Borst, G. C., Michenfelder, H. J., and O'Brian, J. T. Discordant cortisol response to exogenous ACTH and insulin-induced hypoglycemia in patients with pituitary disease. *N. Engl. J. Med.* 306:1462–1464, 1982.
7. Byyny, R. L. Withdrawal from glucocorticoid therapy. *N. Engl. J. Med.* 295:30–32, 1976.
8. Chakmakjian, Z., Nelson, D., and Bethune, J. Adrenocortical failure in panhypopituitarism. *J. Clin. Endocrinol. Metab.* 28:259–265, 1968.
9. Christy, N., Wallace, E., and Jailer, J. Comparative effects of prednisone and of cortisone in suppressing the response of the adrenal cortex to exogenous adrenocorticotropin. *J. Clin. Endocrinol. Metab.* 16:1059–1074, 1956.
10. Dluhy, R. G., Himathongam, T., and Greenfield, M. Rapid ACTH test with aldosterone levels. *Ann. Intern. Med.* 80:693–696, 1974.
11. Editorial. Corticosteroids and hypothalamic pituitary adrenal functions. *Br. Med. J.* 1:813–814, 1980.
12. Graber, A. L., et al. Natural history of pituitary adrenal recovery following long-term suppression with corticosteroids. *J. Clin. Endocrinol. Metab.* 25:11–16, 1965.
13. Grant, S., Forsham, P., and Diraimondo, V. Suppression of 17-hydroxycorticosteroids in plasma and urine by single and divided doses of triamcinolone. *N. Engl. J. Med.* 273:1115–1118, 1965.
14. Greenwood, F., Landon, J., and Stamp, T. The plasma sugar, free fatty acid, cortisol, and growth hormone response to insulin. I. In control subjects. *J. Clin. Invest.* 45:429–436, 1966.
15. Irvine, W. J., and Barnes, E. W. Adrenocortical insufficiency. *Clin. Endocrinol. Metab.* 1:549–594, 1972.
16. Jacobs, H. S., and Nabarro, J. D. N. Tests of hypothalamic-pituitary-adrenal function in man. *Q. J. Med.* 38:475–486, 1969.
17. Harrison, B. D. W., et al. Recovery of hypothalamo-pituitary-adrenal function in asthmatics whose oral steroids have been stopped or reduced. *Clin. Endocrinol.* 17:109–118, 1982.
18. Kehlet, H., and Binder, C. Value of an ACTH test in assessing hypothalamic-pituitary-adrenocortical function in glucocorticoid treated patients. *Br. Med. J.* 2:147–149, 1973.
19. Landon, J., et al. Threshhold adrenocortical sensitivity in man and its possible application to corticotropin bioassay. *Lancet* 2:697–700, 1967.
20. Landon, J., Wynn, V., and James, V. The adrenocortical response to insulin induced hypoglycemia. *J. Clin. Endocrinol. Metab.* 27:183–192, 1963.
21. Liddle, G. W. The adrenal cortex. In D. H. Williams (Ed.), *Textbook of Endocrinology.* Philadelphia: Saunders, 1974. P. 251.
22. Lindholm, J., et al. Reliability of the 30 minute ACTH test in assessing hypothalamic-pituitary-adrenal function. *J. Clin. Endocrinol. Metab.* 47:272–274, 1978.
23. Livanou, T., Ferriman, D., and James, V. Recovery of hypothalamo-pituitary-adrenal function after corticosteroid therapy. *Lancet* 2:856–859, 1967.
24. Meikle, A., and Tyler, F. Potency and duration of action of glucocorticoids. Effects of hydrocortisone, prednisone, and dexamethasone on human pituitary-adrenal function. *Am. J. Med.* 63:200–207, 1977.
25. Nerup, J. Addison's disease—clinical studies. *Acta Endocrinol.* 76:27–141, 1974.
26. Nichols, T., Nugent, C., and Tyler, F. Diurnal variation in suppression of adrenal function of glucocorticoids. *J. Clin. Endocrinol. Metab.* 25:343–349, 1965.
27. Spark, R. F. Simplified assessment of pituitary-adrenal reserve: Measurement of serum 11-deoxycortisol and cortisol after metyrapone. *Ann. Intern. Med.* 75:717–723, 1971.

28. Speckart, P., Nicoloff, J., and Bethune, J. Screening for adrenocortical insufficiency with cosyntropin (synthetic ACTH). *Arch. Intern. Med.* 128:761–763, 1971.
29. Spiegel, R. J., et al. Adrenal suppression after short term corticosteroid therapy. *Lancet* 1:630–633, 1979.
30. Stacpoole, P. W., et al. Isolated ACTH deficiency: A heterogeneous disorder. *Medicine* 61:13–24, 1982.
31. Streck, W. F., and Lockwood, D. H. Pituitary adrenal recovery following short term suppression with corticosteroids. *Am. J. Med.* 66:910–914, 1979.
32. Wood, J. B., et al. A rapid test of adrenocortical function. *Lancet* 1:243–245, 1965.

8   Cushing's Syndrome

William F. Streck

Cushing's syndrome may be defined as a group of clinical and metabolic abnormalities resulting from chronic exposure to excess glucocorticoids [6,10,17]. Four different pathologic mechanisms may lead to Cushing's syndrome: (1) Iatrogenic hypercortisolism may follow the use of exogenous glucocorticoids or adrenocorticotropic hormone (ACTH) in the management of other disease. (2) *Cushing's disease* is that form of the syndrome that is characterized by excessive ACTH secretion by the pituitary, with consequent bilateral adrenal gland hyperplasia. (3) Adrenal disorders (adenoma or carcinoma) may directly produce excess cortisol free of normal feedback constraints. A rare variant of the adrenal disease leading to Cushing's syndrome is nodular adrenal hyperplasia. This disorder may represent a primary adrenal disorder or a secondary process related to ACTH hypersecretion. (4) The ectopic ACTH syndrome consists of the secretion of ACTH by nonpituitary tumors that produce hypercortisolism secondary to adrenal gland hyperplasia.

CLINICAL CONSIDERATIONS

The naturally occurring varieties of Cushing's syndrome are less common than iatrogenic hypercortisolism and more difficult to diagnose, yet a frequent part of a differential diagnosis. The relative approximate incidence of the naturally occurring types of Cushing's syndrome is as follows: Cushing's disease, 70%; adrenal adenoma/carcinoma, 15%; ectopic ACTH, 15%.

Hypercortisolism is the final pathologic mediator in all types of Cushing's syndrome. Variable degrees of excess androgen, estrogen, and mineralocorticoid secretion may accompany the hypercortisolism. Other variables that may modify the presentation of the syndrome include prior physiognomy, rapidity of onset, sex of the patient, and the cause of the syndrome. A prior photograph of the patient may reveal comparative changes not readily appreciated on the initial examination.

Androgen secretion may modify the presentation of hypercortisolism. Excess production of androgens accounts for three of the features most frequently seen in women (hirsutism, menstrual disorders, and acne) [17]. In contrast, testosterone levels are low in men with Cushing's disease, presumably due to inhibition of testicular secretion by androgens of adrenal origin. Decreased libido, impotence, and oligospermia may be present in men with Cushing's syndrome [46].

The signs and symptoms of Cushing's syndrome have been summarized in many studies. The most frequently observed findings are included in Table 8-1. A few useful guidelines emerge from the many studies. Generalized obesity has a strong negative correlation with the

Table 8-1. Clinical Manifestations in Cushing's Syndrome

Weakness
Obesity
Hypertension
Plethora
Decreased glucose tolerance
Menstrual dysfunction
Impotence
Hirsutism and acne
Striae
Osteopenia
Easy bruisability
Emotional disturbances
Edema
Polyuria
Hypokalemia
Hyperpigmentation

presence of Cushing's syndrome. Some clinical features appear to be age related. Striae are more common in younger patients, and weakness and edema in older ones. Men with Cushing's disease had a higher incidence of osteopenia than women in one study [50]. Although various percentages of incidence are assigned to these findings in different studies, in practice such estimates are unnecessary in the florid case and of little help in the subtle case. Since the most discriminating clinical features on a statistical basis are not frequently encountered, it is not surprising that accurate diagnosis on the basis of clinical features alone may be expected in less than 50% of cases [36].

When Cushing's syndrome is present, the cause of the hypercortisolism may be suggested by certain characteristic features [39]. For instance, Cushing's disease is more often a disorder of women, usually affecting those of childbearing age. The excessive ACTH secretion is due to a surgically demonstrable pituitary adenoma in 70 to 80% of cases, although the tumor may be too small (microadenoma) to give evidence of x-ray changes. Recent studies have demonstrated a high incidence of pituitary microadenoma in patients explored by transsphenoidal microsurgery for Cushing's disease [49]. Questions still remain, however, since abnormal neurohypothalamic control of ACTH secretion has been suggested by studies demonstrating improvement in Cushing's disease using cyproheptadine, a serotonin antagonist [22]. In addition, the finding of persistent cortisol-ACTH feedback abnormalities after removal of the pituitary tumor in Cushing's disease that had responded to cyproheptadine suggests a role for higher centers in the pathophysiology of Cushing's disease [24].

Adrenal adenomas may resemble pituitary Cushing's disease in presentation. Adenomas are also more common in women than men and may not produce evidence of virilization since androgen pathways are not usually stimulated but rather suppressed due to decreased ACTH. Adenomas manifest no mass on examination and give no evidence of debilitating malignancy [17]. The natural history of adenomas is quite variable, with fluctuating activity and even spontaneous regression noted [7].

Adrenocortical carcinomas are rare tumors that are usually functional, that is, they produce active hormones that lead to hypercortisolism (50%), virilization (20%), or both (10–15%) [5,19,30]. Feminizing tumors are very rare. Carcinomas that are nonfunctional comprise approximately 10 to 15% of cases of adrenocortical carcinoma [25]. These tumors presumably produce insufficient steroids to elevate basal plasma or urinary steroids or cause endocrinologic syndromes. Adrenal carcinoma is more common in adults in the 50 to 70 age range. However, adrenal carcinoma does occur in young children [16]. As these malignant tumors are less efficient in steroidogenesis, large tumor masses may be present by the time of diagnosis.

A rare adrenal cause of Cushing's syndrome is nodular adrenal hyperplasia [2,31]. This is perhaps a variant of Cushing's disease, with excess ACTH leading to adrenal hyperplasia and subsequent evolution of autonomous adrenal tissue. Pathologic features characteristic of nodular hyperplasia include the presence of one or more nodules in both adrenal glands and diffuse bilateral cortical hyperplasia. Nodular hyperplasia may occur in younger patients, does not predictably respond to dexamethasone suppression, and presents with variable ACTH levels. Consequently, this disorder is difficult to distinguish from other causes of adrenal hypercortisolism by standard stimulation and suppression tests. This variant may account for 10 to 20% of cases of bilateral adrenal hyperplasia not associated with the ectopic ACTH syndrome [2].

Ectopic ACTH production has been demonstrated in many malignancies (Table 8-2). Cushing's syndrome due to excess ectopic ACTH secretion most commonly occurs in tumors of the lung (oat cell) and thymus and in islet cell tumors of the pancreas [37]. Florid symptoms of hypercortisolism are often not apparent. More commonly, Cushing's syndrome due to excess ectopic ACTH production presents as a debilitating illness, with marked hyperpigmentation, a high incidence of edema, and profound hypokalemic alkalosis due to increased levels of desoxycorticosterone (DOC) and corticosterone [44]. Weight loss rather than weight gain characterizes the hypercortisolism due to ectopic ACTH.

DIAGNOSTIC METHODS
Investigation of suspected Cushing's syndrome has two components. First, the presence of hypercortisolism must be established. When

Table 8-2. Tumors Producing Ectopic ACTH

Oat cell carcinoma of the lung
Thymoma
Islet cell tumors of the pancreas
Medullary carcinoma of the thyroid
Carcinoid
Bronchial adenoma
Pheochromocytoma

---

hypercortisolism is confirmed, the second step is the identification of the cause of the syndrome. Different tests are used for these two aspects of the evaluation. More than one test should be required to establish the diagnosis in the less than florid case. The most widely accepted initial studies used to indicate the presence or absence of Cushing's syndrome include overnight (single-dose) dexamethasone suppression, urinary free cortisol determination (μg/24 hours), and low-dose (2-mg) dexamethasone suppression.

Other tests of cortisol dynamics may be abnormal in Cushing's syndrome. These include the diurnal variation of plasma cortisol, the cortisol response to hypoglycemia, and the cortisol secretion rate. However, as initial screening studies, these tests are much less useful than those previously listed. In particular, plasma cortisol levels are not reliable screening studies unless obtained in conjunction with dexamethasone suppression.

Once hypercortisolism has been established, further testing is necessary to define the cause. Tests that are useful in differentiating the causes of established Cushing's syndrome include high-dose (8-mg) dexamethasone suppression, plasma ACTH assay, the metyrapone test, and serum dehydroepiandrosterone-sulfate determination.

Tests to Indicate the Presence of Cushing's Syndrome
OVERNIGHT DEXAMETHASONE SUPPRESSION. The overnight (single-dose) dexamethasone suppression test has been advocated as the best initial screening test for Cushing's syndrome [11,35]. The measurement of urinary free cortisol has also been shown to be a reliable screening test [13]. However, the simplicity of the overnight test is an advantage. The procedure is as follows:

1. A 1-mg dose of dexamethasone is taken orally at 11:00 PM. (A sleeping medication may be administered concurrently.)
2. At 8:00 the next morning, a sample is obtained for determination of plasma cortisol.

A normal response is suppression of plasma cortisol to less than 5 μg/dl. A cortisol level greater than 5 μg/dl indicates the need for further evaluation. As a screening device, this test is very reliable in identifying Cushing's syndrome, with a false-negative incidence of 1 to 2%. False-positive results occur occasionally in obese subjects (10–15%), ill or psychologically stressed patients (30%), or those on estrogens or other drugs [11]. However, since errors are of a false-positive nature, a normal test essentially rules out Cushing's syndrome.

URINARY FREE CORTISOL. The measurement of urinary free cortisol serves as the best urinary discriminator of Cushing's syndrome. Current radioimmunoassay techniques provide an upper limit of normal of 80 to 100 µg per 24 hours. Findings in excess of this level support the diagnosis of Cushing's syndrome.

Although urinary free cortisol has significant advantages over 17-hydroxycorticoids (17-OHCS) or 17-ketosteroids (17-KS) as a screening test, 17-OHCS remains one of the standard suppression tests used in evaluating hypercortisolism. The interpretive value of 17-OHCS measurements may be enhanced by expressing the results in milligrams per gram of creatinine excreted (normal, up to 7 mg/gm creatinine) [48]. However, as a general rule, free cortisol is best used for screening, 17-OHCS (with free cortisol) in dexamethasone suppression tests, and 17-KS to screen for possible carcinoma or to help differentiate between adenoma and pituitary (or ectopic) etiologies.

LOW-DOSE DEXAMETHASONE SUPPRESSION. The low-dose dexamethasone suppression, as initially defined by Liddle, serves as the standard for the identification of Cushing's syndrome [27]. The overnight or single-dose test is a simplified version of the approach. Since the low-dose test often is used to confirm abnormal single-dose or urinary free cortisol results, the protocol is often linked with the higher-dose dexamethasone test for practical reasons. However, the low-dose test simply defines pathologic hypercortisolism; it does not identify the cause of such a disorder. The procedure is as follows:

Days 1, 2   24-hour urine collections for urinary free cortisol, 17-OHCS, and creatinine
Days 3, 4   Dexamethasone, 0.5 mg, administered orally every 6 hours for 48 hours
             24-hour urine collections obtained for urinary free cortisol, 17-OHCS, and creatinine
Day 4   Plasma cortisol obtained at 1600 hours

Normal responses include a 17-OHCS level of less than 4 mg per 24 hours on the second day of dexamethasone administration. Urinary free cortisol should be less than 20 µg per 24 hours. The use of plasma cortisol levels after low- and high-dose dexamethasone suppression has been compared to the standard urinary values in one study [4]. In this study, a serum cortisol value of more than 5 μg/dl at 1600 hours on the second day of dexamethasone administration accurately identified Cushing's syndrome in a manner comparable to that obtained using urine 17-OHCS determinations [4]. Thus, the addition of this cortisol determination may be used to enhance the diagnostic capability of the low-dose test or, in some instances, may prove an alternative to cumbersome urinary collections.

Although a urinary 17-OHCS level of less than 4 mg per 24 hours served as the original discriminatory criterion in this test, a dose of dexamethasone based on 20 μg per kilogram of body weight has been advocated to enhance discrimination [48]. Using this criterion, a normal response is suppression of 17-OHCS to less than 1 mg per gram of creatinine per day. However, studies have confirmed the value of the 4 mg per 24 hour criterion, with a false-negative rate of 3.5% in a recent review [11].

OTHER STUDIES. Other tests used to define Cushing's syndrome have less general application. Studies of diurnal variation of plasma cortisol are subject to many variables. Morning cortisol levels may be normal in Cushing's syndrome. Evening samples may be elevated due to anxiety, depression, heart failure, or drugs. Patients with Cushing's syndrome do not show the normal cortisol rise following insulin-induced hypoglycemia. This occurs even if basal cortisol levels are in the normal range. This test is particularly helpful in those instances in which severe depression is a complicating variable. The insulin tolerance test does not differentiate among the various causes of Cushing's syndrome but may aid in establishing the primary diagnosis. Since patients often have glucose intolerance, 0.2 to 0.3 units of insulin per kilogram of body weight is often required to obtain adequate hypoglycemia.

Tests Used to Determine the Etiology of Established Cushing's Syndrome
HIGH-DOSE DEXAMETHASONE SUPPRESSION. The high-dose dexamethasone suppression test remains the fundamental differential diagnostic tool in the investigation of the etiology of Cushing's syndrome. This test is helpful in distinguishing adrenal hyperplasia due to pituitary hypersecretion of ACTH, in which some degree of feedback responsiveness is maintained, from adrenal tumors or the ectopic ACTH syndrome. The procedure may follow in sequence the low-dose dexamethasone protocol to simplify basal collections or may be as follows:

Days 1, 2   24-hour urine collection for free cortisol, 17-OHCS, and creatinine
Days 3, 4   Repeat urine collections, 2 mg of dexamethasone orally every 6 hours for 48 hours
Day 4   Plasma cortisol at 1600 hours

Suppression of 17-OHCS levels by 40% or more of baseline levels suggests Cushing's disease [26,27]. Suppression of urinary free cortisol values is also expected though less well standardized. This will be found in close to 90% of cases of pituitary-dependent Cushing's disease. Adenomas or carcinomas do not reproducibly suppress, and the ectopic ACTH syndrome and nodular adrenal hyperplasia fail to suppress in 75 to 80% of cases [11]. Plasma cortisol levels on the second day of high-dose dexamethasone have been reported to be comparable to urinary studies in the differential diagnosis of Cushing's syndrome. Patients with Cushing's disease characteristically had suppression of plasma cortisol to less than 10 µg/dl at 1600 hours on the second day of high-dose dexamethasone [4]. As in the low-dose tests, the use of this value may enhance the high-dose test.

PLASMA ADRENOCORTICOTROPIC HORMONE. Now available in commercial laboratories, ACTH determinations show a normal range in most assays of 20 to 100 pg/ml. Several samples may be required to estimate reliably the mean plasma ACTH level since ACTH has a diurnal variation, an episodic secretion, and a short plasma half-life. ACTH is somewhat subject to the vagaries of laboratory processing; it disappears from plasma if left at room temperature and adsorbs to glass containers. Careful collection, prompt separation, and freezing of samples are required. Even with such attention, ACTH measurement is one of the more difficult radioimmunoassays to perform reliably.

Since ACTH is considered part of a precursor molecule, measurement of this larger molecule or another of its components (lipotropin) has been suggested as a means of distinguishing ectopic from entopic production of ACTH [38]. Selective venous sampling for ACTH from the inferior petrosal sinus has been suggested as a useful and reliable procedure in differentiating pituitary from ectopic ACTH hypersecretion in those cases in which clinical and biochemical tests are equivocal [15].

METYRAPONE TEST. The metyrapone test may be useful in distinguishing Cushing's disease from adrenal tumors. Metyrapone blocks cortisol production primarily by inhibiting synthesis at the final step, 11-β-hydroxylation of 11-deoxycortisol to form cortisol. In normals and in patients with Cushing's disease (who have some preservation of feedback inhibition), the resultant lowering of cortisol after metyrapone administration leads to a compensatory increase in ACTH production [20,26]. As a result, urinary 17-OHCS levels, representing the precursors of cortisol, are increased. A normal response is a twofold or 10 mg per day increase in 17-OHCS following metyrapone given as 750 mg every 4 hours in six doses. This requires urine collections the day before, the day of, and the day after administration of the metyrapone (see Chap. 7).

Adrenal adenomas characteristically show either no change or a fall in 17-OHCS excretion after metyrapone since no compensatory ACTH rise occurs. Some overlap has been noted. Thus, as a rule, a normal metyra-pone response makes adrenal tumor unlikely, although not impossible. No response to metyrapone (i.e., no increase in 17-OHCS) rules out Cushing's disease. Short forms of the metyrapone test have also been advocated [32,47]. One recent study demonstrated that the serum 11-deoxycortisol response after metyrapone was superior to the high-dose dexamethasone test in the differential diagnosis of Cushing's syndrome [45a].

DEHYDROEPIANDROSTERONE SULFATE. As discussed earlier, adrenal adenomas characteristically do not produce androgens. Baseline serum levels of the sulfated adrenal androgen dehydroepiandrosterone (DHEA-S) in patients with nonsuppressible Cushing's disease have been shown to be low in patients with adrenal adenomas. This has emerged as a useful means of further characterizing the etiology of established Cushing's syndrome. DHEA-S values of less than 0.4 mg/ml are considered supportive of the diagnosis of adenoma [4].

ADRENOCORTICOTROPIC HORMONE INFUSION. The infusion of 250 μg of synthetic ACTH over 8 hours has been advocated as a test to discriminate adenoma from adrenal carcinoma in Cushing's syndrome. In one series, half of the adenomas showed an increase in 17-OHCS, whereas no carcinomas responded to exogenous ACTH [5]. The reliability and general usefulness of this test have not been established.

Supplementary Studies

Skull films are abnormal in only 10 to 20% of patients with Cushing's disease on initial presentation. Polytomography of the sella will enhance detection of subtle changes of pituitary microadenomas. Computed tomography (CT) has proved accurate and easy to perform in the evaluation of adrenal disease. Results in serial studies indicate that high-resolution CT can accurately differentiate adrenal tumor from hyperplasia [17]. CT of the adrenal gland offers distinct advantages over more difficult procedures such as arteriography and venography [34] in the evaluation of adrenal disease. Although not generally available, adrenal scanning with radioiodinated cholesterol may distinguish between unilateral adenoma and bilateral adrenal hyperplasia [1,28]. Sonography of the adrenal gland has not been shown to be reliable in localizing adrenal masses.

DISCUSSION

The abnormal cortisol dynamics of Cushing's syndrome have been well characterized by extensive studies. Such studies have also provided adequate methods for investigation of the patient who may have this condition. The key to effective diagnosis of Cushing's syndrome is the systematic application of these tests and procedures. The protocols in Figures 8-1 and 8-2 outline three levels of evaluation of suspected Cushing's syndrome.

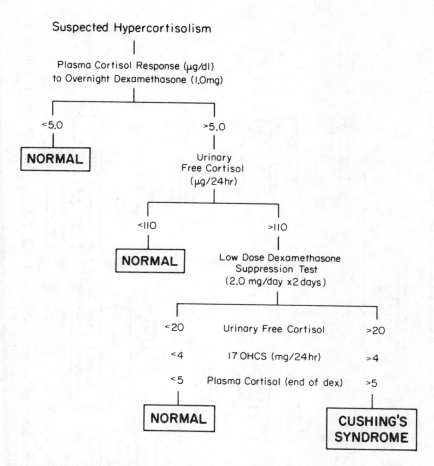

Figure 8-1. Diagnostic protocol: Evaluation of suspected hypercortisolism. 17OHCS, 17-hydroxycorticoids.

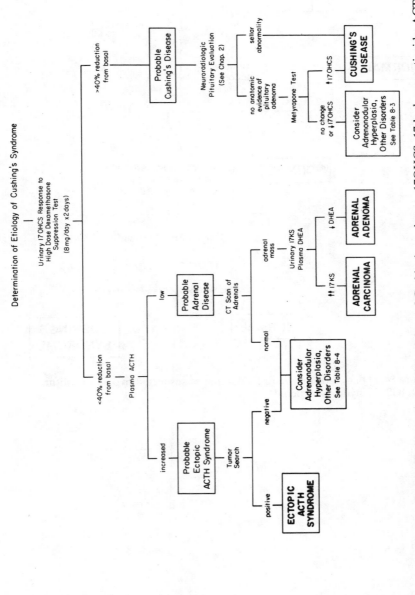

Figure 8-2. Diagnostic protocol: Investigation of the etiology of Cushing's syndrome. 17OHCS, 17-hydroxycorticoids; ACTH, adreno-corticotropic hormone; 17KS, 17-ketosteroids; DHEA, dehydroepiandrosterone.

Screening tests constitute the first step. The overnight dexamethasone suppression test is simple and reliable. In those instances in which obesity or estrogen use may hinder interpretation, determination of urinary free cortisol offers a second reliable initial evaluation. Normal findings in these studies may reasonably end an evaluation. If clinical suspicion remains high, tests may be repeated at a later date. The value of these tests as screening tools is enhanced by the fact that errors are not frequent and are of a false-positive nature when present.

The two-day, low-dose dexamethasone suppression test is the second step in the evaluation sequence. When the overnight dexamethasone test and/or the urinary free cortisol values are abnormal, low-dose dexamethasone suppression may be used. It may be argued that this test is not necessary in cases of florid Cushing's syndrome with markedly abnormal screening responses. In such instances, the high-dose dexamethasone suppression test may be the next step in the evaluation. When the low-dose test is indicated, patients may be hospitalized and basal studies, low-dose, and high-dose dexamethasone suppression performed sequentially.

The use of isolated measurements of 17-OHCS or 17-KS is not recommended as a screening test for Cushing's syndrome. However, measurement of 17-KS may be useful in differentiating the etiology of Cushing's syndrome. If urinary 17-KS are above 50 mg per 24 hours in the presence of Cushing's syndrome, carcinoma of the adrenal gland is likely. If urinary 17-KS are normal with excess 17-OHCS, an adrenal adenoma is likely. In the low-dose dexamethasone suppression test 17-OHCS remain the standard, although free cortisol levels are also useful and may be more informative.

The high-dose dexamethasone suppression test is part of the third level of investigation—determination of the cause of Cushing's syndrome. It is advisable to preserve additional aliquots of urine from each day of the testing protocol until the results have been returned. This ensures that lost samples or technical errors will not negate a study period. The use of urinary free cortisol in this suppression test is also less well standardized than 17-OHCS data, although studies have shown that these two variables do respond in an expected parallel fashion. The critical factor in the high-dose test remains the amount of suppression: 40% reduction of urinary 17-OHCS suggests Cushing's disease, and no suppression suggests adenoma, carcinoma, or ectopic ACTH production. Equivocal suppression (definite decrease in urinary levels, but by less than 40%) keeps alive the possibility of Cushing's disease. This problem may be approached by using higher-dose suppression or extending the duration of the test. Even following such enhanced efforts at suppression, adrenal or ectopic causes of hypercortisolism are not expected to suppress substantially, although exceptions have been noted [3].

Measurement of ACTH in cases of Cushing's syndrome may help to differentiate the causes of hypercortisolism, but such determinations are really helpful only when they are consistent with results from more definitive tests. Undetectable or very low ACTH levels indicate adrenal hypersecretion of cortisol due to adenoma or carcinoma [40]. In contrast, levels above 200 pg/ml will be found in 60 to 70% of cases of ectopic ACTH syndrome [40]. There is overlap in plasma ACTH levels in patients with Cushing's disease and normals [23,41]. Ectopic ACTH production may also be characterized by ACTH levels in the normal range. In cases of nodular adrenal hyperplasia, ACTH levels are unpredictable.

In most instances, the combination of a basal DHEA-S level, high-dose dexamethasone suppression testing, and plasma ACTH assay will differentiate among the causes of Cushing's syndrome [12] (Fig. 8-2). Suppression of urinary 17-OHCS (or plasma cortisol on day 2) by high-dose dexamethasone and a moderately elevated or normal ACTH level support the diagnosis of Cushing's disease. Metyrapone testing may be used as further supportive data. Computed tomography of the sella is a logical next step. Very high ACTH levels and the absence of suppression by high-dose dexamethasone favor the diagnosis of ectopic ACTH production. A chest x-ray to look for ectopic ACTH-secreting lung tumor is indicated. Low ACTH levels and no suppression with high-dose dexamethasone suggest adrenal disease. A low DHEA-S suggests adenoma, as does normal 17-KS with elevated 17-OHCS. Very high 17-KS favors the diagnosis of carcinoma. CT scan of the adrenals should follow.

Exceptions to nearly all the expected results in the evaluation of Cushing's syndrome have been reported [3,29]. Thus, Cushing's disease that apparently regresses spontaneously [18,21], is intermittent [8], or is resistant to standard suppression [3], as well as dexamethasone-suppressible adrenocortical carcinoma, have been reported [42]. Bronchial adenomas may show stimulation and suppression characteristics similar to those seen in Cushing's disease [3]. These variations, however, should not lead to abandonment of the systematic approach to suspected hypercortisolism. Consideration should be given to more extensive studies (i.e., selective ACTH sampling) to define the causes of hypercortisolism in these cases rather than embark upon an incorrect therapeutic course. A list of disorders that may provide atypical responses to standard dexamethasone testing is provided in Table 8-3.

Adrenal nodular hyperplasia has been mentioned as a rare and difficult to diagnose variant of Cushing's syndrome [2]. This particular disorder should be suspected particularly when the plasma ACTH level is detectable, an adrenal mass is noted on CT scan, there is no suppression during high-dose dexamethasone administration, and there is no evidence of an ectopic ACTH syndrome.

Periodic hormonogenesis has been invoked to explain some atypical responses to dexamethasone suppression testing performed in patients with Cushing's syndrome [9]. In periodic hormonogenesis cortisol output varies in a cyclical pattern, with days of high cortisol production alternat-

Table 8-3. Causes of Atypical Responses to Dexamethasone Suppression Tests

Nodular adrenal hyperplasia
Periodic hormonogenesis
Bronchial carcinoid
Depression
Drugs
   Spironolactone
   Estrogen
   Phenytoin
   Alcohol (pseudo-Cushing's syndrome)
Atypical Cushing's disease

ing with days of less production. Cycle lengths have been demonstrated to vary. The key point is that when the cycle is such that the adrenal secretory rate is low, concurrent administration of dexamethasone will appear to produce suppression, although it is in fact a coincidence. The phenomenon of paradoxical dexamethasone stimulation that has been similarly reported in patients with Cushing's syndrome may represent testing performed during an enhanced secretory cycle [14]. The various studies demonstrating episodic secretion [45] emphasize the need to persist with testing when clinical suspicion of Cushing's syndrome is high.

Drugs may cause inappropriate interpretation of stimulation and suppression tests of cortisol dynamics. Estrogen increases cortisol-binding globulin, thereby raising the total cortisol level into the range found in Cushing's syndrome. Use of birth control pills obviously needs to be reviewed in the history. Spironolactone, in contrast, does not raise the plasma cortisol level but may alter its determination in certain assays. Phenytoin has a number of effects on adrenal function [33]. It is most often an interfering agent in the use of the dexamethasone suppression test because of increased dexamethasone metabolism by the liver. Thus, failure to suppress with dexamethasone by a patient taking phenytoin may be explained by drug interactions. However, normal suppression may be considered a reliable test. Excessive alcohol intake has been shown to cause a clinical and biochemical picture consistent with Cushing's syndrome. The abnormalities of this pseudo-Cushing's syndrome revert to normal on ethanol withdrawal [43].

In summary, Cushing's disease, adrenal tumors, and the ectopic ACTH syndrome are the common causes of spontaneous Cushing's syndrome. The selective use of diagnostic methods in most instances will allow confirmation of the presence of the syndrome and delineation of its cause. However, there are complicating variables that may prevent definitive diagnosis. In this instance, variations in dexamethasone metabolism or variants of adrenal disease such as bilateral adrenal nodular hyperplasia should be considered. However, in the long run, the key concept to be kept in mind is that the secretion of cortisol in Cushing's syndrome may not be markedly elevated on every determination. Thus, diagnosis of Cushing's syndrome may well depend as much on tenacity and persistence in obtaining tests when clinical suspicion is high as on the appropriate ordering of any specific test.

REFERENCES

1. Anderson, B. G., and Beierwaltes, W. H. Adrenal imaging with radio-iodocholesterol in the diagnosis of adrenal disorders. *Adv. Intern. Med.* 19:327–343, 1974.
2. Aron, D. C., et al. Pituitary ACTH dependency of nodular adrenal hyperplasia in Cushing's syndrome. *Am. J. Med.* 71:302–306, 1981.
3. Aron, D. C., et al. Cushing's syndrome: Problems in diagnosis. *Medicine* 60:25–35, 1981.
4. Ashcraft, M. W., et al. Serum cortisol levels in Cushing's syndrome after low and high dose dexamethasone suppression. *Ann. Intern. Med.* 97:21–26, 1982.
5. Bertagna, C., and Orth, D. N. Clinical and laboratory findings and results of therapy in 58 patients with adrenocortical tumors. *Am. J. Med.* 71:855–875, 1981.
6. Besser, G. M., and Edwards, C. R. W. Cushing's syndrome. *Clin. Endocrinol.* 1:451–490, 1972.
7. Blau, N., et al. Spontaneous remission of Cushing's syndrome in a patient with adrenal adenoma. *J. Clin. Endocrinol. Metab.* 40:659–663, 1975.
8. Bochner, F., et al. Intermittent Cushing's disease. *Am. J. Med.* 67:507–510, 1979.
9. Brown, R. D., et al. Cushing's disease with periodic hormonogenesis: One explanation for paradoxical response to dexamethasone. *J. Clin. Endocrinol. Metab.* 36:445–451, 1973.
10. Cook, D. M., Kendall, J. K., and Jordan, R. Cushing's syndrome: Current concepts of diagnosis and therapy (medical progress). *West. J. Med.* 132:111–122, 1980.
11. Crapo, L. Cushing's syndrome: A review of diagnostic tests. *Metabolism* 28:955–977, 1979.
12. Dluhy, R. G., and Williams, G. H. Cushing's syndrome and the changing times. *Ann. Intern. Med.* 97:131–133, 1982.
13. Eddy, R. L., et al. Cushing's syndrome: A prospective study of diagnostic methods. *Am. J. Med.* 55:621–630, 1973.
14. Fehm, H. L., et al. Paradoxical ACTH response to glucocorticoids in Cushing's disease. *N. Engl. J. Med.* 297:904–907, 1977.
15. Findling, J. W., et al. Selective venous sampling for ACTH in Cushing's syndrome. *Ann. Intern. Med.* 94:647–652, 1981.
16. Gilbert, M. G., and Cleveland, W. W. Cushing's syndrome in infancy. *Pediatrics* 46:217–229, 1970.
17. Gold, E. M. The Cushing syndromes: Changing views of diagnosis and treatment. *Ann. Intern. Med.* 90:829–844, 1979.
18. Hayslett, J. P., and Cohn, G. L. Spontaneous remission of Cushing's disease. *N. Engl. J. Med.* 276:968–970, 1967.
19. Hutter, A. M., and Kayhoe, D. E. Adrenal cortical carcinoma: Clinical features of 138 patients. *Am. J. Med.* 41:572–580, 1966.
20. Jubiz, W., et al. Plasma metyrapone, ACTH, cortisol, and deoxycortisol levels. *Arch. Intern. Med.* 125:468–471, 1970.

21. Kammer, H., and Barter, M. Spontaneous remission of Cushing's disease. *Am. J. Med.* 67:519–523, 1979.
22. Krieger, D. T., Amorosa, L., and Linick, F. Cyproheptadine-induced remission of Cushing's disease. *N. Engl. J. Med.* 293:893–896, 1975.
23. Krieger, D. T., and Allen, W. Relationship of bioassayable and immunoassayable plasma ACTH and cortisol concentrations in normal subjects and in patients with Cushing's disease. *J. Clin. Endocrinol. Metab.* 10:675–687, 1975.
24. Lankford, H. V., Tucker, H. S. G., and Blackard, W. G. A cyproheptadine reversible defect in ACTH control persisting after removal of the pituitary tumor in Cushing's disease. *N. Engl. J. Med.* 305:1244–1248, 1981.
25. Lewinsky, B. S., et al. The clinical and pathologic features of "non-hormonal" adrenocortical tumors. *Cancer* 33:778–790, 1974.
26. Liddle, G. W., et al. Clinical application of a new test of pituitary reserve. *J. Clin. Endocrinol. Metab.* 19:875–894, 1959.
27. Liddle, G. W. Tests of pituitary-adrenal suppressibility in the diagnosis of Cushing's syndrome. *J. Clin. Endocrinol. Metab.* 20:1539–1560, 1960.
28. Lieberman, L. M., et al. Diagnosis of adrenal disease by visualization of human adrenal glands with [131]I-19-iodocholesterol. *N. Engl. J. Med.* 285:1387–1393, 1971.
29. Linn, J. E., Jr., Bowdoin, B., and Farmer, T. A. Observations and comments on failure of dexamethasone suppression. *N. Engl. J. Med.* 277:403–405, 1967.
30. Lipsett, M. D., Hertz, R., and Ross, G. T. Clinical and pathophysiologic aspects of adrenocortical carcinoma. *Am. J. Med.* 35:374–383, 1963.
31. Meador, C. K., et al. Primary adrenocortical nodular dysplasia: A rare cause of Cushing's syndrome. *J. Clin. Endocrinol. Metab.* 27:1255–1263, 1967.
32. Meikle, A. W., et al. Simplified metyrapone test with determination of plasma 11-deoxycortisol (metyrapone test with plasma S). *J. Clin. Endocrinol. Metab.* 29:985–987, 1969.
33. Meikle, A. W., et al. Effect of diphenylhydantoin on the metabolism of metyrapone and release of ACTH in man. *J. Clin. Endocrinol. Metab.* 29:1553–1558, 1969.
34. Nicolis, G. L., et al. Percutaneous adrenal venography. A clinical study of 50 patients. *Ann. Intern. Med.* 76:899–909, 1972.
35. Nugent, C. A., Nichols, T., and Tyler, F. H. Diagnosis of Cushing's syndrome. Single dose dexamethasone suppression test. *Arch. Intern. Med.* 116:172–176, 1965.
36. Nugent, C. A., et al. Probability theory in the diagnosis of Cushing's syndrome. *J. Clin. Endocrinol. Metab.* 24:621–627, 1964.
37. Odell, W. D., and Wolfsen, A. R. Humoral syndromes associated with cancer. *Ann. Rev. Med.* 29:379–406, 1978.
38. Orth, D. N., et al. Immunoreactive endorphins, lipotropins and corticotropins in a human nonpituitary tumor: Evidence for a common precursor. *J. Clin. Endocrinol. Metab.* 46:849–852, 1978.
39. Plotz, C. M., Knowlton, A. I., and Ragan, C. The natural history of Cushing's syndrome. *Am. J. Med.* 13:597–614, 1952.
40. Ratcliffe, J. G., et al. Tumour and plasma ACTH concentrations in patients with and without the ectopic ACTH syndrome. *Clin. Endocrinol.* 1:27–44, 1972.
41. Raux, M. C., et al. Studies of ACTH secretion control in 116 cases of Cushing's syndrome. *J. Clin. Endocrinol. Metab.* 40:186–197, 1975.

42. Rayfield, E. J., et al. ACTH-responsive, dexamethasone-suppressible adrenocortical carcinoma. *N. Engl. J. Med.* 284:591–592, 1971.
43. Rees, C. H., et al. Alcohol induced pseudo-Cushing's syndrome. *Lancet* 1:726–728, 1977.
44. Schambelan, M., Slaton, P. E., Jr., and Biglieri, E. G. Mineralocorticoid production in hyperadrenocorticism: Role in pathogenesis of hypokalemic alkalosis. *Am. J. Med.* 51:299–305, 1971.
45. Sederberg-Olsen, P., et al. Episodic variation in plasma corticosteroids in subjects with Cushing's syndrome of differing etiology. *J. Clin. Endocrinol. Metab.* 36:906–910, 1973.
45a. Sindler, B. H., Griffing, G. T., and Melby, J. C. The superiority of the metyrapone test versus the high-dose dexamethasone test in the differential diagnosis of Cushing's syndrome. *Am. J. Med.* 74:657–662, 1983.
46. Smals, A. G. H., Kloppenborg, P. W. C., and Benraad, T. J. Plasma testosterone profiles in Cushing's syndrome. *J. Clin. Endocrinol. Metab.* 45:240–245, 1977.
47. Spark, R. F. Simplified assessment of pituitary-adrenal reserve. Measurement of serum 11-deoxycortisol and cortisol after metyrapone. *Ann. Intern. Med.* 75:717–723, 1971.
48. Streeten, D. H. P., et al. The diagnosis of hypercortisolism. Biochemical criteria differentiating patients from lean and obese normal subjects and from females on oral contraceptives. *J. Clin. Endocrinol. Metab.* 29:1191–1211, 1969.
49. Tyrrell, J. B., et al. Cushing's disease. Selective trans-sphenoidal resection of pituitary microadenomas. *N. Engl. J. Med.* 298:753–758, 1978.
50. Urbanic, R. C., and George, J. K. Cushing's disease—18 years' experience. *Medicine* 60:14–24, 1981.

9 Pheochromocytoma

Robert G. Campbell

CLINICAL CONSIDERATIONS
Clinical Manifestations

Pheochromocytomas are catecholamine-secreting tumors of neuroecto-dermal origin derived from chromaffin cells [6]. The clinical manifestations of pheochromocytoma are multiple, extremely variable, and often dramatic. The signs, symptoms, and complications exhibited by patients with these tumors result either from excessive concentrations of catecholamines, namely, norepinephrine or epinephrine, or from the complications of hypertension secondary to the effects of these pressor amines. The major clinical features and manifestations associated with pheochromocytoma are listed in Table 9-1; they are of two patterns, paroxysmal or persistent [13,21,28]. In general, most symptoms are more consistently reported in the paroxysmal form.

In the paroxysmal form, the attacks occur suddenly, usually without warning, concomitant with the presence of excessive circulating catecholamines. Such episodes may occur irregularly. Approximately 75% of the patients have one or more attacks per week, and the remainder have one or more attacks daily. In 50% of the patients, the attacks are short-lived (less than 15 minutes); in 80% of patients, the attacks are less than 1 hour in duration [11,13,17]. A host of factors may initiate an attack, such as change in posture, massage or a blow to the area of the tumor, physical exercise, mental or physical stress, Valsalva maneuver, change in environmental temperature, bladder distention, micturition, and various diagnostic procedures, such as angiography or the administration of various drugs.

The cardinal finding in pheochromocytoma is hypertension. The sustained form of hypertension is seen in over 90% of children. About half of the adult patients with this tumor have sustained hypertension [13,16]. There appears to be no consistent relationship between arterial blood pressure and prevailing levels of circulating catecholamines in patients with pheochromocytoma [2,4].

Marked lability of blood pressure may be observed, often in association with tachycardia or bradycardia, as well as other cardiac arrhythmias that may be aggravated by volume depletion. A strikingly high incidence of orthostatic hypotension has been found, at times accompanied by pronounced reflex postural tachycardia. The etiology of this phenomenon is not yet defined, but it is thought to be due to a defect in peripheral sympathetic vasomotor reflexes rather than significant alterations in blood volume [9,36]. Pallor or other signs of peripheral vasoconstriction may be evident in 50 to 90% of all patients. It has been emphasized that one should question patients specifically regarding such symptoms or signs, as they may be unobserved by the patients themselves.

159

Table 9-1. Clinical Features and Manifestations of Pheochromocytoma

Headaches (severe)
Excessive sweating (generalized)
Palpitations
Postural hypotension
Anxiety or nervousness
Pallor
Hyperglycemia
Tremulousness
Pain in the chest, abdomen (usually epigastric), lumbar regions, lower abdomen, or groin
Retinopathy
Nausea
Weakness, fatigue, prostration
Cholelithiasis
Weight loss (10% of ideal body weight)

Other cardiovascular complications occur in up to 30% of patients. Catecholamine-induced myocardiopathy may be manifested by various tachyarrhythmias, nonspecific electrocardiogram (EKG) changes, and overt congestive heart failure [7].

Some degree of retinopathy, which is indistinguishable from the fundoscopic findings seen in essential hypertension, is present in virtually all patients with sustained hypertension. However, about half of the patients with the paroxysmal form of hypertension have normal ophthalmologic findings [15].

Abnormal carbohydrate tolerance is a frequent finding in pheochromocytoma and is particularly striking in children; 40% of these patients may exhibit either hyperglycemia or abnormal carbohydrate tolerance. However, ketoacidosis is uncommon in such patients, and they rarely require insulin therapy.

The incidence of cholelithiasis in pheochromocytoma is significantly greater than the predicted prevalence of this disease in the United States. There is as yet no explanation for this relationship. It is of clinical importance, as cholecystography is recommended before surgery in order to consider elective cholecystectomy at the time of surgery for removal of the pheochromocytoma [11,36].

Central nervous system manifestations of pheochromocytoma range from mild to severe headaches, which are sometimes relieved upon standing. Marked anxiety states, frank psychosis, and catastrophic cerebrovascular accidents have also been observed [39].

Patterns of Occurrence
Pheochromocytoma may arise from the adrenal medulla or from extraadrenal sites of sympathetic neural tissue. Although the true rate of oc-

Table 9-2. Criteria for Screening Patients for Pheochromocytoma

Unexplained severe hypertension (diastolic, 120 mm Hg)
Symptomatic hypertension (persistent or paroxysmal), the etiology of which is uncertain
Symptomatic hypertension resistant to therapy
Persistent or paroxysmal hypertension with recurrent attacks or features associated with pheochromocytoma (Table 9-1)
A family history of pheochromocytoma, even in the absence of symptomatic hypertension
Normotension with signs and symptoms or associated manifestations of pheochromocytoma
Paradoxic pressor response to hypertensive drugs
Severe pressor response to stress (anesthesia, surgery)
Family history of MEN syndrome

currence of pheochromocytoma is not known, it is estimated that between 0.5 and 0.7% of newly diagnosed hypertensive patients may harbor this tumor [8,21]. This estimate does not, however, indicate the frequency with which the diagnosis must be entertained (Table 9-2).

Pheochromocytoma occurs most frequently between the third and fifth decades; however, approximately 10% occur in children, with over 60% of these occurrences in boys. Virtually all pheochromocytomas are localized in the abdomen, and over 90% are found in the adrenal medulla. Approximately two-thirds of these tumors occur in the right adrenal. Multiple tumors (often bilateral) occur in 15% of adults and 40% of children with the disorder. In the familial form of pheochromocytoma, 75% of patients have bilateral tumors. There is a high incidence of the familial form in children, inheritance being autosomal dominant (21).

Of the 10% of tumors occurring extra-adrenally, the majority arise in the organ of Zuckerkandl, which is located near or below the bifurcation of the aorta. Extra-abdominal pheochromocytomas, constituting less than 2% of cases, involve primarily the thoracic paraganglionic system and, rarely, the carotid bodies in the neck [13,16,21,22]. There is a significantly greater occurrence of malignancy in extra-adrenal pheochromocytoma (28%) than in adrenal pheochromocytoma (11%).

The incidence of malignant pheochromocytomas is approximately 10%, with 70% of the tumors occurring in females. There is a twofold greater incidence of malignancy in familial adrenal pheochromocytoma than in sporadic intra-adrenal pheochromocytoma [31]. Malignant tumors vary in size from 0.5 to 20 cm, averaging about 4.5 cm; however, about 10% of the tumors are less than 3 cm [38]. There appears to be no consistent relationship between severity of symptoms and tumor size and weight.

The complex clinical data regarding pheochromocytoma have been simplified somewhat by the grouping of several characteristic features according to a rough "Rule of Ten": 10% of pheochromocytomas are familial, 10% bilateral, 10% malignant, 10% multiple, 10% extra-adrenal, and 10% occur in children.

Associated Disorders

The coexistence of pheochromocytoma, medullary carcinoma of the thyroid, hyperparathyroidism, with or without mucosal neuromas, and marfanoid habitus is known as the *multiple endocrine neoplasia (MEN) syndrome*. Patients with MEN syndromes constitute about 7% of all patients with pheochromocytoma [20,23,34,37]. These syndromes, usually familial but occasionally sporadic, are rare entities but have certain clinical features that deserve emphasis. Of particular importance is that 85% of patients with either familial or sporadic pheochromocytoma afflicted with medullary throid carcinoma (MEN-II) are normotensive and often asymptomatic. In contrast, over 60% of patients with familial or sporadic pheochromocytoma not associated with medullary carcinoma have sustained hypertension [37].

Another syndrome, considered the result of genetic derangements of neural crest derivatives, has been described in association with familial pheochromocytoma, namely, neurofibromatosis (Von Recklinghausen's disease), retinoangiomatosis (Von Hippel's disease), and angioblastoma of the cerebellum or spinal cord (Lindau's disease) [1].

DIAGNOSTIC METHODS
Assay of Urinary Metabolites of Catecholamines

The definitive diagnosis of the tumor is made by the demonstration of biochemical evidence of increased catecholamines or their metabolites in the plasma or urine. The most widely used diagnostic procedures available to the physician are estimations of urinary catecholamines and their metabolites.

Metanephrine and normetanephrine, together termed *metanephrines* [29], result from the methylation of norepinephrine and epinephrine by the enzyme catechol-O-methyl-transferase (COMT). Metanephrines are then further degraded by monoamine oxidase (MAO), resulting in the major degradation product of metanephrines, vanillylmandelic acid (VMA). Only 1% of circulating catecholamines in normals and 10% in patients with pheochromocytoma are excreted unchanged as urinary catecholamines. Thus, measurement of the degradation product of catecholamines has a distinct advantage over measurement of urinary catecholamines themselves as a consistent index of a functioning tumor.

The determination of urinary metanephrines is the single most reliable screening test for pheochromocytoma because few false-negative tests occur (4%) and measurements are less subject to interference by various drugs and dietary factors when compared to either VMA or catecholamines [5,14,31,36].

The single most important cause of false-negative results is incomplete urine collections. Since completion of urine collections can be estimated fairly accurately by determining creatinine excretion in the absence of significant renal insufficiency, catecholamine assays may be corrected per milligram of creatinine [14]. Similarly, a 12-hour overnight urine specimen for total cathecholamines or a single-voided specimen for metanephrines, when expressed per milligram of creatinine, correlates well with 24-hour urine metanephrine excretion, and can therefore be used in screening for tumors in children or in other clinical situations in which complete 24-hour urine collections may be difficult to obtain [19].

In general, if it is clinically feasible, any hypertensive or vasoconstrictive drugs, narcotics, barbiturates, sedatives, and MAO inhibitors (e.g., pargyline) should be withheld for a period ranging from 48 hours to 1 to 2 weeks before any testing. It is recommended that urinary metanephrines not be measured within 3 days of x-ray procedures using a contrast medium containing methylglucamine (e.g., Renovist, Renografin, or Cardiografin), since this compound will directly interfere with the urinary metanephrine methodology, resulting in decreased values.

Urinary Catecholamine Assay
Urinary catecholamines are less reliable than either VMA or metanephrines in screening for pheochromocytoma, primarily due to technical difficulties in performing these tests. Therefore, they are best reserved for substantiating the diagnosis of pheochromocytoma when either VMA or metanephrine values are equivocal. Urine catecholamines, expressed in micrograms per hour, are a more sensitive reflection of transient changes in catecholamine excretion induced during a spontaneous or provoked attack of symptoms or acute changes in blood pressure [11,17]. Normal values are: total catecholamines, 4 µg per hour; norepinephrine, 3 µg per hour; and epinephrine, 1 mg per hour. Fractionation of urinary catecholamines to determine the predominance of epinephrine may prove helpful. Predominant epinephrine elevations suggest tumor origin from the adrenal gland or the organ of Zuckerkandl, rarely the mediastinum or bladder.

Plasma Catecholamine Assay
Recently, a sensitive and specific radioenzymatic assay for plasma catecholamines has been developed [6,12,26]. This methodology is based on the enzymatic conversion of catecholamines to their respective O-methylated products, allowing both norepineprhine and epinephrine to be measured individually. This assay, although currently expensive and requiring a high degree of technical expertise, has been reported to be the most sensitive diagnostic test for pheochromocytoma [2,4]. The procedure to be followed for screening for a tumor utilizing this assay is as follows: (1) A heparinized indwelling catheter is inserted 20 to 30 minutes prior to sampling in order to avoid the effects of the stress of ven-

ipuncture and to allow stabilization of the cardiovascular status. (2) Plasma samples are collected in the postabsorptive state with the patient in a supine position.

With the appropriate precautions strictly followed, this assay is a better predictor of a functioning tumor than either metanephrines or VMA, particularly in the normotensive patient, in whom, not infrequently, the urinary metabolites are equivocally increased [2]. Furthermore, its use avoids the need for a 24-hour urine collection. Catecholamine levels prior to and following provocative pressor tests may be monitored. Correlation of catecholamine levels with either provoked or spontaneous changes in the cardiovascular state is more easily accomplished. Although postural change and salt depletion will increase plasma catecholamine levels, basal plasma concentrations in patients with pheochromocytoma often exceed 2000 pg/ml. Such levels are rarely seen in any other condition, including essential hypertension [2,18]. Selective vena cava sampling for plasma catecholamines has also proven of value in the diagnosis and localization of a tumor in selected patients with possible multiple tumors or when postoperative tumor recurrence is suspected [24,25].

Even though basal plasma catecholamine levels in patients with pheochromocytoma are generally 5- to 100-fold greater than normal, there exists a wide range of normal values in healthy subjects depending on the particular laboratory performing the procedure. There also exists some overlap in plasma levels in patients with a tumor and those with various forms of hypertension. The interpretation of alterations in plasma catecholamines should be made in close cooperation with the laboratory responsible for doing the assay. In addition, both alpha- and beta-blocking agents, administered either alone or in combination, may elevate plasma catecholamines, particularly in the stressed patient [20a].

Pharmacologic Tests
Because of the currently available specific biochemical assays for measuring urinary and plasma catecholamines, it is generally conceded that the various pharmacologic tests have limited usefulness in the detection of pheochromocytoma. Their use is also restricted by their limited specificity, as evidenced by a high incidence of both false-positive and false-negative responses [11,18,36], and the potentially hazardous side effects associated with the use of some of these agents. Even when both pressor and depressor responsiveness are evaluated in the same patient, only 75% of patients have demonstrated true-positive responses [11,13,36].

Table 9-3 shows study protocols for the clonidine suppression test and the phentolamine adrenergic-blocking vasodepressor test. Correlation of the vascular response to glucagon with alterations in plasma catecholamines has also been used as a diagnostic assay for demonstrating the presence of a tumor [2,35].

Table 9-3. Procedures for Pharmacologic Tests in the Diagnosis of Pheochromocytoma

---

Preparation for Tests
1. Avoid all drugs, especially barbiturates and narcotics, for at least 48 hours before testing. Avoid any hypertensive or vasoconstrictive drugs 1 week prior to testing. Do not perform tests on patients with evidence of renal insufficiency.
2. Insert an indwelling needle into an antecubital vein and keep it patent with normal saline for subsequent drug administration and blood samples for plasma catecholamines.
3. In order to avoid effects of stress of venipuncture, allow the patient to rest in a recumbent position for at least 30 minutes before subsequent testing.

Clonidine suppression test
1. Obtain baseline plasma catecholamine levels.
2. Administer 0.1 to 0.3 mg clonidine orally.
3. Monitor blood pressure and heart rate every 30 minutes.
4. Obtain plasma catecholamine levels at hourly intervals for 3 hours. In pheochromocytoma no suppression of plasma catecholamines is expected.

Vasodepressor test
(Adrenergic blocking may be indicated when blood pressure is greater than 170/110)
1. Study the patient in the recumbent state for 30 minutes following establishment of IV access.
2. Give phentolamine in a 5-mg IV bolus after noting effects of test dose of 0.5 mg. Record blood pressure every 15 seconds for 2 minutes and every 30 seconds for 10 minutes thereafter. A positive response consists of a blood fall of 35 mm Hg systolic and 25 mm Hg diastolic pressure. A peak response usually occurs between 2 and 4 minutes but may be prolonged for 10 minutes or more. In the event of vasomotor collapse, it is essential to have a pressor agent (norepinephrine) and a volume expander readily available.

The alpha-adrenergic blocking test utilizing phentolamine is seldom necessary and is reserved for the hypertensive patient since the normotensive patient without elevated catecholamines will not exhibit a depressor response to this agent. The usefulness of this test in the diagnosis of pheochromocytoma is limited due to the fact that the majority of patients with sustained hypertension have biochemical evidence of a functioning tumor. Therefore, it is usually reserved for the patient with a hypertensive crisis or malignant hypertension, as a preliminary diagnostic test. Vascular collapse has been described in association with phentolamine administration in pheochromocytoma; therefore, appropriate volume expanders and vasoconstrictive agents should be at hand at the time of testing.

The clonidine suppression test has recently been described as useful in the diagnosis of pheochromocytoma [3]. This test is based on the premise that normal, neurologically mediated catecholamine release is suppressible with clonidine, whereas autonomous tumor production of catecholamines is not suppressed. Ten patients with pheochromocytomas were distinguished from 15 patients who had essential hypertension but were suspected of having pheochromocytoma using a single 0.3-mg dose of oral clonidine and measuring serial plasma catecholamine levels for 3 hours. This test is advantageous in the severely hypertensive patient since it lowers rather than elevates the blood pressure. In the volume-depleted or moderately hypertensive patient, a lower dose of clonidine (0.1–0.15 mg) is recommended to avoid excessive hypotensive effects. As more information accumulates, this test may prove more helpful than the other provocative tests for pheochromocytoma. A pentolium suppression test of plasma catecholamines [4] and the measurement of platelet catecholamine content [41] have also recently been shown to aid in the discrimination of pheochromocytoma patients from normal subjects.

Localizing Studies

Intravenous pyelography (IVP) with nephrotomograms is sufficient to detect pheochromocytomas in 30 to 60% of cases [13,17,40]. If there is a high suspicion of extra-adrenal tumors, such as in familial pheochromocytoma and in children, further studies are helpful. Noninvasive techniques such as computed tomography (CT) [10,38] and abdominal sonography [27] for tumor localization detect over 90% of pheochromocytomas. These techniques appear to be highly accurate for detecting tumors over 2 cm in size [38]. With the continued improvement of CT scanning procedures, this is now the preferred noninvasive technique for tumor localization.

Selective arteriography is useful in demonstrating unusually vascular tumors and locating aberrant vessels prior to surgery, as well as in detecting ectopic tumors that may be missed at the time of operation. With the appropriate pharmacologic precautions, namely, alpha blockade before and during the procedure, the risks with arteriography are minimal, but this procedure is best reserved for cases in which CT scanning or sonography fails to locate a tumor.

To exclude the extra-abdominal or ectopic tumor when the procedures described have failed to localize a tumor, it may prove necessary to measure plasma catecholamines in vena cava blood samples from multiple sites. Local increases in catecholamines from veins draining tumor sites have proved to be extremely valuable in the assessment of multiple tumors, small tumors, extra-adrenal and extra-abdominal tumors, and recurrent tumors [8,11,12,24].

DISCUSSION

In the diagnostic approach to the detection of pheochromocytoma, one must first decide which patient should be screened for a tumor and then proceed with the sequence of appropriate diagnostic studies. Table 9-2 provides guidelines for the selection of patients to be screened for pheochromocytoma. It is important to consider screening the patient with classic symptoms even in the absence of hypertension, as over 50% of patients may have normal blood pressure at a time when circulating catecholamines are elevated. It is this patient whose tumor may prove to be the most difficult to detect and who may require more complex tests. However, this is the same patient who undergoes an elective surgical procedure only to have an unexpected operative death.

The sequence of laboratory investigations used to confirm the diagnosis of pheochromocytoma is summarized in the diagnostic protocol (Fig. 9-1). At this time, measurement of urinary metabolites of catecholamines remains the most readily available initial test for patients with suspected pheochromocytoma. However, plasma catecholamine measurements are emerging as sensitive and reliable predictors of pheochromocytoma. Each approach has its advocates [2,4,19,30] for use as a screening test. Urinary determinations are more likely to provide false-negative results, whereas plasma determinations tend toward false-positive results.

As discussed earlier, metanephrines are the most reliable urinary screening test since more than 90% of patients demonstrate elevated values [21,30]. Summary data from five studies [2,9,18,31,33] confirm this impression, with false-negative results using metanephrines being 6%; VMA, 30%; and urinary catechols, 25%.

The primary tests indicated in Figure 9-1 are 24-hour urine collections for metanephrines and appropriately collected plasma catecholamines. If the metanephrines are elevated (>1.0 mg/day or 2.0 μg/mg of creatinine), the diagnosis may be substantiated by the finding of elevated plasma catecholamines. Serial studies may be necessary to confirm the diagnosis, and care must be taken to exclude more common causes of catecholamine elevations such as cardiac failure or the use of cigarettes or drugs. Almost all false-negative tests are the result of either incomplete collections or the failure to withhold drugs known to influence these tests.

In the occasionally symptomatic normotensive patient in whom the initial screening is negative, it may be possible to confirm the diagnosis only by obtaining carefully timed urine collections for catecholamines. Correlation of symptoms may be made with alterations in catecholamines expressed as micrograms per hour.

Plasma catecholamines obtained during and following a spontaneous attack may show a good correlation with the onset of various features characterizing an attack and changes in cardiovascular status. In addition, basal plasma catecholamines may also be strikingly elevated even in the normotensive patient with pheochromocytoma. Plasma catecholamines are particularly valuable in paroxysmal presentations, during selective blood sampling for localization when urinary studies are equivocal, and in the rare instances in which provocative tests are

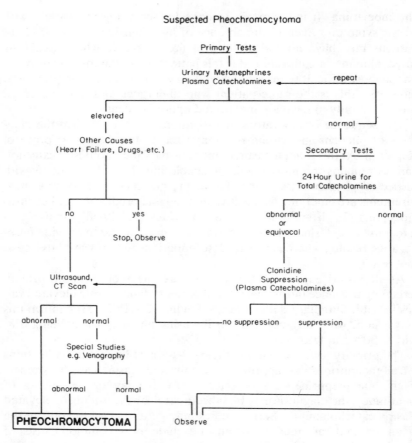

Figure 9-1. Diagnostic protocol: Suspected pheochromocytoma.

employed. It should be emphasized that patients with conditions known to cause spurious elevations in urinary amines or catecholamines, such as congestive heart failure, hypoglycemia, and use of various antihypertensive medications, should be observed rather than subjected to further diagnostic studies. As already mentioned, attempts at tumor localization with CT scanning or ultrasonography are recommended prior to the consideration of selective venographic studies.

If there is a high index of suspicion of a functioning tumor, such as in familial pheochromocytoma associated with MEN syndromes [32,33], and screening tests have been normal, one should proceed with the clonidine suppression test, measuring plasma catecholamine levels. In these instances, the pentolium suppression test [4] or the measurement of platelet catecholamine content [41] may also be considered.

If the findings of these studies are negative and no elective surgery, such as neck exploration for thyroid carcinoma, is indicated, it is reasonable to observe the patient with periodic (every 3–6 months) urinary metanephrine determinations and to instruct the patient to collect attack-related urine specimens for subsequent catecholamine determinations. If, on the other hand, suspicion of the presence of pheochromocytoma remains high and elective neck exploration or other elective surgery is required, it is essential to make further attempts to rule out or localize a tumor. Samples of plasma catecholamines at various levels of vena cava drainage may be collected. To minimize the number of invasive procedures, vena cava plasma catecholamine sampling may be performed just before selective angiography, which permits subsequent correlations of biochemical data with radiologic findings. Adequate volume repletion and appropriate pharmacologic blockade should be instituted prior to such procedures. Only after exhaustive attempts have been made to rule out the presence of a suspected tumor should elective surgery be considered. During the procedure, all appropriate precautions should be taken in case a stress-induced attack occurs.

REFERENCES

1. Atuk, N. O., et al. Familial pheochromocytoma, hypercalcemia, and Van Hippel–Lindau disease. *Medicine* 58:209–218, 1979.
2. Bravo, F. L., et al. Circulating and urinary catecholamines in pheochromocytoma. *N. Engl. J. Med.* 301:682–686, 1979.
3. Bravo, E. L., et al. Clonidine suppression test: A useful aid in the diagnosis of pheochromocytoma. *N. Engl. J. Med.* 305:623–627, 1981.
4. Brown, M. J., et al. Increased sensitivity and accuracy of phaeochromocytoma diagnosis achieved by use of plasma adrenaline estimations and a pentolium suppression test. *Lancet* 1:174–177, 1981.
5. Crout, J. R., Pisano, J. J., and Sjoerdsma, A. Urinary excretion of catecholamines and their metabolites in pheochromocytoma. *Am. Heart J.* 61:375–381, 1961.

6. Cryer, P. E. Physiology and pathophysiology of the human sympathoadrenal neuroendocrine system. *N. Engl. J. Med.* 303:436–444, 1980.
7. DeChamplain, J., et al. Circulating catecholamine levels in human and experimental hypertension. *Circ. Res.* 38:109–114, 1976.
8. DeQuattro, V., and Campese, V. M. Pheochromocytoma: Diagnosis and Treatment. In L. J. DeGroot (Ed.), *Endocrinology*. vol. 2. New York: Grune & Stratton, 1979.
9. Deoreo, G. A., Jr., et al. Preoperative blood transfusion in the safe surgical management of pheochromocytoma: A review of 46 cases. *J. Urol.* 111:715–721, 1974.
10. Egdahl, R. H. CAT scanners and pheos: Diagnostic and policy issues. *N. Engl. J. Med.* 299:475–476, 1978.
11. Engelman, K. Phaeochromocytoma. *J. Clin. Endocrinol. Metab.* 6:769–802, 1977.
12. Engelman, K., and Portnoy, B. A sensitive double-isotope derivative assay for norepinephrine and epinephrine. *Circ. Res.* 26:53–57, 1970.
13. Gifford, R., et al. Clinical features, diagnosis and treatment of pheochromocytoma: A review of 76 cases. *Mayo Clin. Proc.* 39:281–302, 1964.
14. Gitlow, S. E., Mendlowitz, M., and Bertani, L. M. The biochemical techniques for detecting and establishing the presence of a pheochromocytoma. *Am. J. Cardiol.* 26:270–279, 1970.
15. Hollenhorst, R. W. The ocular changes associated with pheochromocytoma. *Am. J. Med. Sci.* 216:226–233, 1948.
16. Hume, D. M. Pheochromocytoma in the adult and in the child. *Am. J. Surg.* 99:458–496, 1960.
17. Juan, D. Pheochromocytoma: Clinical manifestations and diagnostic tests. *Urology* 17:1–12, 1981.
18. Jones, D. H., et al. The biochemical diagnosis, localization and follow-up of pheochromocytoma: The role of plasma and urinary catecholamine measurements. *Q. J. Med.* 49:341–361, 1980.
19. Kaplan, N. M., et al. Single-voided urine metanephrine assays in screening for pheochromocytoma. *Arch. Intern. Med.* 137:190–193, 1977.
20. Khairi, M. R. A., et al. Mucosal neuromas, pheochromocytoma and medullary thyroid carcinoma: Multiple endocrine neoplasia type 3. *Medicine* 54:89–112, 1975.
20a. Lilavivat, W., Brodows, R. G., and Campbell, R. G. Adrenergic influence on glucocounterregulation in man. *Diabetologica* 20:482–489, 1981.
21. Manger, W. M., and Gifford, R. W., Jr. *Pheochromocytoma*. New York: Springer-Verlag, 1977. P. 89.
22. Melicow, M. M. One hundred cases of pheochromocytoma (107 tumors) at the Columbia Presbyterian Medical Center, 1926–1976. *Cancer* 40:1987–2004, 1977.
23. Melvin, K. D. W., Tashjian, A. H., Jr., and Miller, H. H. Studies in Familial (Medullary) Thyroid Carcinoma. In E. B. Astwood (Ed.), *Recent Progress in Hormone Research,* vol. 28. New York: Academic Press, 1977. Pp. 591–603.
24. Mohoney, E. M., et al. Adrenal and extra-adrenal pheochromocytomata: Localization by vena caval sampling and observations on renal juxtaglomerular apparatus. *J. Urol.* 108:4–11, 1972.
25. Mohoney, E. M., and Harrison, J. H. Malignant pheochromocytoma: Clinical course and treatment. *J. Urol.* 118:225–229, 1977.
26. Passon, P. G., and Peuler, J. D. A simplified radiometric assay for plasma norepinephrine. *Anal. Biochem.* 51:618–631, 1973.

27. Pertsemlidis, D., and Gitlow, S. E. Diagnosis of pheochromocytoma by computed axial tomographic scan and other methods. *N. Engl. J. Med.* 299:1469–1471, 1978.
28. Peterson, D. D., et al. Pheochromocytoma: Recent experience with detection and management. *Urology* 10:133–138, 1977.
29. Pisano, J. J. A simple analysis for normetanephrine and metanephrine in urine. *Clin. Chim. Acta* 5:406–414, 1960.
30. Plouin, P. F., et al. Biochemical tests for the diagnosis of pheochromocytoma: Urinary versus plasma determinations. *Br. Med. J.* 282:853–856, 1981.
31. Remine, W. H., et al. Current management of pheochromocytoma. *Ann. Surg.* 179:740–748, 1974.
32. Sheps, S. G., and Maher, F. T. Histamine and glucagon tests in the diagnosis of pheochromocytoma. *J.A.M.A.* 895–899, 1968.
33. Sheps, S. G., Tyce, G. M., and Flock, E. V. Current experience in the diagnosis of pheochromocytoma. *Circulation* 34:473–483, 1966.
34. Sipple, J. J. The association of pheochromocytoma with carcinoma of the thyroid gland. *Am. J. Med.* 31:163, 1971.
35. Siqueira-Filho, A. G., et al. Glucagon blood catecholamine test: Used in isolated and familial pheochromocytoma. *Arch. Intern. Med.* 135:1227–1231, 1975.
36. Sjoerdsma, A., et al. Pheochromocytoma: Current concepts of diagnosis and treatment. *Ann. Intern. Med.* 65:1302–1326, 1966.
37. Steiner, A. L., et al. Study of kindred with pheochromocytoma, medullary thyroid carcinoma, hyperparathyroidism and Cushing's disease: Multiple endocrine neoplasia. *Medicine* 47:371–409, 1968.
38. Stewart, B. H., et al. Localization of pheochromocytoma by computed tomography. *N. Engl. J. Med.* 299(9):400–461, 1978.
39. Thomas, J. E., Roche, E. D., and Kvale, W. F. The neurologist's experience with pheochromocytoma. *J.A.M.A.* 197:100–104, 1966.
40. Zelch, J. V., Meaney, T. F., and Belhobek, G. H. Radiologic approach to the patient with suspected pheochromocytoma. *Radiology* 111:279–284, 1974.
41. Zwiefler, A. J., and Julisus, S. Increased platelet catecholamine content in pheochromocytoma. *N. Engl. J. Med.* 306:890–894, 1982.

10 Primary Aldosteronism

Robert E. Heinig

Primary aldosteronism is ultimately found to be the cause of hypertension in a small segment (1–2%) of unselected hypertensive patients. Despite its relative infrequency, this entity has attracted extraordinary interest since the first case was described in 1954. Numerous journal articles past and present attest to the ongoing interest in this disorder [2,6,8,11,24,34]. Much of the enthusiasm was engendered by the possibility that primary aldosteronism might account for a large percentage of the hypertensive population—namely, the 25% with low-renin hypertension. Clearly, that hypothesis is not valid; however, a steadily increasing body of literature supports the concept that many patients with low-renin hypertension do have excessive mineralocorticoid activity [4,13]. Certainly, it is important to consider primary aldosteronism in any hypertensive evaluation since appropriate medical or surgical management can ameliorate or cure the hypertension and associated metabolic abnormalities in most patients. Proper evaluation has assumed greater import in the past several years with the recognition that there are at least three types of primary aldosteronism and that the responses of these several types to medical and surgical therapy differ considerably.

Secretion of aldosterone by the zona glomerulosa of the adrenal cortex is regulated principally by the renin-angiotensin system primarily in response to alterations in the effective blood volume. Since potassium directly stimulates the secretion of aldosterone, it is important to correct hypokalemia before measuring aldosterone secretion or excretion [19,36]. Adrenocorticotropic hormone (ACTH) plays a relatively minor role in regulating normal secretion. However, in some forms of primary aldosteronism, ACTH exerts a greater effect in regulating aldosterone secretion, a fact of diagnostic importance in the evaluation of a suspected case of primary aldosteronism [22].

The major physiologic action of aldosterone involves the handling of electrolytes in the distal nephron. Aldosterone enhances active sodium reabsorption from the tubular lumen, which is associated with enhanced secretion of potassium and hydrogen ions. Ultimately, excessive aldosterone secretion results in increased total body sodium (and water), and the hypervolemic state that ensues acts to elevate the blood pressure. Despite this sequence of events, patients with primary aldosteronism do not exhibit edema. This apparent paradox is explained by the phenomenon of mineralocorticoid "escape." After a period of positive sodium balance, no further renal sodium retention occurs because sodium reabsorption in aldosterone-insensitive portions of the nephron appreciably diminishes. Patients with primary aldosteronism exhibit this escape phenomenon, whereas patients with secondary aldosteronism (secondary to enhanced renin secretion) do not. Thus, patients with congestive heart failure, hepatic cirrhosis, and the nephrotic syndrome typically reabsorb a high percentage of sodium from both the proximal and distal nephron and thereby become progressivly hypervolemic and edematous.

CLINICAL CONSIDERATIONS

The cardinal features of primary aldosteronism are hypertension, hypokalemia, and low plasma renin levels. Of these, the most helpful clinical clue is hypokalemia. When hypokalemia is unprovoked (i.e., the patient is not on a diuretic), as many as 50% of hypokalemic hypertensive patients can be shown to have primary aldosteronism [20]. On the other hand, hypokalemia in a hypertensive patient taking a diuretic agent has proven to be of little diagnostic significance. Occasionally, a diuretic may induce unusually profound hypokalemia in primary aldosteronism and suggest the correct diagnosis. Brown and colleagues have documented the occurrence of *intermittent* hypokalemia—especially in primary aldosteronism due to adrenal hyperplasia [3,8]. In their series, among 17 patients with bilateral hyperplasia, hypokalemia was intermittent in 10, persistently low in 4, and persistently normal in 3 individuals. Persistently normokalemic primary aldosteronism has also been reported by others. These cases have generally been uncommon, and most have involved bilateral adrenal hyperplasia rather than an adenoma. A recent review found normokalemia (serum potassium ≥ 3.6 mEq/L) in 22% of patients with surgically confirmed primary aldosteronism, including 5 of 37 patients with an adenoma and 6 of 11 with bilateral hyperplasia [34].

Most of the earlier reported patients with primary aldosteronism had adenomas with advanced disease including neuromuscular and/or renal manifestations secondary to severe potassium deficiency [1] (Table 10-1). These patients presented a distinct clinical syndrome with paresthesias, muscle weakness, and polydipsia/polyuria in the majority of cases. A lesser number had tetany or intermittent paralytic symptoms when the potassium depletion (and probably calcium and magnesium deficiency as well) was extreme. Virtually all of these nonhypertension problems were correctable with potassium repletion. In contrast, most individuals diagnosed in recent years have not had severe potassium depletion and consequently have not manifested such striking symptoms and signs (Table 10-2). Instead, these patients usually have had less specific complaints that do not readily differentiate them from the group with essential hypertension. This is especially true for patients with idiopathic adrenocortical hyperplasia (Table 10-3), as both the clinical and biochemical findings of hyperaldosteronism are less striking in this group. Mild hypernatremia and an elevated serum bicarbonate concentration remain helpful clues in all types of primary aldosteronism.

Table 10-1. Electrolyte Abnormalities in Primary Aldosteronism

Reference	Aldosterone-Producing Adenoma (Mean serum electrolytes, mEq/L)				Idiopathic Adrenocortical Hyperplasia			
	No. of Patients	Na+	K+	CO_2	No. of Patients	Na+	K+	CO_2
Ayres et al. [1][a]	16	147	2.0	36				
George et al. [11]	9	146	2.8	33	6	143	3.4	30
Baer[b]	13	146	2.5	32	12	142	3.5	28
Ferriss [8]	62	143	2.7	32	17	141	3.7	26
Weinberger [34]	38	143	3.0		11	142	3.4	

[a]A review of the 16 reported cases, 1955–1957.
[b]Baer, L., Sommers, C. S., and Krakoff, L. R. Pseudo-primary aldosteronism. An entity distinct from true primary aldosteronism. Circ. Res. 26–27 (Suppl. 1):1203, 1970.

Table 10-2. Clinical Characteristics of Patients with Primary Aldosteronism

Cardinal Features	Common Features	Uncommon Features
Hypertension	Hypernatremia; rarely less than 140 mEq/L	Malignant hypertension
Suppressed plasma renin activity	Intermittent or borderline hypokalemia	Severe end-organ disease of retina, heart, kidney
Hypokalemia	Metabolic alkalosis	Paralysis or tetany
Normal 17-hydroxy-steroid and 17-keto-steroid excretion	Muscle weakness Fatigue Nocturia/polyuria	Persistent normokalemia

Table 10-3. Comparison of Clinical Features in Aldosterone-Producing Adenoma and Idiopathic Adrenocortical Hyperplasia

Clinical Features	Aldosterone-Producing Adenoma	Idiopathic Adrenocortical Hyperplasia
Percentage of patients with primary aldosteronism	75%	20%
Average blood pressure, mm Hg	200/110	205/115
Plasma aldosterone response to upright posture	Decrease in 65% of cases	Increase in 50% of cases
Blood pressure response to spironolactone	Decrease to near normal	Little change
Surgical cure*	75%	20%

*Adenomectomy or bilateral adrenalectomy.

A few patients recognize an association between a high-salt diet and symptoms and may notice that symptoms are less severe if salt is avoided. A low salt intake will result in diminished sodium delivery to the aldosterone-responsive distal renal tubule and will thus provide less opportunity for distal tubule sodium/potassium exchange. Variable salt intake may partially explain the intermittent nature of the hypokalemia in some individuals with primary aldosteronism. Serum electrolyte screening of a hypertensive patient is best undertaken when the individual is on a liberal salt intake and off a diuretic agent. Serum potassium values less than 3.6 mEq/L require further investigation (see Fig. 10-1).

Three types of primary aldosteronism have been characterized; however, two types account for almost all cases. The classic type, which presents with the most distinguishing clinical features, is the *aldosterone-producing adenoma* (APA). The second form has been called *idiopathic adrenocortical hyperplasia* (IAH) or *pseudoprimary aldosteronism* and differs in several important ways from the APA syndrome (Table 10-3). Glucocorticoid remedial hyperaldosteronism (GRHA) is the third much less common form.

Aldosterone-Producing Adenoma

In the APA disorder, a single small adenoma of one adrenal gland is usually present, and removal of this benign neoplasm cures the hypertension in the majority of cases. Renal potassium wasting is detectable, and persistent hypokalemia (<3.6 mEq/L) is usually present. Patients with mild hyperaldosteronism may have borderline or normal serum potassium levels but should become hypokalemic in response to an oral salt load. The adenomas are uniquely responsive to ACTH, and it appears that ACTH is the major regulator of aldosterone secretion in these cells [22]. In contrast, the APA responds in a limited fashion to angiotensin II, and this response provides diagnostically helpful information [19]. Since plasma renin is markedly suppressed in the presence of an adenoma, and since the adenoma has a limited response to whatever angiotensin II is produced, the normal increase in plasma aldosterone with upright posture usually does not occur in APA patients. In fact, such individuals typically demonstrate a paradoxic fall in plasma aldosterone levels with standing [10,34]. The use of an aldosterone/PRA ratio has also recently been shown to aid in the identification of APA patients [16]. Finally, treatment with spironolactone for 6 to 8 weeks normalizes the blood pressure, corrects the potassium wasting in most patients, and ameliorates these abnormalities in the remaining patients. In general, the response to spironolactone is predictive of the response to surgical adenomectomy.

Idiopathic Adrenocortical Hyperplasia (Idiopathic Hyperaldosteronism)

As the term *idiopathic adrenocortical hyperplasia* (IAH) implies, this disorder is characterized by hyperplasia of the adrenocortical tissue that

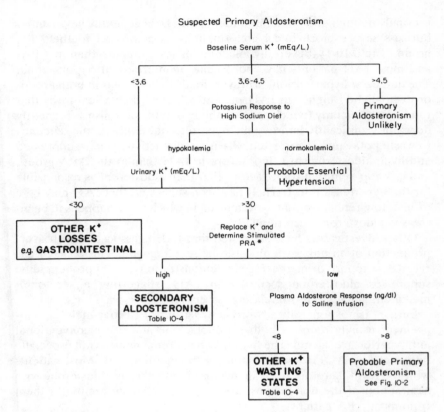

Figure 10-1. Diagnostic protocol: Initial laboratory evaluation of suspected primary aldosteronism. *Plasma renin activity.

is usually nodular and bilateral. Patients with IAH generally have similar but less severe biochemical abnormalities as compared to the APA group (Table 10-1). Severe hypokalemia is less common than in APA, and most IAH patients have borderline or intermittent hypokalemia. The degree of hypertension, however, tends to be similar in both groups or even slightly higher in IAH patients. A remarkable feature is that total adrenalectomy (which corrects the hyperaldosteronism) frequently does not significantly improve the hypertension, although the tendency to waste potassium is corrected. Plasma renin activity is less suppressed and hyperaldosteronism is less severe in IAH than in the APA group, and it is apparent that some factor other than aldosterone is responsible for the hypertension in IAH. It has been suggested that IAH may be a form of low-renin essential hypertension in which there happens to be increased aldosterone secretion [13].

Other investigators have suggested that IAH is associated with overproduction of an unknown aldosterone secretagogue. This concept has received support from the recent demonstration that cyproheptadine suppresses aldosterone secretion in IAH, suggesting a serotonin-mediated, aldosterone-stimulating system [15].

Surgery is not generally advised in this group. Effective medical management usually requires both spironolactone and other conventional antihypertensive agents. The hyperplastic adrenal tissue is not especially influenced by ACTH but is responsive to angiotensin II. Most patients with IAH will therefore have an increase in the plasma aldosterone with assumption of the upright posture—a feature that differentiates them from most APA patients.

Glucocorticoid-Remediable Hyperaldosteronism
(Glucocorticoid-Suppressible Hyperaldosteronism)
Glucocorticoid-remediable hyperaldosteronism (GRHA), an uncommon form of adrenocortical hyperplasia, is more frequently seen in childhood and may be familial [14,29]. The hallmark of GRHA is that administration of small doses of glucocorticoid (0.5–2.0 mg of dexamethasone daily) will reverse all of the clinical and biochemical abnormalities. Cortisol and ACTH production are within the normal range, and it appears that aldosterone secretion is inordinately influenced by normal levels of circulating ACTH [29]. Recent studies have indicated that this form of hyperaldosteronism, as in cases due to adrenal adenoma, may also be characterized by a paradoxic fall in plasma aldosterone after 4 hours of upright posture [9].

DIAGNOSTIC METHODS
When a patient presents with hypertension, moderate or severe unprovoked (not due to diuretic) hypokalemia, and suppressed plasma renin

Table 10-4. Plasma Renin Activity in Hypertensive Disorders

Suppressed *Plasma Renin Activity*	*Increased* *Plasma Renin Activity*

Primary aldosteronism
Deoxycorticosterone (DOC) and
  corticosterone tumors
Cushing's syndrome
Licorice excess
11-Hydroxylase deficiency
17-Hydroxylase deficiency
Liddle's syndrome
	Essential hypertension with diuretic
	  therapy
	Renovascular hypertension
	Malignant hypertension
	Renin-producing tumors
	Sodium-losing renal disease

Source: Modified from R. Horton, Aldosterone: Review of its physiology and diagnostic aspects of primary aldosteronism. *Metabolism* 22:1525–1545, 1973.

activity, the diagnosis of primary aldosteronism is probable and can usually be easily confirmed. Conversely, when normokalemia or intermittent mild hypokalemia is present, extensive testing may be necessary to confirm or deny the diagnosis.

Plasma Renin Activity
As the name implies, *plasma renin activity* (PRA) is a measurement of renin activity and does not directly reflect renin concentration. Renin activity is determined by measuring the rate of angiotensin generation under controlled laboratory conditions. PRA is undetectable or low in primary aldosteronism even when conditions for maximal stimulation are present, that is, volume depletion induced acutely by furosemide or slowly by dietary salt depletion. This test is not specific for primary aldosteronism since suppressed renin secretion is present in approximately 25% of the hypertensive population and only a small fraction of this group has primary aldosteronism. Renin measurement clearly differentiates primary from secondary aldosteronism since the latter is always associated with increased renin production (Table 10-4).

Stimulated Plasma Renin Activity
A number of protocols for stimulating PRA have been successfully used. Since the PRA normally varies depending on the stimulus, the procedure should be standardized in each laboratory. A combination of a low-salt diet for 2 days and the oral administration of 40 mg of furosemide at 1800 and 2400 hours the day before and at 0700 hours the day of testing provides a reliable and quite strong stimulus [4]. A less time-consuming but weaker stimulus consists of administering 40 mg of furosemide intravenously, followed by maintenance of upright posture for 30 to 60 minutes before phlebotomy [21]. Dietary salt depletion requires a 10- to 20-

mEq sodium diet for 5 days, with determination of PRA on day 6 after the patient has been upright for at least 60 minutes. It is advisable to check the urine sodium concentration on day 6 to document the state of sodium balance. Whatever stimulus is used, testing should be conducted in the morning after an overnight fast and with abstinence from tobacco on the test morning.

Plasma Aldosterone Levels

The availability of a sensitive radioimmunoassay for aldosterone has enabled the development of a short-term intravenous saline suppression test suitable for outpatient screening [23]. Plasma aldosterone levels in normal individuals and in most hypertensive patients, including those with secondary elevations of aldosterone, fall promptly after the rapid (over 4 hours) infusion of 2 liters of physiologic saline solution. The test is performed with the subject at bed rest, and the combination of supine posture and saline volume expansion should diminish the plasma aldosterone to less than 8 ng/dl by the end of the infusion. The level may fall in patients with primary aldosteronism, but the suppression is subnormal.

The response of plasma aldosterone to upright posture is determined by obtaining an 8 AM sample after 8 hours in the recumbent posture and another at noon after the patient has been upright for 4 hours (Table 10-3). The plasma concentration usually decreases in patients with APA, whereas the level typically increases in IAH cases and may decrease in cases of GRHA [9].

Aldosterone Excretion and Secretion Measurements

The finding of increased aldosterone production on a high salt intake confirms the diagnosis of hyperaldosteronism [2a]. The aldosterone excretion rate is more commonly used than the more cumbersome aldosterone secretion rate, which measures quantitative adrenal production. The excretion rate approximates about 10% of the secretion rate, and at all ranges of aldosterone secretion this ratio remains constant. During high normal sodium intake (>150 mEq/day), less than 20 μg of aldosterone should be excreted in a 24-hour period. Total urinary creatinine should be determined to ensure the completeness of the collection, and urine sodium needs to be measured to assess the state of sodium balance. Urinary sodium excretion should be at least 150 mEq/day during this testing period.

Computerized Tomography

With computerized tomography (CT) scanning, both adrenal glands can be visualized and characterized by size in 50 to 75% of normal persons. Limited experience suggests that this type of testing will probably localize adenomas larger than 1.5 cm in diameter [25,35]. The utility of

CT scanning in IAH is not known. The noninvasive nature of this testing and the ready availability in most areas are obvious advantages.

Spironolactone Therapeutic Trial
Spironolactone (Aldactone) administered in a dose of 200 to 400 mg per day in divided doses should be effective in limiting renal potassium wasting in all forms of hyperaldosteronism [16,30]. In contrast, the blood pressure response to spironolactone is not uniform among the subtypes of primary aldosteronism (Table 10-3). An appreciable reduction or normalization of blood pressure is the typical response when APA is present. Conversely, many patients with IAH have little or no amelioration of the hypertension with spironolactone. This is a controversial issue, as there are reports indicating excellent responsiveness of IAH patients to both spironolactone and surgery (total adrenalectomy).

Selective Adrenal Venous Sampling During Adrenocorticotropic Hormone Infusion
Selective adrenal venous sampling for determination of aldosterone concentration has been effectively done in experienced centers [7,28]. Anatomic problems may prevent adequate sampling from both adrenal veins. ACTH administration minimizes circadian or episodic changes in plasma aldosterone levels, and ACTH maximizes the aldosterone secretion from an adenoma [22]. Concomitant cortisol measurements should be made to help verify the source of the sample and also to allow the determination of aldosterone/cortisol ratios that further help with localization. The aldosterone concentration of adrenal venous plasma in normal supine subjects ranges from 100 to 450 ng/dl. In APA, the adrenal vein aldosterone level on the involved side averages about 5000 ng/dl, with a wide range from 250 to greater than 15,000 ng/dl. The ratio between the left and right adrenal veins is more critical than the absolute values, and ratios exceeding 10 : 1 (and frequently much higher) should localize the side of the adenoma. Most patients with IAH have bilateral elevations with mean concentrations of approximately 2500 ng/dl (range, 150–>10,000 ng/dl).

Technique of Selective Adrenal Venous Sampling
1. Begin intravenous infusion of synthetic ACTH (cosyntropin), 5 IU (50 μg) per hour.*
2. Perform venous catheterization from the femoral approach.
3. Collect blood from both adrenal veins and from the inferior vena cava below the renal veins. (If the right adrenal vein cannot be catheterized, sample from the inferior vena cava near the orifice of the adrenal vein.)
4. Use gentle aspiration or collect by gravity flow to minimize dilution by nonadrenal venous blood.

*Some investigators advise obtaining both basal and post-ACTH infusion values.

5. Measure aldosterone and cortisol concentrations in all samples and determine aldosterone/cortisol ratios.

As a representative case example, consider a 42-year-old man with right adrenal adenoma. During ACTH infusion, the following values were obtained:

	Right Adrenal Vein	Inferior Vena Cava	Left Adrenal Vein
Plasma aldosterone (ng/dl)	7650	128	160
Plasma cortisol (μg/dl)	380	27	305
Aldosterone/cortisol ratio	20	4.7	0.5

Selective Adrenal Venography
Adrenal venography may be performed at the same time as adrenal vein sampling. Venography has been a reliable localizing technique with adenomas greater than 1.0 cm in diameter, and overall, venography will correctly localize approximately two-thirds of all adenomas [34]. However, several problems have been encountered, including adrenal vein perforation and adrenal hemorrhage and infarction, and the risks of this test must be carefully considered [32]. It appears that venography adds little to the localizing accuracy of selective venous sampling during ACTH infusion.

Adrenal Scintiscan with Iodocholesterol
Isotopic adrenal scanning with [131I]-cholesterol has been used extensively by Conn and others, with a success rate of about 80% in the localization of an adenoma [5,18]. This technique has been generally less successful in other centers for reasons that are not clear. A recent modification involves the addition of dexamethasone to suppress the normal adrenal tissue and highlight an adenoma. Conn finds the modified scan approximately 90% effective in lateralizing an adenoma or predicting bilateral hyperplasia. The uptake of radiocholesterol is early on the side of an adenoma, whereas uptake by the normal contralateral gland is delayed. With IAH, there is bilateral uptake of radioactivity. A new compound, 6-β-iodomethyl-19-norcholesterol (NP-59), is currently being tested and appears to produce better isotopic resolution [33].

DISCUSSION
It is worth emphasizing that persistent hypokalemia with serum values less than 3.6 mEq/L is a hallmark of most patients with APA. Conversely, the types of primary aldosteronism with bilateral adrenal

hyperplasia frequently have intermittently low or borderline low serum potassium levels. Patients with borderline normokalemia should be challenged with a high-salt diet (approximately 250 mEq sodium per day for 5 days). This will induce renal potassium wasting in primary aldosteronism, with a subsequent fall in the serum potassium to less than 3.6 mEq/L in most cases. In order to document the fact that an adequate amount of sodium was ingested and absorbed, a 24-hour urine sample should be collected on the final day to determine the total sodium excretion, which should closely approximate the sodium intake. Analysis of the total potassium in this urine sample is also useful. Excretion of > 30 mEq/L in the presence of hypokalemia suggests renal potassium wasting and is compatible with a diagnosis of primary aldosteronism.

Determination of the stimulated PRA is the next step (Fig. 10-1). If stimulation is attempted by furosemide-induced volume depletion, it is mandatory first to check the serum potassium concentration. If the level is less than 3.8 mEq/L, potassium chloride should be given during the diuretic administration to avoid precipitating marked hypokalemia. If the patient presents with severe unprovoked hypokalemia (serum K^+ < 3.0 mEq/L), it is inadvisable to volume-deplete acutely with furosemide. In such cases, a very low-sodium diet (10–20 mEq/day) should be prescribed before determining the renin activity with upright posture. By the fifth day, sodium balance should be achieved and the total 24-hour urine sodium excretion should approximate 10 to 20 mEq. If the urinary sodium is substantially higher than this, it is probable that the person did not adhere to the vigorous low-salt diet, and a low PRA will be uninterpretable.

Normal levels of PRA vary greatly among laboratories, and it is necessary to know the normal values for the laboratory being used and not to rely on literature values. If patients are studied after a therapeutic trial on spironolactone, it is important to appreciate that this medication generally returns the responsiveness of PRA to normal in spironolactone-responsive hypertension. It has been documented that the PRA may remain relatively elevated for several months after cessation of successful spironolactone therapy, resulting in false-negative responses to the low-renin state [27]. As a general rule, it is recommended that the patient be off all medication for 4 weeks prior to beginning the protocol of study and remain off medication during the evaluation.

The saline infusion test has assumed greater importance in the diagnosis of primary aldosteronism—especially when one considers the relatively large percentage of patients who have normal or near-normal serum potassium concentrations and nondiagnostic urinary aldosterone excretion rates [34]. Patients with baseline severe hypokalemia should first be repleted with potassium chloride before this test is undertaken to ensure safety. The reliability of the laboratory determining the plasma aldosterone concentration assumes great importance. Newer assays for aldosterone have been developed that do not require the laborious techniques necessitated by the older methods. When the test is properly performed, patients with primary aldosteronism will have a mean postinfusion plasma aldosterone level of approximately 35 ng/dl in the adenoma group and 25 ng/dl in IAH. The range is broad, however, and an occasional patient with mild primary aldosteronism may have a postinfusion value as low as 5 to 10 ng/dl.

At this point in the evaluation, patients with probable primary aldosteronism have been identified. Further testing is done in order to confirm the diagnosis and localize the lesion, as illustrated in the second part of the protocol (Fig. 10-2).

There is an extremely broad range of urinary aldosterone excretion, and normal levels are meaningful *only* in relation to the state of sodium balance. Failure to give the patient an adequate salt load is a problem frequently encountered, and after 5 days on the high-salt diet it is essential to document proper salt loading by determining the 24-hour urine sodium excretion. Aldosterone excretion in excess of 20 μg per day on high sodium intake confirms the diagnosis of primary aldosteronism. Suppression of excretion below 20 μg per day may occur, however, in mild cases of primary aldosteronism [32] or in the presence of hypokalemia. It is useful to check changes in serum potassium and 24-hour urine potassium excretion with salt loading to document the presence or absence of potassium wasting. In cases with overall borderline results, it frequently becomes a matter of clinical judgment as to whether to pursue the diagnosis further with invasive tests such as selective adrenal venous sampling.

There is one further noteworthy point regarding the aldosterone excretion rate. Most secreted aldosterone (20–40%) is metabolized in the liver. Approximately 10% is metabolized in the kidney to the acid-labile metabolite aldosterone-18-glucuronide. It is the aldosterone liberated by hydrolysis of the acid-labile metabolite that is commonly measured to determine urinary aldosterone excretion. Thus, the measured excretion rate approximates only 10% of the actual secretion rate. To what extent subtle abnormalities of hepatic or renal function affect the excretion rate has not been well studied. Therefore, minor deviations from normal need to be thoughtfully analyzed [12].

When the urinary aldosterone excretion on a high-salt diet suggests primary aldosteronism, the plasma aldosterone response to upright posture and the spironolactone trial may be used for further assessment. The anomalous fall in plasma aldosterone levels favors the diagnosis of adenoma, although, as has been discussed, a fall may also occur in the much less common form of GRHA. If GRHA is a consideration (suggestive family history), a suppressive trial with glucocorticoids may be used. Dexamethasone (1–2 mg/day) administered for 4 weeks or longer will decrease blood pressure to normal, reduce plasma aldosterone levels, and correct the metabolic abnormalities in GRHA [9].

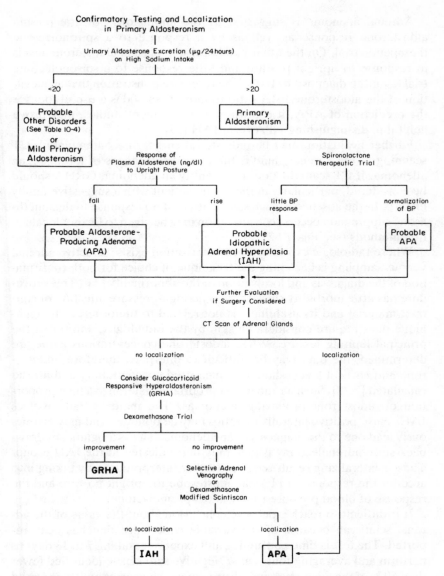

Figure 10-2. Diagnostic protocol: Confirmatory testing and localization in primary aldosteronism.

Adrenal adenoma is suggested by the anomalous postural plasma aldosterone response as well as by a response to a spironolactone therapeutic trial. On the other hand, a rise in plasma aldosterone levels in response to upright posture and little response to a spironolactone trial favor the diagnosis of IAH. The recent demonstration that an elevation of the aldosterone/PRA ratio to more than 400 is a useful tool for the prediction of APA, if confirmed in subsequent studies, may prove helpful in distinguishing APA from IAH [17].

Further evaluation may be indicated if surgery is contemplated. CT scanning of the adrenal gland is the most direct means of localizing an adenoma. If CT scanning does not identify an adenoma, GRHA should be considered, particularly in the young patient with a suggestive family history. In the absence of such suspicions or if no response to dexamethasone suppression occurs, consideration may be given to further localization methods (see Fig. 10-2).

Where radiologic expertise in catheterization exists, selective adrenal venous sampling is becoming the technique of choice for both confirmation of the diagnosis and localization of the abnormality [2a]. This procedure has little morbidity since there is no high-pressure injection of contrast material and its usefulness is not related to tumor size. The technique does require considerable skill by the radiologist, and this is the principal limiting feature. When aldosterone concentrations alone are determined, the data may be difficult to interpret; therefore, aldosterone and cortisol levels should be measured concomitantly and a ratio calculated [7,28]. Such a ratio will appropriately lateralize a high proportion of aldosterone-producing adenomas. The major pitfall involves IAH. False-positive lateralizing ratios may be obtained and may erroneously lead one to the diagnosis of an adenoma. This is a significant drawback since adrenalectomy is generally not indicated in the IAH group. Thus, a lateralizing result requires further interpretation by taking into account the response of plasma aldosterone to upright posture and the response of blood pressure to a trial of spironolactone.

It is difficult to reach a decisive conclusion about the value of the adrenal scintiscan because of the variable experience that has been reported. The test is time-consuming and expensive, taking 7 to 18 days to perform and averaging four scans. Negative series have identified fewer than 50% of the adenomas and, distressingly, have erroneously reported contralateral localization in some patients. In addition, despite the use of dexamethasone, patients with IAH may have lateralizing scans. On the positive side, this procedure is not invasive and has been highly touted by several groups. Whether to localize with selective adrenal vein sampling or scintiscanning seems mostly to be a function of the local expertise with these procedures.

A summary of confirmation/localization approaches suggests the need for a number of tests. It is usually possible to confirm the diagnosis, localize the lesion(s), and differentiate APA from IAH [16,31]. A careful analysis of the degree of renin suppression, the quantity of aldosterone secreted/excreted, the degree of hypokalemia in combination with selective adrenal venous sampling (or iodocholesterol scintiscan), and the plasma aldosterone response to upright posture will lead to the correct diagnosis in most instances. A therapeutic trial of spironolactone should be undertaken in most if not all cases, both to assess the degree of blood pressure improvement and to predict the response to surgery.

The protocol of evaluation outlined is not necessarily indicated in every patient with probable primary aldosteronism. There are many good arguments that can be made for deleting the invasive studies described, proceeding directly with a spironolactone therapeutic trial, and thereafter continuing chronically on spironolactone if the blood pressure is well controlled and the drug is tolerated without severe side effects [26]. The age of the patient, severity of hypertension, local radiologic expertise, and philosophies of the physician and patient must all be taken into consideration in determining how best to proceed with the diagnostic work-up. If surgery is not contemplated, there is little reason to proceed with localization maneuvers, as these tests can be performed at a later time if spironolactone is found to be ineffective or poorly tolerated.

REFERENCES

1. Ayres, P. J., Garrod, O., and Tait, S. A. S. Primary Aldosteronism (Conn(s) Syndrome). In A. F. Muller and C. M. O'Connor (Eds.), *International Symposium on Aldosterone.* Boston: Little Brown, 1958.
2. Biglieri, E. G., Stockigt, J. R., and Schambelan, M. Adrenal mineralocorticoid causing hypertension. *Am. J. Med.* 52:623–632, 1972.
2a. Bravo, E. L., et al. The changing clinical spectrum of primary aldosteronism. *Am. J. Med.* 74:641–651, 1983.
3. Brown, J. J., et al. Plasma electrolytes, renin, and aldosterone in the diagnosis of primary hyperaldosteronism. *Lancet* 2:55–59, 1968.
4. Carey, R. M., et al. The syndrome of essential hypertension and suppressed plasma renin activity. Normalization of blood pressure with spironolactone. *Arch. Intern. Med.* 130:849–854, 1972.
5. Conn, J. W., Cohen, E. O., and Herwig, K. R. The dexamethasone modified adrenal scintiscan in hyporeninemic aldosteronism (tumor vs hyperplasia). A comparison with adrenal venography and adrenal venous aldosterone. *J. Lab. Clin. Med.* 88:841–856, 1976.
6. Conn, J. W., Knopf, R. F., and Nesbit, R. M. Clinical characteristics of primary aldosteronism from an analysis of 145 cases. *Am. J. Surg.* 107:159–172, 1964.
7. Dunnick, N. R., et al. Preoperative diagnosis and localization of aldosteronomas by measurement of corticosteroids in adrenal venous blood. *Radiology* 133:331–333, 1979.
8. Ferriss, J. B., et al. Clinical, biochemical, and pathological features of low-renin ("primary") hyperaldosteronism. *Am. Heart J.* 95:375–388, 1978.
9. Ganguly, A., Grim, C. E., and Weinberger, M. H. Anomalous postural aldosterone response in glucocorticoid suppressible hyperaldosteronism. *N. Engl. J. Med.* 305:991–993, 1981.
10. Ganguly, A., et al. Control of plasma aldosterone in primary aldosteronism: Distinction between adenoma and hyperplasia. *J. Clin. Endocrinol. Metab.* 37:765–775, 1973.

11. George, J. M., et al. The syndrome of primary aldosteronism. *Am. J. Med.* 48:343–356, 1970.
12. Gomez-Sanchez, C. E., and Holland, O. B. Urinary and plasma tetrahydro-aldosterone and aldosterone-18-glucuronide excretion in white and black normal subjects and hypertensive patients. *J. Clin. Endocrinol. Metab.* 52:214–219, 1981.
13. Grim, C. E. Low renin "essential" hypertension. A variant of classic primary aldosteronism? *Arch. Intern. Med.* 135:347–350, 1975.
14. Grim, C. E., and Weinberger, M. H. Familial dexamethasone-suppressible, normokalemic hyperaldosteronism. *Pediatrics* 65:597–604, 1980.
15. Gross, M. D., et al. Suppression of aldosterone by cyproheptadine in idiopathic hyperaldosteronism. *N. Engl. J. Med.* 305:181–185, 1981.
16. Herf, S. M., et al. Identification and differentiation of surgically correctable hypertension due to primary aldosteronism. *Am. J. Med.* 67:397–402, 1979.
17. Hiramatsu, K., et al. A screening test to identify aldosterone-producing adenoma by measuring plasma renin activity. *Arch. Intern. Med.* 141:1589–1594, 1981.
18. Hogan, M. J., McRae, J., and Schambelan, M. Location of aldosterone producing adenomas with [131]I-19-iodocholesterol. *N. Engl. J. Med.* 294:410–414, 1976.
19. Horton, R. Aldosterone: Review of its physiology and diagnostic aspects of primary aldosteronism. *Metabolism* 22:1525–1545, 1973.
20. Kaplan, N. M. Adrenal causes of hypertension. *Arch. Intern. Med.* 133:1001–1006, 1974.
21. Kaplan, N. M., et al. The intravenous furosemide test: A simple way to evaluate renin responsiveness. *Ann. Intern. Med.* 84:639–645, 1976.
22. Kem, D. C., et al. The role of ACTH in the episodic release of aldosterone in patients with idiopathic adrenal hyperplasia, hypertension, and hyperaldosteronism. *J. Lab. Clin. Med.* 88:261–270, 1976.
23. Kem, D. C., et al. Saline suppression of plasma aldosterone in hypertension. *Arch. Intern. Med.* 128:380–386, 1971.
24. Kotchen, T. A., and Guthrie, G. P. Renin-angiotensin-aldosterone and hypertension. *Endocrine Rev.* 1:78–99, 1980.
25. Linde, R., et al. Localization of aldosterone-producing adenoma by computed tomography. *J. Clin. Endocrinol. Metab.* 49:642–645, 1979.
26. Loriaux, D. L., et al. Spironolactone and endocrine dysfunction. *Ann. Intern. Med.* 85:630–636, 1976.
27. Lowder, S. C., and Liddle, G. W. Prolonged alteration of renin responsiveness after spironolactone therapy. A cause of false-negative testing for low-renin hypertension. *N. Engl. J. Med.* 291:1243–1244, 1974.
28. Lund, J. O., et al. Localization of aldosterone-producing tumors in primary aldosteronism by adrenal and renal vein catheterization. *Acta Med. Scand.* 207:345–351, 1980.
29. Oberfield, S. E., et al. Adrenal glomerulosa function in patients with dexamethasone-suppressible hyperaldosteronism. *J. Clin. Endocrinol. Metab.* 53:158–164, 1981.
30. Spark, R. S., and Melby, J. C. Aldosteronism in hypertension. The spironolactone response test. *Ann. Intern. Med.* 69:685–691, 1968.
31. Streeten, D. H. P., Tomycz, N., and Anderson, G. H., Jr. Reliability of screening methods for the diagnosis of primary aldosteronism. *Am. J. Med.* 67:403–413, 1979.
32. Taylor, H. C., Sachs, C. R., and Bravo, E. L. Primary aldosteronism: Remission and development of adrenal insufficiency after adrenal venography. *Ann. Intern. Med.* 85:207–209, 1976.

33. Thrall, J. H., Frietas, J. E., and Beierwaltes, W. H. Adrenal scintigraphy. *Semin. Nucl. Med.* 8:23–41, 1978.
34. Weinberger, M. H., et al. Primary aldosteronism. *Ann. Intern. Med.* 90:386–395, 1979.
35. White, E. A., et al. Use of computerized tomography in diagnosing the cause of primary aldosteronism. *N. Engl. J. Med.* 303:1503–1507, 1980.
36. Williams, G. H., and Dluhy, R. G. Aldosterone biosynthesis: Interrelationship of regulatory factors. *Am. J. Med.* 53:595–605, 1972.

11   Amenorrhea
William T. Cave, Jr.
William F. Streck

Normal menstrual function requires a highly coordinated series of hormonal interactions involving the hypothalamus, pituitary gland, and ovaries. In addition, the normal result of this endocrine process, whether it be menses or pregnancy, requires a morphologically competent uterus and genital tract. Amenorrhea most often results from a dysfunction of some component of the endocrine axis rather than from anatomic or developmental abnormalities of the genital tract.

Conventionally, amenorrhea has been designated as either primary or secondary. The term *primary amenorrhea* describes the failure of a chronologically mature woman to undergo menarche. *Secondary amenorrhea* describes the absence of menses in a woman with previously established menstrual function. The clinical value of this classification of amenorrhea into primary and secondary forms has been seriously questioned by some investigators [10]. However, it is retained in this chapter to emphasize the relative infrequency of primary amenorrhea as opposed to the more common occurrence of secondary amenorrhea. Almost all congenital causes of amenorrhea are associated with the primary group, but it should be recognized that some noncongenital disorders can cause primary amenorrhea (e.g., polycystic ovary disease), and some congenital disorders may occasionally present as secondary cases (e.g., mosaic gonadal dysgenesis).

CLINICAL CONSIDERATIONS
Primary Amenorrhea
The first problem to be faced in the evaluation of any young woman who has not undergone menarche (primary amenorrhea) is to decide if the condition warrants further study [5,11]. In the United States, the mean age of menarche is reported to be 12.6 years, and by 17 years of age, 98% of the female population has initiated menstrual function. In girls, puberty usually begins with a somatic growth spurt and is soon followed by the appearance of breast buds and pubic hair. Normally, within approximately 2 years of these initial changes, menarche, axillary hair development, further public hair growth, and breast development occur. Adequate weight and height for age, however, appear to be necessary in order for menses to begin [8,9]. As a general rule, a girl should be evaluated diagnostically for primary amenorrhea if menstruation has not occurred by age 14 and there is no evidence of the anticipated pubertal changes and skeletal growth, or if menstruation has not occurred by the age of 16.

Obviously, these are broad guidelines, and some degree of individual clinical judgment must be used in each case. For example, a 13-year-old

Table 11-1. Primary Amenorrhea

Constitutional delayed puberty
Chromosomal abnormalities
    Turner's syndrome (XO) and variants (XX)
    Mosaics (XO/XX, etc.)
CNS or pituitary disease
Androgen excess*
    Congenital adrenal hyperplasia
    Drugs (androgens)
    Tumors
Testicular feminization
Resistant ovary syndrome
Hermaphroditism (XX/XY)
Polycystic ovarian disease (rare)
Abnormal development of the genital tract
Exercise/anorexia nervosa

*If this occurs in utero or in infancy, ambiguous genitalia may be present.

girl with no evidence of pubertal development would certainly be of more concern than a 16-year-old girl with only a mild delay in the normal pattern of sexual development. Frequently, however, the mere fact that the patient has sought consultation with a physician for the complaint of amenorrhea indicates that the problem requires attention for medical, family, or social reasons. Some of the disorders that are most commonly associated with primary amenorrhea are listed in Table 11-1. Significantly, genetic abnormalities are present in 40 to 50% of the patients presenting with primary amenorrhea not due to simple delayed puberty.

GONADAL DYSGENESIS. Turner's syndrome is the most common genetic cause of primary amenorrhea. It occurs once in every 3000 newborn females and is characterized by a karyotype that has a chromosome number of 45 due to the absence of one of the sex chromosomes (45 XO). In the absence of this genetic information, the ovaries are replaced by fibrous stroma. As a result, these individuals develop phenotypically as females. Their serum estrogen levels remain low throughout life, and their gonadotropin levels rise into the castrate range after 9 to 10 years of age.

This diagnosis should be suspected in any young woman with primary amenorrhea who has a short stature, sparse pubic or axillary hair, and absent secondary sexual characteristics. Likewise, the presence of micrognathia, epicanthal folds, low-set ears, and a square, shield-like chest with microthelia may also be diagnostically helpful. Other commonly observed abnormalities include webbing of the neck (40%), coarctation of the aorta (10–20%), congenital lymphadema of the hands and feet at birth (30%), a short fourth metacarpal (50%), and renal abnormalities

(60%). Diabetes mellitus, Hashimoto's thyroiditis, and red-green color blindness are also noted more frequently in these patients [5,18].

Approximately 20% of patients with typical ovarian pathology of gonadal dysgenesis have a 46 XX karyotype. This situation is thought to be due either to a structural abnormality in one of the X chromosomes or to an XO/XX chromosome mosaicism. The karyotype may also detect deletions of the long or short arm of the X chromosome. The former may present with either primary or occasionally secondary amenorrhea. Interestingly, in patients with chromosome mosaicism, the ultimate degree of ovarian dysgenesis observed appears to be related to the ratio of the XO primitive germ cells to the normal XX ones. These patients are not invariably short, nor do they exhibit many of the somatic anomalies often seen in the classic XO phenotype. They usually have normal-appearing female internal and external genitalia, but due to the ovarian dysgenesis that is present, their genital structures tend to remain immature and their serum gonadotropins become elevated. Virilization in a patient with Turner's syndrome suggests that some male chromatin material is present as part of an XO/XY mosaic pattern. This is an important observation since patients with Y chromosomal material and abnormal intra-abdominal gonads require gonadectomy because of an increased incidence of gonadoblastomas and dysgerminomas.

EXERCISE/ANOREXIA NERVOSA. Menarche may be delayed in adolescent women who exercise strenuously and regularly [8,9]. This is an increasingly recognized syndrome and one that may be suspected in the otherwise healthy, lean adolescent with primary amenorrhea. In a similar fashion, the malnourished individual with early-onset anorexia nervosa may present with a delay in menarche. The presumed pathophysiology of these disorders is discussed in more detail in the subsequent section on secondary amenorrhea.

HYPOTHALAMIC-PITUITARY DISEASE. Primary amenorrhea may result from the congenital absence or pathologic destruction of any component of the hypothalamic-pituitary axis that is responsible for normal gonadotropin secretion. Such varied lesions as tumors, infiltrative diseases, infections, aneurysms, and congenital central nervous system (CNS) malformations have all been reported to be capable of producing this result. The clinical presentations of these patients, however, differ greatly and depend significantly on the age of onset and number of associated hormone deficiencies. Characteristically, when an isolated gonadotropin deficiency occurs, there is an absence of secondary sexual development, a delay in epiphyseal closure, and a eunuchoid habitus. Such features in a patient with anosmia or hyposmia are consistent with the diagnosis of Kallman's syndrome [28]. Hyperprolactinemia may present as primary amenorrhea [19]. This topic is discussed in more detail in the subsequent section on secondary amenorrhea.

CONGENITAL ADRENAL HYPERPLASIA. A congenital deficiency of either the 21- or 11-hydroxylase enzymes in the adrenal glands will cause hyperandrogenism. Since abnormally high androgen levels interfere with the normal hypothalamic pituitary regulation of ovarian function, amenorrhea and infertility are common features of these disorders. Hirsutism, virilization, and short stature may be present.

TESTICULAR FEMINIZATION OR PARTIAL ANDROGEN INSENSITIVITY. Testicular feminization is a distinctive hereditary disorder that occurs in genetic males and is characterized by an apparent resistance of the tissues to circulating testosterone. Available experimental evidence suggests that there is a genetically determined qualitative or quantitative abnormality of the cytoplasmic androgen receptors in these patients [15]. Since these receptors are considered necessary for the transport of testosterone, or its derivative dihydrotestosterone, into the nucleus where hormone action is initiated, patients with this disorder are unable to induce normal tissue responses to androgen. They therefore develop as phenotypic females. However, even though their external genitalia are feminine, their vaginas are often shallow and end in a blind pouch. This is because their testes have müllerian-inhibiting factor, which inhibits the growth of müllerian structures (uterus, tubes, upper third of the vagina). Normal female breast development usually occurs in these patients at adolescence due to unopposed estrogen effects, but their pubic and axillary hair growth is generally quite scant and in a significant percentage is completely absent. Interestingly, the Leydig cells within the intra-abdominal testes found in these individuals remain functional and produce an amount of testosterone that is sufficient to maintain the plasma level within the normal or elevated range.

RESISTANT OVARY SYNDROME. Patients with resistant ovary syndrome present as phenotypic females with hypoplastic ovaries containing unstimulated follicles. Their serum estrogen levels are low in spite of the fact that their serum gonadotropin levels are elevated. Apparently, the pathologic abnormality in these individuals is an ovarian insensitivity to the pituitary gonadotropins, because even when exogenous gonadotropins are administered, the gonad usually fails to respond appropriately [30]. This disorder may also present as secondary amenorrhea.

TRUE HERMAPHRODITISM. True hermaphroditism is defined as the presence of both ovarian and testicular tissue in either the same or opposite gonads. The cells of these patients are probably derived embryologically from a doubly fertilized ovum or from the fusion of two normally fertilized ova. On physical examination, the external genitalia of these patients are often ambiguous, although they can in some patients be distinctly male or female. Significant breast development occurs in the majority, and a uterus is present in virtually all patients. Menstruation will occur in over half of them.

DEVELOPMENTAL ABNORMALITIES OF THE GENITAL TRACT. The most common examples of patients with primary amenorrhea due to genital tract abnormalities are those with an imperforate hymen or obstruction to the cervical or vaginal canal. Occasionally, however, developmental anomalies such as the absence or dysplasia of the uterus, fallopian tubes, or vagina may occur. The detection of these latter types of abnormalities is clinically important because they are frequently associated with urinary tract abnormalities (20–50%). This is presumably due to the common embryologic derivation of these organs from the urogenital ridge.

Secondary Amenorrhea
Although *secondary amenorrhea* may be strictly defined as the absence of any menstrual period in a woman who has previously experienced normal menses, it is the persistent absence of menses that is of true clinical concern. Ideally, the menstrual period should occur regularly every 24 to 35 days until menopause, unless interrupted by pregnancy. In reality, however, women may normally have some slight abnormality in as many as 20% of their cycles, and the occasional absence of a menstrual period is not uncommon. Therefore, it has been generally considered reasonable to wait until the amenorrhea has persisted for at least 4 months before considering it significant enough to warrant an exhaustive search for a pathologic etiology.

Once pregnancy has been excluded, polycystic ovary disease, hypothalamic dysfunction usually secondary to exercise, weight loss, or stress, hyperprolactinemia, and the amenorrhea occurring after the discontinuation of oral contraceptive use represent the most frequent causes of secondary amenorrhea [16,27] (Table 11-2).

POLYCYSTIC OVARIAN DISEASE (PCOD). Polycystic ovarian disease may be considered a steady state of tonic subthreshold ovarian stimulation by the gonadotropins [2,14,24]. The low but not totally suppressed follicle-stimulating hormone (FSH) levels found in these patients allow follicular growth to continue, whereas elevated luteinizing hormone (LH) levels stimulate continued hormonal production from the stromal cells. The net result is that many follicles proceed to various stages of development and produce a hormonal steady state that limits ovulation while maintaining increased steroid production. This syndrome can occur spontaneously or within a familiar pattern (autosomal dominant with variable penetrance). Its primary etiology is not clearly established; both adrenal and ovarian dysfunction have been suggested.

The endocrinologic consequences seem to be perpetuated by an ina-

Table 11-2. Secondary Amenorrhea

Pregnancy
Polycystic ovarian disease
Exercise induced
Hypothalamic-nutritional amenorrhea
Emotional stress
Anorexia, starvation
Hyperprolactinemia
Drugs (post-pill amenorrhea)
Ovarian failure
Premature menopause
Chemotherapy/radiation
Destructive CNS lesion
Ovarian tumors
Endocrine disorders
Adrenal
Thyroid
Uterine disease
Oophorectomy

bility of the hypothalamus to regulate ovarian function in the normal manner. Typically, these patients have unusually high LH : FSH ratios, and their serum estrone/estradiol ratios are often elevated. Their ovaries eventually become thickened and enlarged with numerous follicles, cysts, and atretic follicles, and as outlined in the section on hirsutism, mild increases in testosterone production routinely occur (see Chap. 12). As a consequence of this hyperandrogenism, these patients are often hirsute, but very rarely do they become severely virilized. Anovulation is a constant feature, and menstrual abnormalities ranging from prolonged amenorrhea to oligomenorrhea with episodes of menometrorrhagia frequently occur. Obesity and enlarged ovaries, although frequently identified as common manifestations of this disorder, are not invariably present in all cases [33].

EXERCISE-INDUCED AMENORRHEA. Exercise-induced amenorrhea may be considered under the broader category of hypothalamic-nutritional causes of amenorrhea. The disorder may be of the primary form, particularly in young girls who participate in vigorous, sustained physical training (e.g., ballet, gymnastics) [8,9]. Secondary amenorrhea is more common and has been reported as a consequence of many vigorous activities, including running, swimming, ballet, and rowing. Studies have suggested that the amenorrhea is in part a consequence of altered estrogen metabolism due to a failure to maintain a critical lean/fat ratio, as well as stress-induced changes in hypothalamic function [3,7–9]. In several studies, amenorrhea has been noted to develop more frequently in nulliparous than in parous runners [3,7]. Menses characteristically resume with discontinuation of training [32] and/or increased weight gain with modest increases in fat stores. The age of menarche and subsequent menstrual cyclicity may be influenced by the age at which the individual began intensive athletic training [8].

HYPOTHALAMIC-NUTRITIONAL CAUSES OF AMENORRHEA. Hypothalamic-nutritional factors include some of the most common causes of secondary amenorrhea in young women. Usually, these patients are not hirsute, but they do have a history of either severe psychologic stress or excessive weight loss. It is postulated that any of these stresses, alone or in combination, may produce amenorrhea by disrupting the normal hypothalamic regulatory mechanisms responsible for gonadotropin release [9,31]. As a result, the definitive conclusion that amenorrhea is due to one of the disorders in this category is largely dependent on the systematic exclusion of all other possible causes.

Anorexia nervosa and the amenorrhea of starvation are two typical representatives of the disorders in this group. Interestingly, anorexia nervosa patients have not only low basal gonadotropins but also elevated growth hormone levels and thermoregulatory deficiencies. Exactly how this disorder modifies hypothalamic function is unknown, but when the patient is given adequate nutritional replacement, the gonadotropins often return to normal. As noted, anorexia nervosa that is manifested before menarche may delay the onset of menses or present with primary rather than secondary amenorrhea.

HYPERPROLACTINEMIA. The availability of reliable radioimmunoassays for prolactin has allowed recognition of the fact that hyperprolactinemia is frequently associated with amenorrhea. Hyperprolactinemia apparently interferes with positive estrogen feedback, thus inhibiting ovulatory surges of LH and FSH and often leading to anovulation. Present data indicate that approximately one-third of patients with secondary amenorrhea, two-thirds or more of patients with amenorrhea and galactorrhea, and one-third of patients with post-pill amenorrhea have a demonstrable elevation in serum prolactin [25,26]. When patients with hyperprolactinemia and amenorrhea are evaluated, it can be shown that 40 to 50% present after the discontinuation of birth control pills, 20 to 40% present with spontaneous onset of symptoms, and 5 to 15% present within the postpartum period [26]. The presence of galactorrhea in a patient with normal menstrual function is usually not indicative of hyperprolactinemia [21].

In all patients with hyperprolactinemia, the possibility of a prolactin-secreting pituitary adenoma should be seriously considered, even when the standard anatomic investigative techniques demonstrate no definitive evidence of tumor. In the absence of drug therapy or pregnancy, a serum prolactin level greater than 100 ng/ml is often strong presumptive evidence of the presence of a pituitary tumor [20], because, as a general rule, the height of the serum prolactin level correlates with the likelihood of tumor presence. Prolactin levels less than 100 ng/ml do not exclude the presence of an adenoma, but other causes, such as hypothalamic pituitary dysfunction, are more frequently found in this patient group. Obviously, the diagnosis of a prolactin-secreting pituitary adenoma is most secure when both marked hyperprolactinemia and abnormal sellar tomography are present [26]. Those patients who have marginally elevated prolactin levels and no anatomic evidence of tumor presence may be followed with serial prolactin assays, and lateral skull films should be repeated periodically until the diagnosis becomes more apparent or the hyperprolactinemia resolves.

DRUG-INDUCED AMENORRHEA. Amenorrhea following the discontinuation of birth control pills occurs in approximately 2% of pill users [13] and accounts for approximately 30% of the cases of secondary amenorrhea [26]. Of this group, one-third will have hyperprolactinemia [26], and many will have a history of previous menstrual irregularity [13]. At present, it is postulated that this persistent amenorrhea is due to a continued suppression of the hypothalamic centers involved in the control of gonadotropin secretion [29]. In general, spontaneous recovery can be anticipated unless a pituitary adenoma is present.

Psychotropic drugs of the phenothiazine family have also been associated with amenorrhea. This condition is believed to be the result of either a direct effect of the drug at the hypothalamic level or a secondary effect of the hyperprolactinemia induced by the drug.

Finally, in addition to the more common causes of secondary amenorrhea already listed, there remain several less frequent, but medically important, etiologies. The following sections will outline the characteristics of some of these disorders. It should, of course, also be remembered that certain forms of gonadal dysgenesis may also present as secondary amenorrhea, particularly in the younger patient.

PREMATURE MENOPAUSE. In the United States the average age of spontaneous ovarian failure, or menopause, is estimated to be 48 years. If it occurs prior to age 40, it is considered to be premature. The exact pathogenesis of premature ovarian impairment is uncertain, but probably several different processes are capable of producing this end result [34]. A limited number of cases appear to represent late manifestations of various forms of gonadal dysgenesis. Immunologic mechanisms may also be responsible for certain cases, since some patients with idiopathic Addison's disease have also been reported to have primary ovarian failure associated with autoantibodies directed against the cells of the corpus luteum and the theca interna [17]. However, there is little likelihood that autoimmunity is the major cause of premature menopause because such antiovarian antibodies are rarely found in the absence of other systemic signs of autoimmune disease. In the patient less than 30 years of age, the karyotype may reveal mosaic Turner's syndrome.

CHEMOTHERAPY AND RADIOTHERAPY. It should always be borne in mind that patients undergoing therapy with agents such as cyclophosphamide or those receiving abdominal radiation are susceptible to secondary amenorrhea on the basis of ovarian cell death. Older patients appear to be more susceptible to this form of amenorrhea [6].

OVARIAN TUMORS. Ovarian tumors producing excessive levels of androgen or estrogen can cause amenorrhea by suppressing the hypothalamic-pituitary axis. Rare androgen-producing ovarian tumors include arrhenoblastomas, hilus cell tumors, and luteomas. The predominant estrogen-producing neoplasm is the granulosa-theca cell tumor, which accounts for 15 to 20% of all solid ovarian tumors [18]. Eighty percent of patients with this tumor have a palpable ovarian mass on pelvic examination, and most have symptoms of polymenorrhea or irregular bleeding alternating with periods of amenorrhea.

DESTRUCTIVE LESIONS OF THE HYPOTHALAMIC-PITUITARY AXIS. As indicated in the discussion of primary amenorrhea, any process capable of destroying the part of the hypothalamic-pituitary axis responsible for gonadotropin secretion can result in amenorrhea. In adults, tumors, granulomas and postpartum necrosis are the most frequent causes of pituitary destruction, whereas neoplastic and infiltrative processes account for most hypothalamic lesions.

ADRENAL DISORDERS. Any adrenal disorder capable of increasing circulating androgens may alter the hypothalamic regulation of gonadotropin release and thereby produce amenorrhea. Adrenal neoplasms, congenital adrenal hyperplasia, Cushing's disease, and ectopic adrenocorticotropic hormone (ACTH) syndrome all represent disorders in which amenorrhea may be present.

Chronic adrenal insufficiency has also been reported to cause amenorrhea. The mechanism responsible for this dysfunction remains unclear, but it may be due in part to the accompanying malnutrition that often occurs in this disease. In general, this amenorrhea can be easily reversed by adequate corticosteroid therapy. However, sometimes when adrenal disease is due to autoimmune adrenal failure, there is an accompanying destruction of the ovary as well [17].

THYROID DISORDERS. Thyrotoxicosis is often associated with a decrease in the volume of menstrual flow, and in severe cases, amenorrhea may be observed. Hypothyroidism, in contrast, usually is associated with menorrhagia resulting from anovulatory breakthrough bleeding.

INTRAUTERINE LESIONS. Secondary amenorrhea may occur following uterine curettage or postabortal or postpartum endometritis. Interestingly, total obliteration of the endometrial cavity does not always have to be present for amenorrhea to occur. In many cases, simple lysis of the adhesions can restore normal menstrual flow, although the prognosis for fertility is not good.

DIAGNOSTIC METHODS
Progesterone Test
The progesterone test consists of giving the patient 100 mg of progesterone intramuscularly, or a course of 10 mg of medroxyprogesterone acetate orally for 5 days and observing if menstrual bleeding occurs within the following week. If withdrawal bleeding occurs, it indicates not only that the endometrium is sensitive to hormonal changes but also that enough estrogen has been present to stimulate the endometrium so that progesterone withdrawal results in detectable vaginal bleeding. Moreover, withdrawal bleeding also implies that the pituitary-hypothalamic axis is capable of stimulating the ovary to produce estrogen. A positive withdrawal response, therefore, verifies the integrity of the entire system, short of ovulation, and suggests that the complex hormonal interactions required for ovulation are functionally disordered.

Estrogen-Progesterone Test
The estrogen-progesterone test is usually reserved for those nonpregnant patients who fail to have menstrual bleeding following the progesterone test. It is designed to evaluate the functional capacity of the uterine endometrium. The test consists of the oral administration of 0.1 mg of ethinyl estradiol or 1.25 mg of conjugated estrogen daily for 20 days and then medroxyprogesterone acetate, 10 mg daily, for 5 days. If withdrawal bleeding occurs within a week following this course of therapy, it indicates that the previous lack of response to progesterone alone was due to ovarian or pituitary failure. If no withdrawal bleeding occurs following the estrogen-progesterone therapy, an endometrial abnormality is present.

Prolactin
Radioimmunoassay (RIA) values for prolactin normally range from 0 to 30 ng/ml. Levels greater than 200 ng/ml are very suggestive of the presence of prolactin-secreting tumor, 100 to 200 ng/ml are suggestive, and 30 to 100 ng/ml are equivocal. There is no major diurnal variation.

Gonadotropins
RIA has proved to be a sensitive and precise method of measuring gonadotropins in the serum and urine of both adults and children. RIA results are expressed in terms of standards obtained from purified extracts of pituitaries or urine from postmenopausal women. It is important to recognize that the diagnostic value of a random single serum gonadotropin sample is often limited by the considerable fluctuation in gonadotropin levels that occurs throughout the day [12]. This variation occurs because the pituitary has an episodic secretion pattern. For this reason, many investigators recommend that a 24-hour urine collection for gonadotropins be obtained instead [1], whereas others favor two to four serum samples drawn at 15- to 20-minute intervals.

Estrogens
Sensitive, precise immunoassays are now also available for measuring plasma estradiol [23]. If an assessment of the daily estrogen secretion rate is needed, however, a 24-hour urine measurement of total estrogens can also be obtained.

Buccal Smear
Buccal smears provide a readily accessible source of somatic cells that can be stained to determine the chromosomal sex of an individual. Cells with more than one X chromosome will have a detectable chromatin mass (Barr body) on the inner surface of the nuclear membrane. Patients with only one X chromosome will have no Barr body evident. Normal females will have Barr bodies evident in at least 25% of the nuclei in a buccal smear.

Fluorescent Y Test
The Y chromosome, when present, can also be specifically identified in mucosal cells by fluorescent staining with quinacrine. Using the buccal smear in this manner, one can categorize patients with primary amenorrhea into three major groups: (1) Barr body positive and Y chromatin negative (XX), (2) Barr body negative and Y chromatin negative (XO), and (3) Barr body negative and Y chromatin positive (XY).

Chromosome Analysis (Karyotype)
A karyotype is the systematized arrangement of metaphase chromosomes from a single cell. In contrast to the buccal smear, karyotyping provides a precise morphologic characterization of the individual chromosome and allows more subtle genetic defects to be detected.

H-Y Antigen
The H-Y antigen is a cell surface antigen that reliably indicates the presence of Y chromosomal material. This antigen may be useful in genetic

disorders in which virilizing features are present in the absence of an identifiable Y chromosome.

Clomiphene Stimulation Test

Clomiphene is an antiestrogen that blocks feedback of estrogen at the hypothalamus, leading to stimulation of LH release by the pituitary. It is useful in determining the integrity of the hypothalamic-pituitary-ovarian axis. Clomiphene is administered orally in doses of 50 mg twice daily for 7 days. Patients with a normal hypothalamic-pituitary axis will demonstrate markedly increased LH and FSH levels after the course of therapy. A lack of response suggests pituitary or hypothalamic disease.

Gonadotropin-Releasing Hormone Stimulation Test

Gonadotropin-releasing hormone (GnRH), also known as luteinizing hormone–releasing hormone (LHRH), is a decapeptide secreted by the hypothalamus that stimulates LH and, to a lesser degree, FSH release from the pituitary. Synthetic GnRH is administered intravenously at a dose of 100 μg, with blood samples obtained at − 10, 0, 30, and 60 minutes. Normal patients exhibit a 5- to 10-fold rise in LH. Patients with pituitary disease show no response. Patients with hypothalamic disease show a rise in LH but this may require repeated injections in patients with long-standing disease.

DISCUSSION

The rational selection and interpretation of diagnostic studies in the evaluation of amenorrhea are largely dependent on information gained from the history and physical examination. Since most cases of amenorrhea encountered clinically are of the secondary type (Fig. 11-1), the patient's history should help identify any previous drug or hormone therapy, nutritional abnormalities, or psychiatric problems. Details regarding neurologic deficiencies, visual field defects, galactorrhea, or acral changes may be particularly useful in characterizing organic CNS lesions. The obstetric and gynecologic history may be invaluable in determining the etiology of various endometrial disorders. Finally, the family history may identify certain diseases, such as congenital adrenal hyperplasia and PCOD, which often occur as inherited disorders.

The extragenital portion of the physical examination should clearly establish the nutritional status of the patient, as well as identify specific features such as temporal balding, hirsutism, hyperpigmentation, breast atrophy, thyromegaly, centripetal obesity, and striae. The pelvic examination should begin with a careful evaluation of the external genitalia and should specifically note whether clitoromegaly is present. The uterus and adnexae should be palpated with sufficient care to diagnose an unsuspected pregnancy, PCOD, or an ovarian tumor. The use of ultrasonography may aid in the identification of ovarian enlargement. On sub-

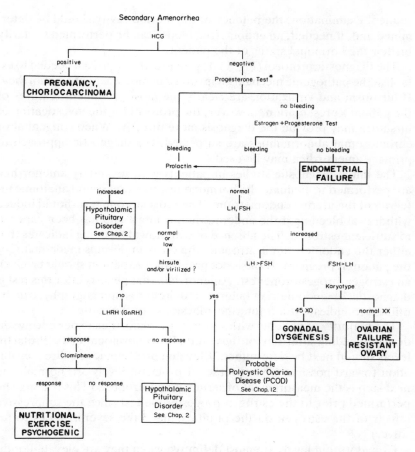

Figure 11-1. Diagnostic protocol: Secondary amenorrhea. HCG, human chorionic gonadotropin; LH, luteinizing hormone; FSH, follicle-stimulating hormone; LHRH, luteinizing hormone-releasing hormone; GnRH, gonadotropin-releasing hormone. *Obtain LH, FSH.

sequent examination, the patency of the uterine cavity should be determined and, if needed, an endometrial biopsy can be performed to clarify further the hormonal status of the patient.

The diagnostic protocol (Fig. 11-1) provides the approach needed to establish the pathogenic mechanism involved in most cases of amenorrhea. If hirsutism and virilization are clearly the most prominent features of the patient's presentation, however, the protocol for the investigation of hirsutism may provide the diagnosis more directly. When congenital or chromosomal abnormalities are suspected, the diagnostic approach to primary amenorrhea may be used.

The initial diagnostic studies in patients with secondary amenorrhea are performed to evaluate the hormone responsiveness and anatomic integrity of the uterine endometrium. The progesterone test should induce withdrawal bleeding if the endometrium is intact and has been exposed to sufficient estrogen. The absence of withdrawal bleeding indicates that either the endometrium is atrophic, the estrogen level is inadequate, or the patient is pregnant. If she is not pregnant, the patient should be given an estrogen-progesterone test. Amenorrhea that persists after this test is diagnostic of endometrial failure, and hysterosalpingography can be utilized to indicate if intrauterine adhesions are the cause.

The majority of patients with secondary amenorrhea experience withdrawal bleeding after one of these initial two hormonal tests. Prolactin levels should next be determined. Elevated prolactin levels direct evaluation toward possible CNS disease. If prolactin levels are normal, the next step is the measurement of serum gonadotropins. (This test may be performed prior to the estrogen-progesterone test since the suppressive effects of the estrogen on the pituitary may take several weeks to resolve.)

Gonadotropin levels are most definitive when they are elevated, indicating ovarian failure [22]. Most patients with secondary amenorrhea, however, have gonadotropin levels that are low or normal [16,27]. If there is also clinical evidence of hyperandrogenism, a search for PCOD or other causes of androgen excess should be initiated. If hyperandrogenism is not present, the possibility of a pituitary tumor should be considered, particularly if there is simultaneous evidence of other endocrine dysfunction. Only when all of these diagnoses have been excluded and there is documented evidence of normal adrenal (17-ketosteroids [17-KS], pregnanetriol, and cortisol levels), thyroid, and pituitary function (prolactin) can a diagnosis of hypothalamic-nutritional cause be considered and investigated using LHRH and clomiphene stimulation (Fig. 11-1).

Clinically, primary amenorrhea (Fig. 11-2) tends to present much less frequently than does secondary amenorrhea. However, when it does occur, the history and physical examination must be modified to encompass the congenital or genetic causes of amenorrhea discussed earlier in this chapter.

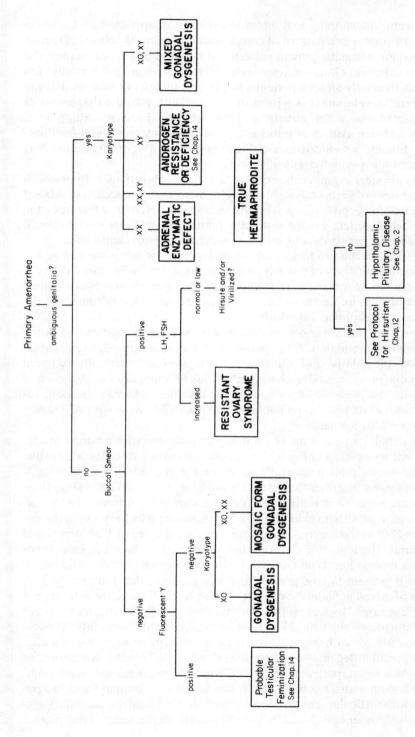

Figure 11-2. Diagnostic protocol: Primary amenorrhea. LH, luteinizing hormone; FSH, follicle-stimulating hormone.

Careful questioning may provide evidence of specific familial endocrine disorders or a pattern of constitutionally delayed puberty. Data on the patient's somatic growth pattern and pubertal development may also prove valuable. Gonadal dysgenesis, hypopituitarism, and hypothyroidism all distinctly affect a patient's height and skeletal growth. A delay in pubertal development is typical of patients with gonadal dysgenesis or ovarian failure. Alternatively, a history of normal breast development, despite absent axillary or pubic hair growth, suggests testicular feminization. Finally, a well-documented history of hirsutism or virilization may point to a hyperandrogenic disorder.

On physical examination, one of the major objectives is to establish the amount of secondary sexual development that has occurred. Absent or deficient secondary sexual features are characteristic of most of the gonadal disorders except testicular feminization. Conversely, clinical evidence of breast development, together with pubic and axillary hair, suggests that the production of gonadal steroids is adequate and makes constitutional delay of puberty or a local vaginal or endometrial disorder more likely. Nonsexually related physical findings of importance include the short stature and somatic anomalies of Turner's syndrome and the anosmia of Kallman's syndrome.

Last, but perhaps most important, are the findings that can be noted on pelvic examination. If the pelvic examination is normal, vaginal aplasia, uterine aplasia, and testicular feminization can be virtually excluded from diagnostic consideration. Ambiguous or anomalous genitalia often indicate the presence of an androgenic disorder, whereas a normal vagina and cervix without palpable ovaries are highly suggestive of gonadal dysgenesis or agenesis.

Gonadal dysgenesis may be initially investigated with a buccal smear. A positive smear confirms the female genotype, whereas a negative smear necessitates a careful search for the possible presence of a Y chromosome by either fluorescent Y analysis or formal karotyping. Both tests are negative in patients with classic Turner's syndrome. In the virilized patient with no evidence of a Y chromosome by karyotype, the use of the H-Y antigen may serve to confirm the presence of Y chromosomal material. Evidence for the X chromosome may be found in individuals with a mosaic karotype (XO/XX), whereas evidence of the Y chromosome is present in true genetic males (e.g., testicular feminization). A form of mixed gonadal dysgenesis with an XO/XY karotype is found but is characterized by ambiguous external genitalia. Such information is not only diagnostically valuable but also has significant therapeutic implications. Patients with mixed gonadal dysgenesis are at high risk of malignant gonadal degeneration, whereas those with Turner's syndrome are not. As a result, patients with mixed gonadal dysgenesis are usually subjected to immediate gonadectomy, whereas the abdominal testes in a patient with testicular feminization are not removed until the secondary sexual development produced by the estradiol from the testes is complete.

The presence of ambiguous genitalia or clitoromegaly in an amenorrheic patient requires an aggressive investigation as outlined. The initial objective is to identify the genetic sex of the patient. In the genetic female, adrenal causes of ambiguous genitalia should then be investigated. Urinary 17-KS, 17-hydroxysteroids and pregnanetriol values, and plasma 17-hydroxyprogesterone levels are determined to evaluate adrenal function (see Chap. 12). If any of these values are elevated, investigation for a specific enzymatic abnormality of steroid synthesis should be initiated. These data, when combined with the information obtained from the visualization and biopsy of the gonad [4], should be sufficient to determine whether the patient has mixed gonadal dysgenesis, partial androgen insensitivity, or true hermaphroditism.

REFERENCES

1. Abraham, G. E., et al. Simultaneous radioimmunoassay of plasma FSH, LH, progesterone, 17-OH progesterone and estradiol 17-B during the menstrual cycle. *J. Clin. Endocrinol. Metab.* 34:312–318, 1972.
2. Baird, D. T., et al. Pituitary ovarian relationship in polycystic ovary syndrome. *J. Clin. Endocrinol. Metab.* 45:798–809, 1977.
3. Bauer, E. R., et al. Female runners and secondary amenorrhea: Correlation with age, parity, mileage, and plasma hormonal and sex-hormone binding globular concentrations. *Fertil. Steril.* 36:183, 1981.
4. Black, W. P., and Govan, A. D. T. Laparoscopy and gonadal biopsy for assessment of gonadal function in primary amenorrhea. *Br. Med. J.* 1:672–675, 1972.
5. Braunstein, G. D. Female Reproductive Disorders. In J. M. Hershman (Ed.), *Endocrine Physiology*. Philadelphia: Lea & Febiger, 1977. Pp. 147–175.
6. Chapman, R., Sutcliff, S., and Malpas, J. Cytotoxic-induced ovarian failure in women with Hodgkin's disease. *J.A.M.A.* 242:1877–1881, 1979.
7. Dole, E., Gerlack, D. J., and Wilhite, H. L. Menstrual dysfunction in distance runners. *Obstet. Gynecol.* 54:47–53, 1979.
8. Frish, R. E., et al. Delayed menarche and amenorrhea of college athletes in relation to age of onset of training. *J.A.M.A.* 246:1559–1563, 1981.
9. Frisch, R. F., Wyshak, G., and Vincent, L. Delayed menarche and amenorrhea in ballet dancers. *N. Engl. J. Med.* 303:17–19, 1980.
10. Ginsburg, J., Scadding, G., and Havard, C. W. H. Primary amenorrhea: The ambiguous non-entity. *Br. Med. J.* 2:32–35, 1977.
11. Giusti, G., et al. Classification and Procedure for the Evaluation of Amenorrhea: The Clinician's View. In V. H. T. James, M. Serio, and G. Giusti (Eds.), *The Endocrine Function of the Human Ovary*. New York: Academic Press, 1976. Pp. 267–273.
12. Goldenberg, R. L., et al. Gonadotropins in women with amenorrhea. *Am. J. Obstet. Gynecol.* 116:1003–1007, 1973.
13. Golditen, L. M. Post contraceptive amenorrhea. *Obstet. Gynecol.* 39:903–908, 1972.
14. Greenblatt, R. M., and Mahesh, V. B. The androgenic polycystic ovary. *Am. J. Obstet. Gynecol.* 125:712–726, 1976.
15. Griffin, J. E., and Wilson, J. D. The syndromes of androgen resistance. *N. Engl. J. Med.* 302:198–209, 1980.
16. Hirvonen, E. Etiology, clinical features and progress in secondary amenorrhea. *Int. J. Fertil.* 22:69–76, 1977.

17. Irvine, W. J., and Barnes, E. W. Addison's disease, ovarian failure and hypoparathyroidism. *Clin. Endocrinol. Metab.* 4:379–434, 1979.
18. Kase, N. G., and Speroff, L. The Ovary. In P. K. Bondy and L. E. Rosenberg (Eds.), *Metabolic Control and Disease.* Philadelphia: Saunders, 1980. Pp. 1598–1608.
19. Kenmann, E., and Jones, J. R. Hyperprolactinemia and primary amenorrhea. *Obstet. Gynecol.* 54:692–694, 1979.
20. Keye, W. R., et al. Prolactin secreting pituitary adenomas. III. Frequency and diagnosis in amenorrhea-galactorrhea. *J.A.M.A.* 244:1329–1332, 1980.
21. Kleinberg, D., Noel, G., and Frantz, A. Galactorrhea: A study of 235 cases, including 48 with pituitary tumors. *N. Engl. J. Med.* 296:579–600, 1977.
22. Kletzky, O. A., Davajan, V., and Nakamura, R. M. Classification of secondary amenorrhea based on distinct hormonal patterns. *J. Clin. Endocrinol. Metab.* 41:660–668, 1975.
23. Korenmann, S. G., et al. Estradiol radioimmunoassay without chromatography: Procedure, validation and normal values. *J. Clin. Endocrinol. Metab.* 38:718–720, 1974.
24. Rebar, R., Judd, H. L., and Yen, S. S. C. Characterization of the inappropriate gonadotropin secretion in polycystic ovary syndrome. *J. Clin. Invest.* 57:1320–1329, 1976.
25. Rowe, T. C., Shearman, R. P., and Fraser, I. S. Antecedent factors and outcome in amenorrhea and galactorrhea. *Obstet. Gynecol.* 54:535–543, 1979.
26. Schlechte, J., et al. Prolactin secreting pituitary tumors in amenorrheic women: A comprehensive study. *Endocrine Rev.* 1:295–308, 1980.
27. Smith, R. A. Investigation and classification of oligomenorrhea and amenorrhea. *Med. Clin. North. Am.* 56:931–936, 1972.
28. Spitz, I. M., Diamant, Y., and Rosen, E. Isolated gonadotropin deficiency: A heterogeneous syndrome. *N. Engl. J. Med.* 290:10–15, 1974.
29. Van Campenhout, J., et al. Amenorrhea following the use of oral contraceptives. *Fertil. Steril.* 28:728–736, 1977.
30. Van Campenhout, J., Van Clair, R., and Maraghi, K. Gonadotropin resistant ovaries in primary amenorrhea. *Obstet. Gynecol.* 40:6–12, 1972.
31. Vigersky, R. A., et al. Hypothalamic dysfunction in secondary amenorrhea associated with simple weight loss. *N. Engl. J. Med.* 297:1141–1145, 1977.
32. Warren, M. P. The effect of exercise on pubertal progression and reproductive functions in girls. *J. Clin. Endocrinol. Metab.* 51:1150–1157, 1980.
33. Yen, S. S. C. Polycystic Ovary Syndrome. In S. S. C. Yen and R. B. Jaffe (Eds.), *Reproductive Endocrinology.* Philadelphia: Saunders, 1978. Pp. 306–319.
34. Zarate, A., et al. Premature menopause. *Am. J. Obstet. Gynecol.* 106:110–114, 1970.

12   Hirsutism

William T. Cave, Jr.
William F. Streck

CLINICAL CONSIDERATIONS

The quantity and distribution of hair in women vary widely with family and ethnic backgrounds. What is considered excessive hair growth for one woman may be quite normal for another. A definition of *hirsutism,* then, must be a relative one, yet provide some guidelines for clinical decision making. A pragmatic approach is to define hirsutism as either excessive hair growth at normal sites (face, periareolar areas) or the presence of hair growth at abnormal sites (chin, chest, lumbosacral area). Even this definition must be modified to include the perception of the patient. A woman presenting with complaints of excessive hair requires evaluation, as the process has reached a stage abnormal to her body image. Whatever the initial stimulus for evaluation, on a statistical basis hyperandrogenism is the most common cause of hirsutism. Common causes of hirsutism are listed in Table 12-1.

Virilization is a clinical syndrome of which hirsutism is one component. In addition to excess hair, other signs and symptoms of masculinization are present. Such findings include temporal balding, clitoromegaly, increased muscle mass, and deepening of the voice. Conversely, feminine features are diminished, with breast atrophy and amenorrhea often present.

Initially, during the history one should attempt to exclude the possibility that the patient's increased hair is either the result of some recent drug therapy (e. g., Dilantin, diazoxide, minoxidil, adrenocorticotropic hormone [ACTH], anabolic steroids, or progestational agents) or the expression of a familial trait. Any documented family history of pathologic hirsutism, however, deserves serious attention, as diseases such as polycystic ovarian disease (PCOD) and congenital adrenal hyperplasia (CAH) often follow distinct genetic patterns [21].

The type and pattern of hair growth should be characterized in detail. Specific information should be sought regarding the age of onset, rapidity of progression, and association with virilizing features. Rapidly progressive hirsutism with severe virilization suggests the presence of an adrenal or ovarian tumor. Slowly progressive hirsutism beginning at puberty usually reflects a less severe disorder such as idiopathic hirsutism, PCOD, or CAH.

The physical examination should be used to substantiate and amplify the descriptive information obtained from the history. Observations on the presence or absence of such signs of virilization as a male pattern of pubic hair, clitoromegaly, breast atrophy, and deepening of the voice will provide a reasonable estimate of the level of androgen excess. Similarly, other physical findings may predict the location of the pathologic

Table 12-1. Causes of Hirsutism

Idiopathic hirsutism
Ovarian androgen excess
  Polycystic ovarian disease (PCOD)
  Ovarian stromal hyperplasia
  Ovarian hilus cell hyperplasia
  Ovarian tumors
Adrenal androgen excess
  Late-onset congenital adrenal hyperplasia (CAH)
  Adrenal tumors
  Increased ACTH secretion
Drug-induced hirsutism
Other disorders
  Porphyria
  Starvation

---

lesion. For example, hypertension associated with centripetal obesity and striae may signal the presence of Cushing's syndrome. An adnexal mass noted on pelvic examination may establish the existence of an ovarian lesion.

The hormonal evaluation of hirsutism focuses on the two organ systems that produce androgens—the ovaries and the adrenals—and three major androgenic hormones—testosterone, androstenedione, and dehydroepiandrostenedione (DHEA). Normally in the female, approximately 25% of the testosterone is of adrenal origin and 25% of ovarian origin. The remaining 50% is a result of approximately equal ovarian and adrenal secretion of prehormones, primarily androstenedione, with subsequent conversion to testosterone [1,7,11]. DHEA and its conjugate (DHEA-S) are predominantly of adrenal origin. Increased androgen production from either or both sources may result in saturation of hepatic mechanisms for androgen metabolism with consequent metabolism of androgens at extrahepatic sites such as the skin [24,28].

Diagnostic evaluation is initially directed at determining the most likely site of androgen overproduction. The three most common causes of hirsutism are idiopathic disease, PCOD, and adrenal disease. These three conditions form a continuum of disordered production of androgens in women. At one end are the ovarian diseases, characterized by excess production of testosterone and its precursors. PCOD serves as a model for this disorder. At the other end of the continuum, adrenal diseases such as CAH account for the androgen excess. Idiopathic hirsutism lies somewhere between these two, more closely approximating the ovarian overproduction disorders in most studies [14,15,27].

Idiopathic or Benign Hirsutism

Idiopathic or *benign hirsutism* is a term used to describe the large group of hirsute women with normal or minimally elevated urinary 17-ketosteroid (17-KS) values, normal cortisol levels, no ovarian enlargement, and no evidence of an adrenal or ovarian tumor. The fact that most of these patients have slightly elevated plasma levels of "free" androstenedione and/or testosterone, however, suggests that they do have some form of androgen dysfunction [5,11]. Furthermore, direct metabolic studies show that these patients actually have excessive testosterone production rates, and in most patients the ovary is the dominant androgen source [14,15,27]. This disorder, which accounts for most cases of hirsutism, may be diagnosed only after the exclusion of other causes.

Polycystic Ovarian Disease

From the earlier description of a clinical syndrome of sterility, amenorrhea, and hirsutism in women with enlarged cystic ovaries (by Stein-Leventhal), a concept of overlapping ovarian and adrenal dysfunction with variable clinical features has emerged. This broader syndrome is recognized as PCOD, a small proportion of which meets the classic Stein-Leventhal criteria.

The clinical symptoms vary. The onset may follow normal menarche and an interval of normal menstruation. The most frequent features are sterility, hirsutism, and amenorrhea or oligomenorrhea. True virilization is possible but not common. The patient is often a young woman with a recent history of menstrual irregularity who seeks advice because of sterility or worsening hirsutism. The irregular menses may serve to distinguish these individuals from those with idiopathic hirsutism. Late-onset CAH, Cushing's syndrome, and virilizing adrenal or ovarian tumors must be considered.

Excess production of androstenedione and testosterone characterizes the laboratory picture. Data suggest that these active androgens are primarily of ovarian origin. The exact cause of this androgenic dysfunction is not clear; however, specific gonadotropin abnormalities are involved in its perpetuation [16,30]. Free testosterone levels, when measured, are high. Androstenedione, estrone, and luteinizing hormone (LH) levels may also be elevated. The increased LH and lower follicle-stimulating hormone (FSH) levels provide the abnormal LH : FSH ratio ($>2 : 1$) that has been described in this syndrome. Urinary 17-KS are variably increased.

Late-Onset Congenital Adrenal Hyperplasia

A small number of hirsute women have been discovered to have a defect in cortisol synthesis due to an inherited deficiency of either one of two enzymes: 21-hydroxylase or 11-hydroxylase. The resulting mild cortisol deficiency that occurs in these patients induces an increase in ACTH secretion that ultimately results in the overproduction of 17-hydroxy (17-

OH) pregnenolone, 17-OH progesterone, and its metabolite, pregnane-triol.

Interestingly, in spite of the presumed genetic etiology of this defect, its clinical expression is delayed until after puberty, when these patients typically experience a slowly progressive form of hirsutism commonly associated with oligomenorrhea [6,10]. Laboratory testing reveals that these patients have elevated plasma levels of testosterone and androstenedione. Increased 24-hour urinary pregnanetriol excretion is diagnostic of this disorder. Cortisol blood levels, however, are usually normal, indicating that the defect is mild and has been well compensated. The androgenic abnormalities can be readily corrected by pituitary suppression with low-dose dexamethasone.

Severe virilization, marked elevations of serum testosterone levels, or very high urinary 17-KS values should raise the question of ovarian or adrenal tumors.

Ovarian Tumors

Pathologically, the most common androgen-secreting ovarian tumors are arrhenoblastomas, hilus cell tumors, and lipoid cell tumors [13,22]. These very rare tumors usually synthesize large amounts of testosterone, and severe virilization is commonly produced. Normally, these tumors are neither ACTH nor gonadotropin dependent; however, rare cases of ovarian tumors responding to exogenous estrogen (gonadotropin suppression) have been reported.

Ovarian Stromal Hyperplasia

Ovarian stromal hyperplasia, a postmenopausal disorder, is associated with ovarian hyperplasia and androgen excess. The pathogenesis of this dysfunction is unclear, but it may be related to the rise in LH levels that occurs with menopause. This lesion, like PCOD, appears to be gonadotropin dependent [7].

Adrenal Tumors

Both benign and malignant tumors of the adrenal cortex are capable of producing hyperandrogenism [22]. Hirsutism and virilization are often rapidly progressive in patients with such tumors. Laboratory studies characteristically show marked elevations in urinary 17-KS (see Chap. 8).

Bilateral Adrenal Hyperplasia (Cushing's Disease)

The hypothalamic-pituitary dysfunction of Cushing's disease alters the sensitivity of the normal feedback system responsible for regulating ACTH production. The subsequent rise in ACTH to inappropriately high levels causes adrenocortical hyperfunction. Symptoms of androgenic, glucocorticoid, and mineralocorticoid hormone excess result (see Chap. 8).

Other Disorders
A number of drugs are associated with the production of hirsutism. These drugs may be subdivided into those that produce predictable effects, such as anabolic steroids, ACTH, and progestational agents, and those such as minoxidil and phenytoin that produce hirsutism for unknown reasons. In addition, there are a number of disorders associated with increased hair growth in which a direct cause-and-effect relationship has not been established. These disorders include porphyria, starvation, malabsorption, and hypertrichosis lanugosa. The last disorder technically should not be included under hirsutism since it applies to a generalized increase in hair growth without terminal hair production.

DIAGNOSTIC METHODS
Urinary 17-Ketosteroids
Weak androgens possessing a keto group on carbon-17 such as androstenedione and DHEA are measured as 17-KS. These 17-KS normally provide an index of combined adrenal and ovarian androgenic activity. It must be remembered that urinary testosterone is not included in this measurement. Measurement of 17-KS alone is not an adequate screen for suspected hyperandrogenism [12,19].

Urinary 17-Hydroxycorticosteroids and 17-Ketogenic Steroids
Urinary 17-hydroxycorticosteroids (17-OHCS) and 17-ketogenic steroids (17-KGS) measure nonandrogenic steroids possessing a hydroxyl group on carbon-17. Certain steroids (e.g., 17-OH progesterone and pregnanetriol) included in the 17-KGS determination are excluded from the 17-OHCS analysis by the Glenn Nelson method (see Chap. 7). Patients with CAH due to 21-hydroxylase deficiency, therefore, characteristically have elevated 17-KGS but normal 17-OHCS. In contrast, patients with Cushing's syndrome (hypercortisolism) have elevations in both their 17-KGS and 17-OHCS values.

Urinary "Free" Cortisol
Urinary free (unconjugated) cortisol, like 17-OHCS and 17-KGS, measures adrenocortical function. This free cortisol reflects the nonprotein-bound cortisol in the plasma and correlates well with the cortisol secretion rate. Elevation of urinary free cortisol is usually considered a very specific indicator of pathologic hypercortisolism (Cushing's syndrome) [4].

17-Hydroxyprogesterone—Basal/Stimulated
Normally, 17-hydroxyprogesterone (17-OHP) is metabolized by 21-hydroxylase to 11-desoxycortisol, the immediate precursor of cortisol. In classic CAH with 21-hydroxylase or 11-hydroxylase deficiency, the basal levels of 17-OHP are elevated.

The use of ACTH infusions and the measurement of the 17-OHP response have now demonstrated that a certain percentage of hirsute women, though having normal basal 17-OHP levels, manifest dramatic 17-OHP elevations after ACTH administration [3,10,18]. This diagnostic tool has been used to identify the most commonly encountered adult form of CAH, late-onset 21-hydroxylase deficiency. The 17-OHP response in this disorder contrasts to the elevated basal levels in classic CAH or the milder abnormalities seen in 21-hydroxylase deficiency heterozygotes, idiopathic hirsutism, or the PCOD syndrome [3,18].

Normal 17-OHP levels range from 60 ng/dl in the follicular phase to 300 ng/dl in the luteal phase. Following ACTH stimulation using 0.25 mg of synthetic ACTH as an intravenous bolus, most normal subjects will have a 17-OHP peak of less than 300 ng/dl at 30 and 60 minutes [3,18].

Urinary Pregnanetriol
Pregnanetriol is a metabolic derivative of 17-OH progesterone. Elevated urinary levels of this metabolite are often helpful in identifying patients with CAH due to either 11- or 21-hydroxylase deficiency.

Dexamethasone Suppression Test
In the investigation of hirsutism, the standard low-dose (2 mg per day) dexamethasone test has been modified by extending the drug administration to 4 [12] to 7 [11] days. This low dose of dexamethasone is sufficient to suppress ACTH secretion and will normalize the elevated 17-KS and pregnanetriol characteristic of CAH. However, in other forms of hirsutism, studies have shown that dexamethasone suppression of 17-KS does not correlate well with suppression of plasma androgens [12]. For this reason, measurement of plasma androgens is suggested before and after the dexamethasone suppression test. The criteria for normal suppression are not clearly established. Some authors have used 50% suppression [14], whereas others suggest that after 7 days of dexamethasone, serum free testosterone should be less than 8 pg/ml and total testosterone less than 60 ng/dl [11]. Those patients who do not have suppression of plasma androgens are considered to have ovarian hyperandrogenism (PCOD and variants).

Plasma Testosterone
Plasma testosterone as measured by radioimmunoassay (RIA) is 99% protein bound, primarily to testosterone-estrogen binding globulin (TeBG). A direct measurement of the TeBG binding capacity, or the dialyzable testosterone, may be needed to determine the amount of physiologically active or free testosterone actually present [23,25,26]. Since androgens may decrease TeBG (as estrogens may increase it), the hyperandrogenic female may have a normal testosterone, a lower TeBG, and a consequent increase in the free or active testosterone level.

This free or unbound testosterone shows an excellent correlation with the testosterone production rate. The free testosterone determination has emerged as the best single laboratory assessment of androgen production in women [23].

Plasma Androstenedione
Plasma androstenedione can be measured by RIA. Due to its mixed adrenal-ovarian origin, it shows both a diurnal variation and a mid-cycle surge [1]. Knowledge of the plasma androstenedione level is diagnostically helpful because a large proportion of both testosterone and dihydrotestosterone is derived from the peripheral conversion of androstenedione.

Dehydroepiandrosterone (DHEA)/DHEA-S
The adrenal glands produce 80% of DHEA, most of which is found in the circulation in the sulfate conjugate DHEA-S. Plasma DHEA levels in normal women range from 200 to 500 ng/dl. A diurnal rhythm in secretion is found, as with other adrenal hormones. Increased DHEA levels in hirsute women are suggestive of adrenal disease, although in some instances of PCOD increased DHEA levels have been noted in ovarian venous drainage [7].

Ovarian Suppression Test
Analogous to the dexamethasone suppression test, the ovarian suppression test is designed to evaluate the degree of hypothalamic-pituitary involvement in the hypersecretion of androgenic steroids. The test consists of giving an oral contraceptive in a standard cyclic manner and then obtaining a repeat plasma testosterone and androstenedione level during the third week of therapy [8]. In patients with gonadotropin-dependent hyperandrogenism (i.e., PCOD), the plasma androgen levels may fall into the normal range, whereas in patients with adrenal disorders or autonomous hormone-secreting lesions, no significant response will be noted even after repeated cycles. Caution is warranted in interpretation, however, since estrogen may induce a net increase in TeBG, so that the resultant total testosterone may be unchanged. The biologically active free testosterone is, however, lowered [8,9].

Serum Luteinizing Hormone and Follicle-Stimulating Hormone
The gonadotropins LH and FSH can be measured directly in the serum by RIA. They are often particularly useful in characterizing certain types of gonadal dysfunction, such as PCOD, in which, typically, the LH levels are high and the FSH levels are low.

DISCUSSION
Current concepts of hormone action indicate that it is the amount of dihydrotestosterone synthesized intracellularly and available to the hair

follicles that ultimately regulates the androgenic stimulation of hair growth [24,28,29]. At present, it is not clinically feasible to measure intracellular dihydrotestosterone; therefore, the circulating adrenal and ovarian steroid precursors essential for dihydrotestosterone synthesis are measured instead. Hirsutism due to hyperandrogenism is always associated with the increased production of at least one of these precursor androgens (i.e., testosterone, androstenedione, or DHEA) [5,7,11,16], whereas urinary 17-KS levels are often normal [19].

In this context, plasma androgens are more reliable indicators of subtle hyperandrogenism (Fig. 12-1). Although some suggest that 17-KS are not necessary in the first phase of evaluation [11], it is often advisable to be thorough in the initial evaluation rather than to prolong the investigation. Since the diagnosis of idiopathic hirsutism requires the exclusion of the less common disorders, including Cushing's syndrome and adrenal tumors, measurement of urinary 17-KS and 17-OHCS (or free cortisol) is reasonably added to plasma androgen determinations. If all studies (testosterone, androstenedione, 17-KS, 17-OHCS) fall in the normal range, there is little likelihood of a serious androgenic disorder, and idiopathic hirsutism becomes the most probable diagnosis.

Because excess androgens may lower the TeBG, the total testosterone level may not accurately reflect the amount of free or active hormone [2,20]. The measurement of free testosterone or TeBG may, however, be used to detect these subtle androgen abnormalities [11,26]. Recent studies have emphasized that free testosterone values are almost always elevated in hirsutism, whereas total testosterone values are increased only 40 to 50% of the time [11,23].

The normal fluctuation in plasma androgen levels must also be considered when studying the hirsute female. The variability of plasma testosterone levels may be greater in hirsute women than in normals. Rosenfield demonstrated that any single total testosterone level fell within only 38% of the 24-hour mean level for a given individual. The best short-term estimate of the 24-hour plasma testosterone level was obtained from the mean of four samples over a 3-hour period [26]. The estimates for free and total testosterone were not significantly different; however, free testosterone levels were more consistently elevated.

Although PCOD is clearly the most frequent cause of ovarian hyperandrogenism, other etiologies must always be considered (see Fig. 12-1). Androgen-producing ovarian tumors do occasionally occur and may be associated with greatly elevated plasma testosterone (>250 ng/dl) and/or androstenedione (>800 ng/dl) levels. Normally, such patients will have clinically apparent virilization at the time of diagnosis.

Adrenal dysfunction is not a frequent cause of hyperandrogenism, but of those adrenal diseases that are associated with hirsutism, late-onset CAH probably is the one most frequently observed [3]. Generally, the biochemical defects involved in this disorder are relatively mild and well

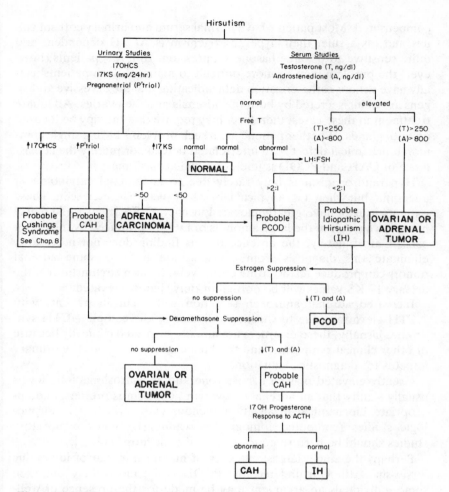

Figure 12-1. Diagnostic protocol: Hirsutism. 17OHCS, 17-hydroxycorticoids; 17KS, 17-ketosteroids; FSH, follicle-stimulating hormone; LH, luteinizing hormone; CAH, congenital adrenal hyperplasia; PCOD, polycystic ovarian disease; ACTH, adrenocorticotropic hormone.

compensated. Most patients have normal serum and urinary cortisol values and, as a rule, their hyperandrogenism is ACTH dependent and quite sensitive to dexamethasone suppression. In a few patients, however, the problem may be more difficult to manage. Such patients usually have venous catheterization data indicating that the excessive androgens are being secreted by both the adrenals and the ovaries. Adequate treatment in these cases, therefore, may require that therapy be focused on both glands. Whether patients with such problems have a single common biochemical defect, two interrelated defects, or merely the coexistence of CAH and PCOD is undetermined at this time.

Hyperandrogenism is only rarely due to an adrenal carcinoma or adenoma, but when it is, a typical laboratory picture is often seen. These patients usually have greatly elevated urinary 17-KS levels (>50 mg/24 hours) as a result of the large amounts of DHEA produced by the tumor cells. Unfortunately, the absence of this finding does not necessarily eliminate this diagnosis from consideration because some adrenal tumors can produce testosterone exclusively. In such circumstances, the urinary 17-KS values will be normal or only slightly elevated.

Increased adrenal androgen secretion will occur in patients with ACTH elevations due to Cushing's disease or the ectopic ACTH syndrome. Usually, these disorders are already suspected clinically because of other clinical symptoms, and the hirsutism per se is not the primary impetus for diagnostic evaluation.

Greatly elevated plasma testosterone and/or androstenedione levels usually signify that an adrenal or ovarian neoplasm is present, and appropriate biochemical localization (venous catheterization), morphologic studies (computed tomography scanning), and/or exploratory studies should be performed to confirm the diagnosis [14,15].

Perhaps the single largest category of hirsutism is that of idiopathic hirsutism. Although undetectable PCOD is the most likely cause, in some individuals an argument may be made for the presence of well-compensated CAH. The fact that an etiology is often not determined may well represent a lack of sensitivity and specificity of the laboratory studies available rather than the lack of an endocrinopathy per se. Since most cases are presumably due to excess androgen production by the ovaries, the estrogen suppression test may often serve as a reasonable first diagnostic trial. In PCOD [8] and idiopathic hirsutism [9], the use of oral contraceptives has been associated with decreased levels of testosterone and androstenedione. Unless a distinction between these disorders may be made on other grounds (LH : FSH ratio, laparoscopy), it may not be possible to make a diagnosis that is more definite than gonadotropin-dependent hyperandrogenism.

If, after two 3-week trials of oral contraceptives, no suppression of testosterone or androstenedione levels is noted, dexamethasone suppression may be used. This is necessary to assess for the possibility of a nonsuppressible ovarian or adrenal tumor and to investigate for possible mild adrenal hyperplasia. Successful suppression of plasma androgens may be further investigated by assessing the 17-OH progesterone response to ACTH. If an identifiable defect in adrenal steroid synthesis does not emerge, the diagnosis of idiopathic hirsutism again arises. In this instance, long-term therapy with dexamethasone may be considered, whereas such therapy appears to be of limited value in PCOD [17].

There are several pitfalls in the laboratory work-up of hirsutism that should be kept in mind. First, elevations in urinary 17-KS are not always a reflection of adrenal hyperandrogenism because several ovarian conditions (e.g., stromal hyperplasia, luteoma of pregnancy) can be associated with this laboratory abnormality as well. Second, it is important to remember that normal urinary 17-KS values do not exclude the presence of a testosterone-secreting adrenal tumor. Third, suppression tests must be interpreted cautiously since dexamethasone has been observed to suppress testosterone and androstenedione secretion in women with ovarian hyperandrogenism, and a few adrenal adenomas have been reported to respond to gonadotropin suppression.

When exogenous obesity is also present in patients with hirsutism, it is important to recognize that this obesity may make the interpretation of certain endocrine tests more difficult. Normal obese people, for example, frequently have elevated urinary 17-OHCS values, and therefore a urinary free cortisol value is often needed to estimate accurately adrenal function. Likewise, obese patients often have decreased serum TeBG levels with subsequently reduced total testosterone values, even when the "free" hormone fraction in the plasma is increased. In such patients, a plasma free testosterone test may be required since the total testosterone value may underestimate the amount of functional androgen present [11].

In summary, hirsutism is a common disorder in which some form of endocrinopathy is frequently present. Many cases are eventually classified as idiopathic, but this may simply reflect the current inability to define some of the more subtle endocrine abnormalities that may be present. Most of these probably represent a mild form of PCOD, but it is also quite likely that some are additional cases of unrecognized mild adrenal hyperandrogenism. The results of hormone suppression with either birth control pills or glucocorticoid therapy may be diagnostically helpful and can provide a rational basis for subsequent therapy.

REFERENCES

1. Abraham, G. E. Ovarian and adrenal contribution to peripheral androgens during the menstrual cycle. *J. Clin. Endocrinol. Metab.* 39:340–346, 1974.
2. Bardin, C. W., and Lipsett, M. D. Testosterone and androstenedione blood production rates in normal women and women with idiopathic hirsutism and polycystic ovaries. *J. Clin. Invest.* 46:891–902, 1967.

3. Crousus, G. P., et al. Late onset 21-hydroxylase deficiency mimicking idiopathic hirsutism or polycystic ovarian disease. *Ann. Intern. Med.* 96:143–148, 1982.
4. Eddy, R. L., et al. Cushing's syndrome: A prospective study of diagnostic methods. *Am. J. Med.* 55:621–630, 1973.
5. Farber, M., et al. Diagnostic evaluation of hirsutism in women. *Clin. Obstet. Gynecol.* 20:1–9, 1977.
6. Gabrilove, J. L., Sharma, D. C., and Dorfman, R. I. Adrenocortical 11-β-hydroxylase deficiency and virilism first manifest in the adult woman. *N. Engl. J. Med.* 272:1189–1194, 1965.
7. Givens, J. R. Hirsutism and hyperandrogenism. *Adv. Intern. Med.* 21:221–247, 1976.
8. Givens, J. R., et al. Dynamics of suppression and recovery of plasma FSH, LH and androstenedione and testosterone in polycystic ovarian disease using an oral contraceptive. *J. Clin. Endocrinol. Metab.* 38:727–735, 1974.
9. Givens, J. R., et al. The effectiveness of two oral contraceptives in suppressing plasma androstenedione, testosterone, LH, and FSH, and in stimulating testosterone-binding capacity in hirsute women. *Am. J. Obstet. Gynecol.* 124:333–341, 1976.
10. Guthrie, G. P., et al. Adrenal androgen excess and defective 11-hydroxylation in women with idiopathic hirsutism. *Arch. Intern. Med.* 142:729–735, 1982.
11. Hatch, R., et al. Hirsutism: Implications, etiology, and management. *Am. J. Obstet. Gynecol.* 140:815–830, 1981.
12. Judd, H. L., et al. Correlation of the effects of dexamethasone administration on urinary 17 ketosteroid and serum androgen levels in patients with hirsutism. *Am. J. Obstet. Gynecol.* 128:408–415, 1977.
13. Killinger, D. W. Hirsutism. In C. Ezrin, J. O. Godden, and P. G. Walfish (Eds.), *Clinical Endocrinology.* New York: Appleton-Century-Crofts, 1977. Pp. 296–310.
14. Kirschner, M. A., and Jacobs, J. B. Combined ovarian and adrenal vein catheterization to determine the site(s) of androgen overproduction in hirsute women. *J. Clin. Endocrinol. Metab.* 33:199–209, 1971.
15. Kirschner, M. A., Zucker, I. R., and Jespersen, D. Idiopathic hirsutism— an ovarian abnormality. *N. Engl. J. Med.* 294:637–640, 1976.
16. Lachelin, G. C. L., et al. Adrenal function in normal women and women with the polycystic ovary syndrome. *J. Clin. Endocrinol. Metab.* 49:892–898, 1979.
17. Lachelin, G. C. L., et al. Long term effects of nightly dexamethasone administration in patients with polycystic ovarian disease. *J. Clin. Endocrinol. Metab.* 55:768–773, 1982.
18. Lobo, R. A., and Goebelsmann, V. Adult manifestation of congenital adrenal hyperplasia due to incomplete 21-hydroxylase deficiency mimicking a polycystic ovarian disease. *Am. J. Obstet. Gynecol.* 138:720–726, 1980.
19. Maroulis, G. B., Manlimos, F. S., and Abraham, G. E. Comparison between urinary 17 ketosteroids and serum androgens in hirsute patients. *Obstet. Gynecol.* 49:454–458, 1977.
20. Mathur, R. S., et al. Plasma androgens and sex hormone binding globulin in the evaluation of hirsute females. *Fertil. Steril.* 35:29–35, 1981.
21. Muller, S. A. Hirsutism: A review of the genetic and experimental aspects. *J. Invest. Dermatol.* 60:457–474, 1973.
22. Osborn, R. H., and Vannone, M. E. Plasma androgens in the normal and androgenic female: A review. *Obstet. Gynecol. Survey* 26:195–228, 1971.

23. Paulsen, J. D., et al. Free testosterone concentration in the serum: Elevation is the hallmark of hirsutism. *Am. J. Obstet. Gynecol.* 128:851–857, 1977.
24. Price, V. H. Testosterone metabolism in the skin. *Arch. Dermatol.* 111:1496–1502, 1975.
25. Rosenfield, R. L. Plasma testosterone binding globulin and indexes of the concentration of unbound plasma androgens in normal and hirsute subjects. *J. Clin. Endocrinol. Metab.* 32:717–728, 1971.
26. Rosenfield, R. L. Plasma free androgen patterns in hirsute women and their diagnostic implications. *Am. J. Med.* 66:417–421, 1979.
27. Rosenfield, R. L., Erlich, E. N., and Cleary, R. E. Adrenal and ovarian contributions to the elevated free plasma androgen levels in hirsute women. *J. Clin. Endocrinol. Metab.* 34:92–98, 1972.
28. VanScott, E. J. Physiology of hair growth. *Clin. Obstet. Gynecol.* 7:1062–1074, 1964.
29. Wilson, J. D. Recent studies on the mechanism of action of testosterone. *N. Engl. J. Med.* 287:1284–1291, 1972.
30. Yen, S. S. C. Chronic Anovulation due to Inappropriate Feedback System. In S. S. C. Yen and R. B. Jaffe (Eds.), *Reproductive Endocrinology.* Philadelphia: Saunders, 1978. Pp. 297–323.

13 Male Hypogonadism and Infertility

John M. Amatruda
William F. Streck

In the fetus, sexual differentiation spontaneously takes a female orientation. The presence of testicular tissue is necessary to direct differentiation along masculine pathways [38]. In the male fetus with a normal XY karyotype, the presence of Y chromosomal material initiates the hormonal changes that lead to testicular development and the male phenotype. Even in cases in which the Y chromosome is apparently lacking, as in 46 XX males, the presence of Y chromosomal material is indicated by the presence of H-Y antigen, a cell surface antigen coded by genes on the Y chromosome [16]. In fact, the presence of the H-Y antigen is the best correlate known for the mammalian male gonad [16,55,58].

This genetically determined formation of the testes serves two major functions in the fetus. First, the testes produce the müllerian regression factor, which suppresses the müllerian ducts and prevents development of the uterus, cervix, upper third of the vagina, and fallopian tubes [28]. Second, the fetal testes secrete androgens that induce development of the male reproductive organs. It is now postulated, based on studies of male pseudohermaphrodites, that the development of the seminal vesicles, vas deferens, and epididymis is testosterone (T) dependent and that of the scrotum, penis, and prostate is dihydrotestosterone (DHT) dependent [26,27,37].

In the normal adult male, the hypothalamic-pituitary-gonadal axis and the control of spermatogenesis are controlled by complex negative feedback actions of androgens and estrogens [34,41,57]. Both androgen and estrogen receptors are present in the anterior pituitary, hypothalamus, and preoptic area. However, responses to these hormones vary. For instance, pure androgens do not suppress secretion of luteinizing hormone (LH) in agonadal men, whereas estrogens do suppress. This suggests that short-term effects of pure androgens may be due to displacement of testosterone from testosterone binding globulin (TeBG), with subsequent conversion to suppressive estrogen. The importance of estrogens in central regulation of LH in the male is further illustrated when the antiestrogen, clomiphene, is used to block feedback at the hypothalamic-pituitary level. Under these conditions, neither estradiol nor testosterone infusion will decrease gonadotropin levels [57]. It now appears that although both androgens and estrogens are capable of exerting independent effects on LH secretion, most LH suppression can be accounted for by conversion of testosterone to suppressive estrogens.

Follicle-stimulating hormone (FSH), as opposed to LH, is thought to be controlled through a protein made in Sertoli cells, variously referred to as *inhibin* or *Sertoli cell factor* [46], which is thought to act primarily at the pituitary level [57]. This protein is found in animal seminal plasma, rete testis fluid, and follicular fluid, and does not bind steroids. Antisera to inhibin lead to an increase in FSH levels, with no effect on serum LH. FSH also stimulates the production of androgen-binding protein in the Sertoli cells and increases receptors for LH in Leydig cells.

A unifying concept of the hypothalamic-pituitary-gonadal axis in males proposes that androgens and estrogens are secreted by the Leydig cells of the testis and that estrogens are also synthesized by peripheral conversion of androgens. These hormones interact at the hypothalamic (androgens) and pituitary (estrogens) levels to decrease LH. FSH increases the sensitivity of the Leydig cell to LH by increasing the receptor number, which perhaps increases testosterone synthesis. In addition, FSH stimulates the Sertoli cell to make androgen-binding protein, which transports the androgen to sperm precursors for development. Inhibin, in turn, feeds back on the pituitary (? hypothalamus) to decrease FSH.

CLINICAL CONSIDERATIONS

Hypogonadism, infertility, and impotence are distinct disorders of male sexual function that may be present to variable degrees in a given patient. The overlapping nature of these problems often complicates evaluation, the investigation of one necessitating consideration of the others.

Hypogonadism in the male may be defined as testicular failure with retardation of sexual development and/or function and may result from primary diseases of the testes or may be secondary to other disorders (Table 13-1). Hypogonadism may present with different manifestations depending on when hormonal failure occurred. Androgen deficiency occurring during early embryogenesis may present with developmental abnormalities, including ambiguous genitalia, or variable phenotypic presentations ranging from female to nearly normal male. Androgen deficiency occurring after birth but before puberty presents with less dramatic phenotypic alterations and is difficult to distinguish from simple delay in normal pubertal development in the young male.

Leydig cell failure occurring prior to puberty is manifested by a eunuchoid habitus in the adult. Because of continued long bone growth in such patients, they tend to be tall with disproportionately long legs. Other eunuchoid features include sparse or absent beard growth, decreased body, pubic, and axillary hair, failure of growth of the penis, scrotum, testis and prostate, a high-pitched voice, and failure of the temporal hairline to recede. In contrast, once secondary sexual characteristics are established, they are slow to recede if secondary hypogonadism appears. Decreased libido, potency, and spermatogenesis may become apparent. However, slowed hair growth and other signs of hypovirilization may be very subtle.

Table 13-1. Causes of Male Hypogonadism

Hypothalamic
  Kallman's syndrome
  Laurence-Moon-Biedl syndrome
  Prader-Willi syndrome
  Fröhlich's syndrome
  Isolated LH deficiency—fertile eunuch syndrome
Pituitary
  Hyperprolactinemia
  Postpubertal—partial or complete pituitary failure
    Tumor
    Surgery
    Irradiation
    Granulomatous disease
    Empty sella syndrome
    Infarction: postpartum, diabetes mellitus
    Other: vascular malformation, trauma, hemochromatosis
  Prepubertal—pituitary dwarfism
    Partial
    Complete
  Constitutional delay of puberty
Testicular
  Chromosomal abnormalities
    Klinefelter's syndrome (seminiferous tubule dysgenesis)
    XYY syndrome
    Pseudo-Turner's syndrome (Noonan's syndrome)
  Sertoli cell only syndrome
  Adult seminiferous tubule failure
  Infections of the genitourinary tract
  Myotonia dystrophica
  Congenital anorchia
  Physical agents
Defective hormone action or synthesis
  Male pseudohermaphroditism
Mixed
  Drugs
  Uremia
  Chronic alcoholism

Infertility describes a state in which a male is unable to induce conception (Table 13-2). Endocrine abnormalities are uncommon causes of infertility, ranging in incidence from 2 to 8% in two large series [13,53]. Most cases of infertility are of the idiopathic variety, characterized by sperm counts below those associated with fertility.

Impotence describes the inability of the male to have an erection or complete intercourse. Impotence is an obvious cause of infertility and a frequent accompaniment of hypogonadism. However, impotence, like

Table 13-2. Causes of Male Infertility

Idiopathic oligospermia
Immunologic infertility
Varicocele
Hypogonadism
Systemic disease
Drug exposure
Impotence
Cryptorchidism
Febrile illness or heat
Infections
Immobile cilia syndrome
Androgen resistance

Table 13-3. Causes of Impotence

Psychologic
Drugs
Surgery
Vascular disease
Diabetes
Hypogonadism
Neurologic disease

infertility, is more often due to nonendocrine disorders (Table 13-3). Historically, psychologic disorders have been invoked to explain most cases of impotence. However, recent studies have emphasized the need to look for hormonal disorders in impotent men [45].

Gynecomastia, an increase in male mammary tissue, is not a disease but rather a sign of an underlying disturbance in androgen-estrogen dynamics [56]. Gynecomastia may result from a decrease in testosterone formation or action with a subsequent alteration in the testosterone/estrogen ratio or from increased estrogen production. The causes of gynecomastia are outlined in Table 13-4.

Feminization, the induction or development of female sexual characteristics in the male, presents with gynecomastia as a part of the syndrome. However, feminization is usually associated with more extensive clinical features, including loss of libido, atrophy of the testes, and a change in body configuration. Gynecomastia is a relatively common clinical finding. Feminization, usually due to adrenocortical carcinoma, is rare.

In recognition of the overlapping nature of many of these problems, this discussion will focus on endocrine-related causes of sexual dysfunction. The discussion will be divided into five general sections: (1)

Table 13-4. Causes of Gynecomastia and Feminization

Physiologic
  Neonatal, pubertal

Decreased testosterone production
  Primary testicular failure (Klinefelter's syndrome, etc.)
  Secondary testicular failure (pituitary disease)
  Congenital defects in testosterone synthesis

Androgen resistance (testicular feminization and variants)

Increased estrogen production
  Tumors producing hCG (testicular, lung)
  Tumors secreting estrogen (testicular)
  Tumors producing estrogen precursors (adrenal)
  Diseases with increased androgen availability for conversion to estrogen
    (adrenal hyperplasia, liver disease, thyrotoxicosis, starvation)

Drugs
  Inhibition of testosterone synthesis or action (spironolactone, cimetidine)
  Estrogens (androgens)
  Gonadotropins
  Others (digitalis, tricyclic antidepressants)

___

hypogonadism, (2) delayed pubertal development, (3) gynecomastia and feminization, (4) infertility, and (5) disorders due to defective hormone action or synthesis.

Hypogonadism
From the detailed list in Table 13-1, some of the more commonly encountered causes of hypogonadism may be selected. The following disorders should warrant early consideration in the investigation of the hypogonadal male: chromosomal abnormalities, systemic diseases, pituitary disease, and hyperprolactinemia.

CHROMOSOMAL ABNORMALITIES. The major chromosomal abnormalities are Klinefelter's syndrome and its variants and the XYY syndrome. Klinefelter's syndrome (seminiferous tubule dysgenesis) is the most common chromosomal abnormality and is characterized by an extra X chromosome, low testosterone, elevated gonadotropins, eunuchoid habitus, small firm testes, gynecomastia, and hyalinized seminiferous tubules with clumping of Leydig cells. Infertility is usually present. It is important to recognize that variations in Leydig cell function occur with variable expression of the classic phenotype. This is especially true in patients with mosaicism if an XY cell line is present, for example, XXY/XY. Also, chromosomal abnormalities may be localized to the testes. The usual chromosomal pattern in Klinefelter's syndrome is 47 XXY.

SYSTEMIC DISEASES AND DRUGS. Of particular interest, from a medical standpoint, are the consequences of chronic renal failure and acute and chronic alcohol administration.

Uremic men tend to have abnormal spermatogenesis, testicular atrophy, impotence, and decreased libido [31]. Testicular biopsies frequently show spermatogenic arrest. Leydig cell dysfunction with reduced levels of testosterones and elevated LH and FSH levels are found in most patients [24,42]. Responses to gonadotropin-releasing hormone (GnRH) and clomiphene may be normal [42], but subnormal responses to human chorionic gonadotropin (hCG) have been demonstrated [24]. The site of the defect may be both testicular and hypothalamic. Hemodialysis does not usually correct the defects in Leydig cell and germinal cell functions, but such defects may be reversed by successful transplantation. Recently, impotence in uremia has been related to increased levels of parathyroid hormone [35]. In some patients, zinc therapy has resulted in improved potency and increases in plasma testosterone [6], and in another recent series bromocryptine treatment resulted in decreased plasma prolactin and improved libido and sexual function [7].

Acute alcohol administration in men leads to decreased testosterone production, increased testosterone metabolism, decreased TeBG, and an increase in testosterone degradation [17]. These combine to decrease mean plasma testosterone. There is no change in estrogen levels or conversion of androgens to estrogens. The levels of gonadotropins are inconsistent. Indeed, there is a decreased LH response to GnRH after acute alcohol ingestion, suggesting a pituitary defect. Acutely, alcohol's effect may be due to decreased testosterone synthesis. Also, alcohol has a 50-fold greater affinity for the dehydrogenase that oxidizes retinol to retinal, which is needed for spermatogenesis [48].

Chronic ethanolism is associated with impotence, sterility, testicular atrophy, gynecomastia, and decreased body hair [2]. In chronic alcoholism with liver disease, mean plasma gonadotropins are elevated; yet, in any given patient, they can be normal [50]. Total testosterone and free testosterone are decreased and estradiol (E) levels are normal to elevated, leading to a decrease in the $T : E_2$ ratio [10]. Estrone levels are increased. These changes may be due in part to decreased clearance of estrogens by the liver and enhanced peripheral conversion of androgens to estrogens. Both testicular unresponsiveness to hCG and hypothalamic-pituitary unresponsiveness to clomiphene have been demonstrated [51,52]. The latter defect may reside in the pituitary since some authors have demonstrated a decreased response to GnRH. Elevations in prolactin, TeBG, and estrogen-dependent neurophysin have been shown in some chronic alcoholics with liver disease.

PITUITARY DISEASE. Postpubertal pituitary failure can be due to any of the causes listed in Table 13-1. All of these patients have low gonadotropin and testosterone levels, with no response to GnRH or clomiphene. Pituitary causes of male hypogonadism are usually related to structural or vascular lesions of the pituitary. Many patients formerly thought to have partial or complete prepubertal pituitary failure probably have hypothalamic dysfunction. These patients are usually diagnosed in childhood, and tests of pituitary function are variably impaired. Given chronic stimulation with hypothalamic factors, many of these patients will respond, indicating intact pituitary function.

HYPERPROLACTINEMIA. Hyperprolactinemia [8,40,43,45] is associated with hypogonadism and infertility in men as well as women. Low testosterone, oligospermia, and impotence are commonly present. Treatment with bromocriptine leads to increases in serum testosterone and sperm count, which are associated with major clinical improvement. Pituitary tumors may or may not be demonstrable. There is evidence of both hypothalamic and primary testicular dysfunction in the presence of elevated prolactin. Hyperprolactinemia is increasingly recognized as an important cause of male sexual dysfunction [8,45].

Less Common Causes of Hypogonadism
Hypogonadotropic hypogonadism may be associated with a variety of central nervous system (CNS), somatic, and genital defects. For example, patients with Kallman's syndrome have anosmia or hyposmia due to complete or partial absence of the olfactory lobes and can have 8th nerve deficits, color blindness, cleft lip and palate, unilateral renal agenesis, ichthyosis, seizure disorders, and short metacarpals. Both male and female family members can have the somatic abnormalities previously discussed. Patients with Laurence-Moon-Biedl syndrome have retinitis pigmentosa, mental deficiency, ataxia, polydactyly, and obesity. Those with Prader-Willi syndrome are obese, diabetic, mentally retarded, and hypotonic. In Fröhlich syndrome, hypothalamic damage leads to both obesity and decreased gonadotropins, infantile genitalia, and a pituitary that is responsive to GnRH. However, because of the chronic absence of GnRH, the pituitary may not respond acutely but instead may require repeated stimulation with exogenous GnRH to restore responsiveness. The fertile eunuch syndrome is characterized by normal FSH levels, varying degrees of spermatogenesis, and low LH with low testosterone levels. Many patients have gynecomastia.

Noonan's syndrome is characterized by webbed neck, short stature, ptosis, hypogonadism, and congenital heart disease. The karyotype is normal, and the mode of genetic transmission is autosomal dominant.

Delayed Puberty or Pubertal Failure
In 95% of males, puberty commences between 9.5 and 13.5 years, with a mean age of onset of 11.6 years. The pubertal process takes a mean of 3 years with peak height velocity occurring at a mean age of 14.1 years.

During puberty there is an increase in the size of the penis and scrotum with the development of scrotal rugal folds, growth of body and facial hair, development of the diamond-shaped male escutcheon, some recession of the hairline, accelerated linear growth, development of the prostate, seminal vesicles, and vas deferens, deepening of the voice, and development of libido and sexual competence. The male patient who has no evidence of sexual development at age 14 to 15 years most commonly represents a benign constitutional variant in development, with an associated reduced growth rate and slow skeletal development. Constitutional delay of puberty is a diagnosis of exclusion. Frequently, delayed puberty is associated with systemic illness, such as uremia, regional enteritis, or ulcerative colitis. Endocrine causes of delayed sexual development include hypothyroidism, poorly controlled diabetes mellitus, and selective growth hormone deficiency, as well as those causes of hypogonadism listed in Table 13-1. Unfortunately, there is no single test or group of tests to distinguish adequately patients with constitutional delay of puberty from those with nondetectable hypothalamic or pituitary lesions. A recent study has suggested that the prolactin (PRL) response to thyrotropin releasing hormone (TRH) may prove useful in differentiating isolated gonadotropin deficiency from delayed puberty [45a]. Frequently, a family history of delayed maturation is obtained. The earliest detectable change, as a child enters puberty, is a sleep-associated increase in LH levels [19]. Physically, the earliest change is an increase in testicular size.

Gynecomastia and Feminization

Gynecomastia may be found in many of the hypogonadal disorders listed in Table 13-1. Increased breast tissue in the male may, however, be a normal physiologic finding in neonates due to placental estrogens and in adolescent boys and older men due to altered testosterone/estradiol ratios. Pathologic gynecomastia may result from three primary processes—deficient testosterone production or action, increased estrogen production, or drugs. The disorders to be considered under each of these categories are outlined in Table 13-4.

Frank feminization in the male is usually a result of adrenocortical carcinoma. In these cases, increased production of androgen precursors presumably provides substrate for increased peripheral estrogen formation. In a major review of this topic, 41 of 52 patients had adrenal gland carcinoma and 7 had adenomas; in 4 cases, the diagnosis was doubtful [15]. Testicular tumors and carcinoma may produce feminization by secretion of hCG, which stimulates estradiol and testosterone production by the uninvolved testes. Seminomas, choriocarcinomas, and embryonal cell carcinomas may produce gynecomastia in this fashion, whereas Leydig cell or Sertoli cell tumors may secrete estrogens directly.

The most commonly encountered causes of pathologic gynecomastia, usually not associated with marked feminization, are those due to liver disease, drugs, thyrotoxicosis, or Klinefelter's syndrome.

Infertility

The presence of sperm that are adequate in quantity and quality does not ensure fertility. As has been increasingly emphasized in the literature, fertility is best evaluated by considering the couple as a unit. Thus, there must be documentation of ovulation, mechanical aspects of intercourse, and adequate endometrial tissue, as well as adequacy of sperm. When investigation points toward a possible male cause for infertility, the following disorders are most likely to be encountered: idiopathic oligospermia, anatomic abnormalities, hypogonadism, and drugs or systemic illness.

IDIOPATHIC OLIGOSPERMIA. As the name implies, idiopathic oligospermia, which accounts for most cases of male infertility, is not well understood. Endocrine studies are normal but sperm quantity is below that necessary to accomplish fertilization, usually less than 20 million/ml. Specific defects have been noted in certain cases of previously unexplained infertility. Immunologic mechanisms including antisperm antibodies have been demonstrated [21,23], as well as defects in androgen metabolism [3], subtle cytogenic abnormalities in the testes of infertile individuals [12], and decreased protein-carboxylmethylase in immotile spermatozoa [16]. The pathophysiologic mechanisms discovered to date suggest that this general category of idiopathic disease will undergo further classification and clarification in the future. Recently, androgen resistance has been postulated as a common cause of oligospermia in infertile but otherwise normal males. These patients have normal to increased testosterone and gonadotropin levels, oligospermia, and a decreased number of androgen receptors [3].

It is worth noting that in patients with infertility alone there is little correlation between the degree of oligospermia and the level of FSH. However, studies have demonstrated a strong correlation between FSH levels and stages of spermatogenesis determined by testicular biopsy. FSH levels are usually elevated when complete hyalinization is present, but with lesser degrees of impairment FSH levels are normal. LH levels are normal, reflecting the normal testosterone levels usually found in infertility.

ANATOMIC ABNORMALITIES. Varicoceles have been reported in up to 39% of infertile men in one series [13]. Although this estimate may be high, impaired sperm motility and increases in immature and tapered forms are often found in cases of varicocele. The pathophysiology of this disorder is not well understood, but improvement in fertility following high ligation of varicoceles suggests that increased blood flow and stasis around the testis may somehow decrease spermatogenesis.

Ductal obstruction is usually a consequence of infection. Most commonly seen in one series was epididymal obstruction due to previous epididymitis with gonorrhea or tuberculosis [13]. Azoospermia is a characteristic of total obstruction. Before ductal obstruction may be invoked to explain azoospermia, a testicular biopsy may be required to confirm that spermatogenesis is present.

HYPOGONADISM. As discussed in the previous section, testicular failure of a primary or secondary nature may result in infertility.

DRUGS OR SYSTEMIC ILLNESS. Heat may limit spermatogenesis, with consequent infertility. Tight clothing may increase intratesticular temperatures. A febrile illness may lead to a decreased sperm count for 25 to 55 days after an illness before recovery occurs [33].

Drugs (Table 13-5) may cause infertility through many mechanisms. Direct injury to the testes may occur (cyclophosphamide), or normal hypothalamic-pituitary-gonadal relationships may be suppressed (testosterone). Cimetidine recently has been demonstrated to alter gonadotropic responses to clomiphene [49]. The immotile cilia syndrome provides a model of a specific illness associated with infertility [14]. Hyperthyroidism is an endocrine disorder that may present with infertility not associated with hypogonadism.

IMPOTENCE. The inability to complete intercourse is an obvious explanation for infertility. Impotence is most often due to psychogenic disorders. The other causes listed in Table 13-3 are apparent on the basis of the history or physical examination. Antihypertensive drugs are commonly implicated as a cause of impotence.

Impotence due to hypogonadism may occur in all forms of androgen deficiency. Characteristically, the hypogonadal male is often unaware of the functional change since his libido has diminished as well. Other endocrine disorders, including hyperthyroidism or hypothyroidism and diabetes mellitus, may present with features of impotence. In diabetes, infertility is usually due to impotence secondary to an autonomic neuropathy [29]. Retrograde ejaculation may be present even when adequate spermatogenesis occurs.

TESTICULAR FAILURE. Males with the XYY karyotype [25,54] are characteristically tall and have nodulocystic acne and skeletal anomalies, such as radioulnar synostoses. Although only a small percentage of these males manifest antisocial behavior, their prevalence in criminal institutions is greater than that in the general population. Most are normally masculinized, have normal testosterone and gonadotropin levels, and are fertile, although varying degrees of testicular damage and spermatogenic arrest can be present.

The Sertoli cell only syndrome [36] represents a congenital absence of germ cells and usually presents with infertility and normal masculiniza-

Table 13-5. Drugs and Chemicals Affecting Gonadal Function

Busulfan (Myleran)
Triethylenemelamine (TEM)
Chlorambucil
Cyclophosphamide
Methotrexate
Cyclic combination chemotherapy [9]
Colchicine
Dilantin [47]
Aspirin
Diethylstilbestrol (DES) during pregnancy
Marijuana [30]
Lead poisoning
Arsenic
Nitrofurantoin
Testosterone
Cimetidine [49]
Monoamine oxidase (MAO) inhibitors
Spironolactone [32,39]
Methadone [11]
Antihypertensives

tion. These patients frequently have normal to slightly decreased testosterone, normal LH with azoospermia, and elevated FSH. The diagnosis is confirmed by testicular biopsy, which shows normal Leydig cells and tubules with markedly reduced to absent germ cells.

Adult seminiferous tubule failure leads to decreased sperm counts, and most patients have normal LH, FSH, and testosterone values. The cause of such tubular failure is usually unknown, although it occasionally can be traced to a previous infection with mumps or gonococcal orchitis.

Myotonic dystrophy [22] is a familial disorder manifested by myotonia, frontal baldness, lenticular cataracts, and small, soft testes associated with oligospermia, elevated LH and FSH, and low testosterone levels. Pathologically, the testes are similar to those in patients with Klinefelter's syndrome. These patients are normally masculinized, with testicular failure and infertility occurring after puberty.

Congenital anorchia [1] is a syndrome of obscure etiology characterized by the absence of testes and subsequent lack of sexual development. The presence of a male phenotype, in the absence of testes and female internal genitalia, indicates that müllerian regression was normal and that testes were present during fetal development. In patients seen after the expected time of puberty, FSH and LH are markedly elevated, and testosterone levels are very low.

Defective Hormone Action or Synthesis
Disorders of gonadal development due to defective hormone action or
synthesis are rare. Such disorders have, however, provided major ad-
vances in the understanding of gonadal development and function.

ENZYMATIC ABNORMALITIES IN ANDROGEN PRODUCTION. Enzymatic defects of steroid synthesis may limit the production of sex
steroids, glucocorticoids, or mineralocorticoids to varying degrees [20].
In those instances in which androgen production is interrupted with consequent androgen deficiency, infants have ambiguous genitalia or are
phenotypic females depending on the severity of the defect. The more
severe defects (due to 20,22-desmolase, 3β-dehydrogenase, or 17-hy-
droxylase) occur early in the steroid synthetic pathway and present with
decreased cortisone production as well as the consequences of androgen
deficiency. Selective deficiencies in the androgen pathway (e.g., 17-
ketosteroid reductase) may result in inadequate virilization and ambiguous genitalia. Male pseudohermaphroditism, that is, a genetic male with
varying degrees of feminization, may result from these defects.

The syndrome resulting from a deficiency of the enzyme 5-alpha-re-
ductase may also cause male pseudohermaphroditism (familial incomplete male pseudohermaphroditism type II) [26,27]. This syndrome is
described in 46 XY males and is characterized by a clitoral-like phallus,
bifud scrotum, and urogenital sinus at birth. The testes are in the inguinal canal or labioscrotal folds. Wolffian structures are normally differentiated, and there are no müllerian structures. At puberty, a male habitus
develops, with growth of the phallus and scrotum, voice change, and no
gynecomastia. The testes are normal. Plasma testosterone is higher and
dihydrotestosterone lower than normal, and the abnormal T : DHT
ratio persists after hCG stimulation. LH and FSH levels are high, and
the conversion of testosterone to dihydrotestosterone is less than 1%.
Inheritance is autosomal recessive, with sisters showing the same
biochemical defect and carrier parents an intermediate defect.

DEFECTIVE ANDROGEN ACTION. Defective androgen action [18] can
be due to a decreased number of androgen receptors or a postreceptor
defect in androgen action. Partial androgen insensitivity of mixed etiology may also be encountered.

Patients with such partial androgen insensitivity, or type I familial incomplete male pseudohermaphroditism, have been described as the
Lubs, Gilbert-Dreyfus, Reifenstein, and Rosewater syndromes, ranging
from the most to the least severe [5]. The physical findings range from
fused labioscrotal folds with hypospadias in Lubs syndrome to gynecomastia and sterility as the only abnormal findings in Rosewater syndrome. These males have a 46 XY karyotype with incomplete virilization
at puberty. The phenotype is indistinguishable from that produced by a

variety of enzyme defects mentioned previously. However, plasma testosterone is normal or elevated, suggesting a defect in androgen responsiveness. LH and FSH levels are high, reflecting an impairment of the
negative feedback regulation of androgens on the hypothalamic-pituitary axis. These hormonal findings are similar to those in the complete
androgen insensitivity syndrome; however, the presence of incomplete
virilization indicates that patients with Reifenstein's syndrome have a
partial androgen insensitivity syndrome.

Patients with the complete androgen insensitivity syndrome (testicular
feminization) [18] are genotypic males (46 XY) who are phenotypic
females. The inheritance is X-linked recessive or male-limited autosomal
dominant. In an affected sibship, all of the females are normal and half
of the males are affected. The testes may be intra-abdominal, or in the
labia majora or inguinal canal, and contain immature seminiferous
tubules. There are no müllerian structures. Leydig cells tend to become
hyperplastic after adolescence, and malignant degeneration occurs in approximately 10% of cases. External genitalia are female with a blind vaginal pouch. In one-third of patients, there is no pubic and axillary hair,
and it is scanty in the remainder. At puberty, female secondary sexual
characteristics appear. Testosterone levels are in the range of normal
males, but LH levels are high. All organs are resistant to testosterone,
which fails to decrease LH or to masculinize and has no protein anabolic
effects, that is, nitrogen or phosphorus retention. Estrogen levels are in
the lower range for normal females, but are unopposed by androgens.

DIAGNOSTIC MEASURES
Testicular Size
The normal adult testis measures 4.6 cm in length (3.6–5.5 cm).

Span/Height Ratio and Upper/Lower Segment Ratio
In normal adult men, the span/height and upper/lower segment ratios
are 1.0. A eunuchoid habitus is characterized by a span more than 5 cm
greater than the height and by a distance from the soles to the symphysis
that is more than 5 cm greater than the distance from the symphysis to
the head, that is, a floor-to-symphysis span more than 5 cm greater than
the height minus the floor-to-symphysis span.

Semen Analysis
Specimens must be collected by masturbation only in a sterile container
and delivered to the laboratory at room temperature within 1 hour. Normal men are usually fertile with sperm counts greater than 20 million per
milliliter, greater than 60% motility, and greater than 50% normal morphology.

Luteinizing Hormone and Follicle-Stimulating Hormone (LH and FSH)
LH and FSH are determined by radioimmunoassay. Normal values vary depending on the assay used but usually range from 4 to 20 mIU/ml for both hormones in the male.

Serum Testosterone
Serum testosterone is determined by radioimmunoassay. Normal values depend on the laboratory, but are usually greater than 300 ng/dl in adult males.

Estrogen
Both estrone and the more potent estradiol are produced in the normal male. Most production of these estrogens can be accounted for by peripheral conversion from androstenedione and testosterone. Normal levels for estradiol are approximately 10 to 35 pg/ml by radioimmunoassay in the male.

Human Chorionic Gonadotropin
Levels of hCG are usually very low to nondetectable in the normal male. Cross-reactivity of this hormone with LH is high, and a specific measurement of the beta subunit of hCG in the plasma is required. Use of hCG levels is helpful in the evaluation of suspected testicular tumors (seminoma or teratoma) in which very high hCG levels may cause hyperestrogenemia and feminization. Tumors of lung, stomach, and liver have also been shown to secrete hCG.

Prolactin
Normal prolactin levels in the male are usually less than 20 pg/ml.

Chromosome Analysis
BUCCAL SMEAR. A normal male is XY in all tissues and Barr body negative, that is, less than 5% of cells from a buccal smear have Barr bodies, depending on the quality of the technique. The Barr body represents an inactive X chromosome that is present whenever there is more than one X chromosome in a cell. It is seen as a dark-staining area at the periphery of the nucleus of buccal epithelial cells.

FLUORESCENT Y TEST. The presence of the Y chromosome can be identified by fluorescent staining with quinacrine. This may serve as a simple confirmatory test of male genetic sex and may complement data obtained in the buccal smear.

KARYOTYPE. Normal males are XY. Occasionally, peripheral leukocytes may have an XY chromosomal pattern with chromosomal abnormalities occurring in the testes, as in some variants of Klinefelter's syndrome.

Gonadotropin-Releasing Hormone Stimulation Test

GnRH is a decapeptide secreted from the hypothalamus that stimulates the secretion and synthesis of both LH and FSH by the pituitary. In males with hypogonadism and normal or low gonadotropins, the GnRH stimulation test is useful in distinguishing hypothalamic from pituitary dysfunction. The test is performed by administering 250 μg of GnRH intravenously as a bolus injection, with blood samples obtained at −10, 0, 30, 60, and 90 minutes. A normal response is a 100–250 to 900% increase in LH and a 25 to 400% increase in FSH. In patients with hypothalamic hypogonadism, prolonged stimulation with GnRH may be necessary. Prepubertal males do not respond to GnRH.

Clomiphene Stimulation Test

Clomiphene is an antiestrogen that works at the hypothalamic level to stimulate LH release. It is useful in determining the integrity of the hypothalamic-pituitary-testicular axis [56]. For a normal LH and FSH response, both the hypothalamus and the pituitary gland must be functional, and for a normal testosterone response, the testes must be functional as well. The test is performed by administering clomiphene, 50 μg twice a day for 7 days. A normal response is an increase over control levels of at least 30% for LH, 22% for FSH, and 25% for testosterone.

Human Chorionic Gonadotropin Stimulation Test

Human chorionic gonadotropin stimulates testosterone production by the Leydig cell through interaction with the LH receptor. The test determines the ability of the testes to respond to LH. The test is performed by the administration of 5000 IU of hCG intramuscularly every morning for 4 days. A normal response is a doubling of plasma testosterone on the morning of the fifth day.

Urinary 17-Hydroxycorticoids, 17-Ketosteroids, and Pregnanetriol

These studies may be indicated for patients suspected of having enzymatic abnormalities in androgen production. They may also be used to investigate acquired excess of androgen metabolites, which is suggestive of adrenal or testicular tumor.

H-Y Antigen

The H-Y antigen is a cell surface antigen detectable by the cytotoxic effect upon mouse sperm of antiserum raised in mice. This is a difficult test and is available in only a limited number of research laboratories.

DISCUSSION

Hypogonadism, infertility, and impotence may be found in various overlapping clinical presentations. As discussed, hypogonadal men are likely to have associated impotence and infertility, whereas infertile or impotent men are more frequently hormonally intact. Hormonal dysfunction may, however, be quite subtle in men presenting with complaints of sexual dysfunction. Thus, hypogonadism should not be ruled out by a history of occasional early morning erections or infrequently successful sexual intercourse. Physical examination may fail to suggest hormonal deficiency: testes may not be dramatically decreased in size, and hair loss may be subtle. The evaluation of the patient presenting with sexual dysfunction should therefore include a hormonal assessment.

A normal habitus and testes of adult size suggest gonadal failure occurring after puberty, and the evaluation sequence in the first protocol may be followed (Fig. 13-1). A eunuchoid habitus indicates prepubertal testicular hypofunction or injury, whereas feminization of male features provides a second clinical clue to possible hormonal disorders. The approach to these clinical presentations is presented in Figure 13-3.

As outlined in Figure 13-1, measurement of serum testosterone levels provides an assessment of the end product of the hypothalamic-pituitary-gonadal axis in the male with a normal habitus. Several determinations should be obtained since levels vary throughout the day. Consistently low testosterone levels indicate hypogonadism. Prolactin levels emerge as an early test in the evaluation of hypogonadal, infertile, or impotent males since variable degrees of hypothalamic pituitary dysfunction may result from hyperprolactinemia. In the presence of normal prolactin levels, gonadotropin levels distinguish primary testicular disease from secondary hypothalamic-pituitary disorders. In most cases of Leydig cell dysfunction of endocrine or chromosomal etiology, gonadotropins are elevated. Low or normal gonadotropin levels in combination with a low testosterone level suggest secondary failure since compensatory elevation of the hormones would be expected. In this instance, further evaluation is outlined in Figure 13-2. Low gonadotropin levels are not easily defined since normal values may be as low as 4 to 5 mIU/ml. It is the level of gonadotropins relative to the testosterone level that is important.

Consistently normal testosterone levels in the hypogonadal or infertile male are reassuring but do not rule out an endocrine disorder. In particular, hyperprolactinemia has been associated with impotence and infertility even in the presence of normal testosterone levels [39]. If both prolactin and testosterone levels are normal, hypogonadism is probably not the major problem. In this instance, infertility may better serve as the focus for investigation (Table 13-2).

Semen analysis provides the most useful information in the infertile male without apparent endocrine or chromosomal disorders. Semen analysis, like testosterone level tests, should be performed more than once before conclusions are drawn [44]. As a general rule, total sperm counts below 20×10^6/ml or abnormal morphology in 50% of sperm are associated with infertility. A relatively low sperm count with all other studies normal leads to a diagnosis of idiopathic infertility. Although

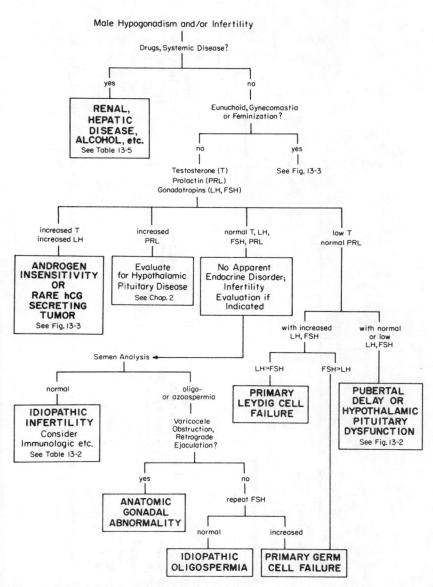

Figure 13-1. Diagnostic protocol: Male hypogonadism and/or infertility. LH, luteinizing hormone; FSH, follicle-stimulating hormone; hCG, human chorionic gonadotropin.

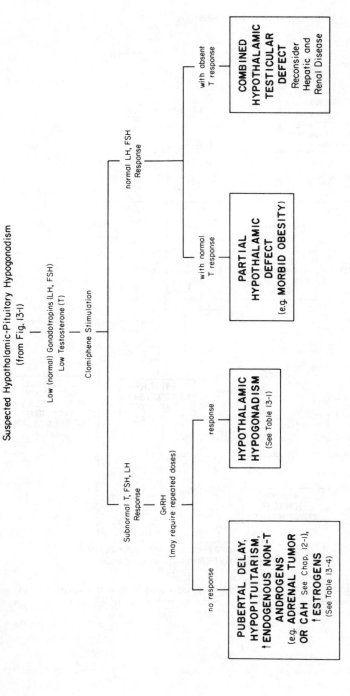

Suspected Hypothalamic-Pituitary Hypogonadism
(from Fig. 13-1)

Low (normal) Gonadotropins (LH, FSH)
Low Testosterone (T)

Clomiphene Stimulation

Subnormal T, FSH, LH
Response

GnRH
(may require repeated doses)

no response

response

**PUBERTAL DELAY,
HYPOPITUITARISM,
↑ENDOGENOUS NON-T
ANDROGENS**
(e.g. ADRENAL TUMOR
OR CAH See Chap. 12-1),
↑ESTROGENS
(See Table 13-4)

**HYPOTHALAMIC
HYPOGONADISM**
(See Table 13-1)

normal LH, FSH
Response

with normal
T response

with absent
T response

**PARTIAL
HYPOTHALAMIC
DEFECT**
(e.g. MORBID OBESITY)

**COMBINED
HYPOTHALAMIC
TESTICULAR
DEFECT**
Reconsider
Hepatic and
Renal Disease

13-2. Diagnostic protocol: Suspected hypothalamic-pituitary hypogonadism. LH, luteinizing hormone; FSH, follicle-stimulating hormone; GnRH, gonadotropin-releasing hormone; CAH, congenital adrenal hyperplasia.

studies have suggested subtle cytogenic abnormalities [12,13], immunologic factors [21], and defects in androgen metabolism in some instances, most cases remain unexplained. Oligospermia with abnormal forms suggests possible variocele, whereas azoospermia suggests obstruction, retrograde ejaculation, or the Sertoli cell only syndrome, the last usually characterized by elevated FSH levels.

As indicated in Figure 13-2, low testosterone levels in combination with low or normal gonadotropins may be further investigated with the clomiphene stimulation test. A total lack of response in levels of gonadotropins and testosterone indicates hypothalamic-pituitary disease, suppression of this axis with exogenous hormones, or endogenous suppression such as may be found in various adrenogenital syndromes. The cause of an absent response may be further investigated by use of the GnRH stimulation test. Whereas clomiphene blocks at the hypothalamic level and thus indirectly assesses pituitary function, GnRH directly stimulates the pituitary. A normal GnRH response in combination with an abnormal clomiphene response suggests hypothalamic disease. Repeated doses of GnRH may be necessary to elicit a response in the quiescent pituitary that accompanies chronic loss of hypothalamic stimulation.

A clear-cut gonadotropin rise after clomiphene that is not accompanied by a testosterone elevation provides evidence of both primary testicular failure and some deficiency in hypothalamic function since LH levels should be elevated. Such combined defects may be found in chronic alcoholism or renal disease.

A normal response to clomiphene stimulation in the man with low to normal basal levels of gonadotropins and low testosterone is difficult to explain. However, such cases do occur, particularly in massively obese males [4,4a,17a]. The presumed disorder, a hypothalamic one, can be further supported by a normal GnRH stimulation test. The hypothalamic disorder in such a case must be subtle since pituitary failure does not accompany it. When such subtle hypothalamic defects are present in the absence of massive obesity, evaluation should exclude intracranial tumors, aneurysms, and other lesions that might impinge on the hypothalamic area.

The hypogonadal or infertile male with eunuchoid features requires investigation for prepubertal or chromosomal diseases (Fig. 13-3). Testicular examination further defines the causes of the eunuchoid habitus. If testes are not present, cryptorchidism or congenital anorchia are suggested. Infantile testes are suggestive of hypothalamic or pituitary disease in the adult and simple delayed puberty in the adolescent. Small, very firm testes are characteristic of Klinefelter's syndrome. The presence of a Barr body will support this diagnosis. Eunuchoid features and small testes with an absent Barr body suggest prepubertal testicular disease or the XYY variant.

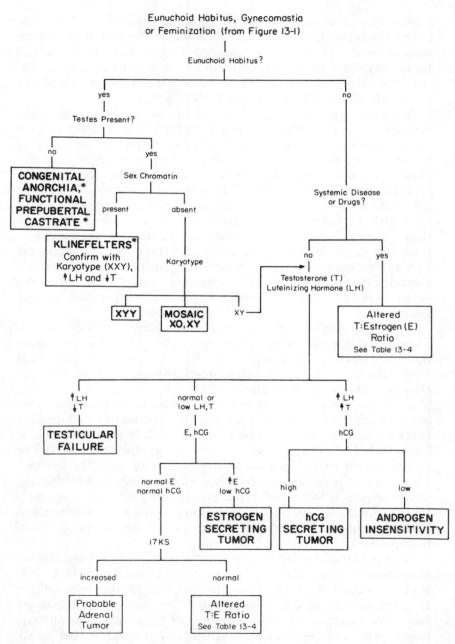

Figure 13-3. Diagnostic protocol: Eunuchoid habitus, gynecomastia, or feminization. hCG, human chorionic gonadotropin; 17KS, 17-ketosteroids. *May have gynecomastia.

Gynecomastia, redistribution of body fat, or other evidence of estrogen excess should raise the question of chronic alcoholism, drug ingestion, or rare feminizing tumors. On a practical basis, the more common disorders associated with feminine features may be ascertained by the history (drug use) and routine laboratory tests and x-rays (thyroid, renal, or lung disease). In the clearly feminized male, a tumor producing hCG, estrogen, or estrogen precursors should be considered. At this juncture, urinary 17-ketosteroids, plasma estradiol levels, and hCG levels may be measured. Elevation of 17-ketosteroids points toward adrenal disease (probably carcinoma), whereas increased estradiol levels may result from testicular or other neoplasms (see Table 13-4).

If these studies do not suggest excess estrogen production, the subsequent protocol may be followed. It should be borne in mind that gynecomastia may be a component of several hypogonadal disorders, and although this may provide some clues to the etiology, more often it may reflect the altered testosterone/estradiol ratio associated with primary or secondary testicular failure.

Finally, the rare disorders due to defective androgen synthesis or action should be considered in the adult male presenting with ambiguous genitalia. These disorders of androgen resistance characteristically show elevated testosterone and LH levels. Complete androgen insensitivity (testicular feminization) represents the end product of such a process of hormone resistance. The elevated LH levels distinguish these disorders from those due to the enzymatic defects of forms of congenital adrenal hyperplasia in which high androgen production suppresses LH secretion.

REFERENCES

1. Abeyaratne, M. R., Aherne, W. A., and Scott, J. E. S. The vanishing testis. *Lancet* 2:822–824, 1969.
2. Adlercreutz, H. Hepatic metabolism of estrogens in health and disease. *N. Engl. J. Med.* 290:1081–1083, 1974.
3. Aiman, J., et al. Androgen insensitivity as a cause of infertility in otherwise normal men. *N. Engl. J. Med.* 300:223–227, 1979.
4. Amatruda, J. M., et al. Depressed plasma testosterone and fractional binding of testosterone in obese males. *J. Clin. Endocrinol. Metab.* 47:268–271, 1978.
4a. Amatruda, J. M., et al. Hypothalamic and pituitary dysfunction in obese males. *Int. J. Obesity* 6:183–189, 1982.
5. Amrhein, J. A., et al. Partial androgen insensitivity: The Reifenstein syndrome revisited. *N. Engl. J. Med.* 297:350–356, 1977.
6. Antoniou, L. D., et al. Reversal of uremic impotence by zinc. *Lancet* 2:895–898, 1977.
7. Bommer, J., et al. Improved sexual function in male hemodialysis patients on bromocryptine. *Lancet* 2:496–497, 1979.
8. Carter, J. N., et al. Prolactin-secreting tumors and hypogonadism in 22 men. *N. Engl. J. Med.* 299:847–852, 1978.
9. Chapman, R. M., et al. Cyclical combination chemotherapy and gonadal function. *Lancet* 1:285–289, 1979.
10. Chopra, I. J., Tulchinsky, D., and Greenway, F. L. Estrogen-androgen imbalance in hepatic cirrhosis. *Ann. Intern. Med.* 79:198–203, 1973.

11. Cicero, T. J., et al. Function of the male sex organs in heroin and methadone users. *N. Engl. J. Med.* 292:882–887, 1975.
12. deKretser, D. M., et al. Hormonal, histological and chromosomal studies in adult males with testicular disorders. *J. Clin. Endocrinol. Metab.* 35:393–401, 1972.
13. Dublin, L., and Amelar, R. D. Etiologic factors in 1294 consecutive cases of male infertility. *Fertil. Steril.* 22:469–474, 1971.
14. Ellasson, R., et al. The immotile-cilia syndrome: A congenital ciliary abnormality as an etiologic factor in chronic airway infections and male sterility. *N. Engl. J. Med.* 297:1–6, 1977.
15. Gabrilove, J. L., et al. Feminizing adrenocortical tumors in the male: A review of 52 cases including a case report. *Medicine* 44:37–51, 1965.
16. Gagnon, C., et al. Deficiency of protein-carboxylmethylase in immotile spermatozoa of infertile men. *N. Engl. J. Med.* 306:821–825, 1982.
17. Gerald, P. S. The H-Y antigen and male sexual development. *N. Engl. J. Med.* 300:788–789, 1979.
17a. Glass, A. R., et al. Low serum testosterone and sex hormone binding globulin in massively obese men. *J. Clin. Endocrinol. Metab.* 45:1211–1219, 1977.
18. Griffin, J. E., and Wilson, J. D. The syndromes of androgen resistance. *N. Engl. J. Med.* 302:198–209, 1980.
19. Grumbach, M. M., et al. In M. M. Grumbach et al. (Eds.), *The Control of the Onset of Puberty.* New York: Wiley, 1974. Pp. 115–181.
20. Grumbach, M. M., and Van Wyk, J. J. Disorders of Sexual Differentiation. In R. H. Williams (Ed.), *Textbook of Endocrinology.* Philadelphia: Saunders, 1974. Pp. 480–484.
21. Haas, G. G., Jr., Cines, D. B., and Schreiber, A. D. Immunologic infertility: Identification of patients with antisperm antibody. *N. Engl. J. Med.* 303:722–727, 1980.
22. Harper, P., et al. Gonadal function in males with myotonic dystrophy. *J. Clin. Endocrinol. Metab.* 35:852–855, 1972.
23. Hendry, W. F., et al. Steroid treatment of male subfertility caused by antisperm antibodies. *Lancet* 2:498–500, 1979.
24. Holdsworth, S., Atkins, R. C., and deKretser, D. M. The pituitary-testicular axis in man with chronic renal failure. *N. Engl. J. Med.* 296:1245–1249, 1977.
25. Hope, K., Phillip, A. E., and Loughran, J. M. Psychological characteristics associated with XYY sex-chromosome complement in a state mental hospital. *Br. J. Psychiatry* 113:496–498, 1967.
26. Imperato-McGinley, J., and Peterson, R. E. Male pseudohermaphroditism: The complexities of male phenotypic development. *Am. J. Med.* 61:215–272, 1976.
27. Imperato-McGinley, J., et al. Androgens and the evolution of male gender identity among male pseudohermaphrodites with 5 alpha reductase deficiency. *N. Engl. J. Med.* 300:1233–1237, 1979.
28. Josso, N., Picard, J. Y., and Tran, D. The antimullerian hormone. *Recent Prog. Hormone Res.* 33:117–167, 1977.
29. Kolodny, R. C., et al. Sexual dysfunction in diabetic men. *Diabetes* 23:306–309, 1974.
30. Kolodny, R. C., et al. Depression of plasma T levels after chronic intensive marihuana use. *N. Engl. J. Med.* 290:872–874, 1974.
31. Lim, V. S., and Fang, V. S. Gonadal dysfunction in uremic men. *Am. J. Med.* 58:655–662, 1975.

32. Loriaux, D. L., et al. Spironolactone and endocrine dysfunction. *Ann. Intern. Med.* 85:630–636, 1976.

33. MacLeod, J., and Hotchkiss, R. S. The effect of hyperpyrexia upon spermatozoa counts in men. *Endocrinology* 28:780–784, 1941.

34. Marynick, S. P., et al. Evidence that testosterone can suppress pituitary gonadotropin secretion independently of peripheral aromatization. *J. Clin. Endocrinol. Metab.* 49:396–398, 1979.

35. Massary, S., et al. Impotence in patients with uremia: A possible role for parathyroid hormone. *Nephron* 19:305–310, 1977.

36. Odell, W. D., and Swerdloff, R. S. Abnormalities of gonadal function in men. *Clin. Endocrinol.* 8:149–180, 1978.

37. Ohno, S. Sexual differentiation and testosterone production. *N. Engl. J. Med.* 295:1011–1012, 1976.

38. Oshima, H., and Troen, P. Endocrine and environmental influences on sexual roles. *Am. J. Med.* 70:1–3, 1981.

39. Rose, L. I., et al. Pathophysiology of spironolactone induced gynecomastia. *Ann. Intern. Med.* 87:398–403, 1977.

40. Sardi, K., Wenn, R. V., and Sharif, F. Bromocryptine for male infertility. *Lancet* 1:250–251, 1977.

41. Santen, R. J. Independent Effects of Testosterone and Estradiol on the Secretion of Gonadotropins in Man. In P. Troen and H. N. Nankin (Eds.), *The Testis in Normal and Infertile Men.* New York: Raven Press, 1977. Pp. 197–211.

42. Schalch, D. S., et al. Plasma gonadotropins after administration of LH-releasing hormone in patients with renal or hepatic failure. *J. Clin. Endocrinol. Metab.* 41:921–925, 1975.

43. Segal, S., Polishuk, W. Z., and Ben-David, M. Hyperprolactinemic male infertility. *Fertil. Steril.* 27:1425–1427, 1976.

44. Sherins, R. J., Brightwell, D., and Sternthal, P. M. Longitudinal Analysis of Semen of Fertile and Infertile Men. In P. Troen and H. N. Nankin (Eds.), *The Testis in Normal and Infertile Men.* New York: Raven Press, 1977. Pp. 473–488.

45. Spark, R. F., White, R. A., and Connolly, P. B. Impotence is not always psychogenic: Newer insights into hypothalamic-pituitary-gonadal dysfunction. *J.A.M.A.* 243:750–755, 1980.

45a. Spitz, I. M., Hirsch, H. J., and Trestian, S. The prolactin response to thyrotropin-releasing hormone differentiates isolated gonadotropin from delayed puberty. *N. Engl. J. Med.* 308:575–579, 1983.

46. Steinberger, A., and Steinberger, E. Inhibition of FSH by a Sertoli Cell Factor In Vitro. In P. Troen and H. N. Nankin (Eds.), *The Testis in Normal and Infertile Men.* New York: Raven Press, 1977. Pp. 271–279.

47. Stewart-Bentley, M., et al. Effect of Dilantin on FSH and spermatogenesis. *Clin. Res.* 24:101, 1976.

48. VanThiel, D. H., Gavaler, J., and Lester, R. Ethanol inhibition of vitamin A metabolism in testes: Possible mechanism for sterility in alcoholics. *Science* 186:941–942, 1974.

49. VanThiel, D. H., et al. Hypothalamic pituitary gonadal dysfunctions in men using cimetidine. *N. Engl. J. Med.* 300:1012–1015, 1979.

50. VanThiel, D. H., and Lester, R. Alcoholism: Its effect on hypothalamic pituitary gonadal function. *Gastroenterology* 71:318–327, 1976.

51. VanThiel, D. H., Lester, R., and Sherins, R. J. Hypogonadism in alcoholic liver disease: Evidence for a double defect. *Gastroenterology* 67:1188–1199, 1974.

52. VanThiel, D. H., Lester, R., and Vaitukaitis, J. Evidence for a defect in pituitary secretion of luteinizing hormone in chronic alcoholic men. *J. Clin. Endocrinol. Metab.* 47:499–502, 1978.
53. Van Zyl, J. A., et al. Oligospermia: A seven-year survey of the incidence, chromosomal aberrations, treatment and pregnancy rate. *Int. J. Fertil.* 20:129–132, 1975.
54. Vorhees, J. J., et al. The XYY chromosomal complement and nodulocystic acne. *Ann. Intern. Med.* 73:271–276, 1970.
55. Watchel, S. D., et al. Serologic detection of a Y-linked gene in XX males and XX true hermaphrodites. *N. Engl. J. Med.* 295:750–754, 1976.
56. Wilson, J. D., Aiman, J., and MacDonald, P. C. The pathogenesis of gynecomastia. *Adv. Intern. Med.* 25:1–32, 1980.
57. Winters, S. J., et al. Studies on the role of sex steroids in the feedback control of gonadotropin concentration in cancer. II. Use of the estrogen antagonist clomiphene citrate. *J. Clin. Endocrinol. Metab.* 48:222–227, 1979.
58. Winters, S. J., et al. H-Y antigen mosaicism in the gonad of a 46 XX true hermaphrodite. *N. Engl. J. Med.* 300:746–749, 1979.

14 Hyperlipidemia

Robert G. Brodows
William F. Streck

At the simplest level, *hyperlipidemia* is defined as an elevation of serum cholesterol, triglycerides, or both. However, the implications of such elevations are often not clear [1]. The more rigorous the effort to classify disorders, the less practical the distinctions may become in clinical practice. Lipid elevations may be classified on the basis of lipoprotein phenotype [10], genetic patterns of expression [25], or pathophysiologic mechanisms [4]. In addition, lipid disorders may be classified as primary diseases with familial or sporadic occurrence [25] or may be secondary to diet, drug therapy, underlying disease, or all three. These various approaches to classification reflect the heterogeneity of lipid disorders and the lack of specificity of triglyceride and cholesterol elevations.

Cholesterol and triglycerides do not circulate independently in the plasma. Rather, these lipids, in combination with various phospholipids, circulate as lipoproteins [9,25]. These lipoprotein complexes contain various distributions of cholesterol, triglyceride, phospholipid, and protein. The measurement of cholesterol and triglyceride assesses the total lipid content distributed throughout these lipoprotein groups. Overproduction or underremoval of specific lipoproteins may affect cholesterol and triglyceride levels to different degrees.

The characteristics of the various lipoproteins have been defined by electrophoretic and ultracentrifugation techniques.

1. Chylomicrons, the largest and lightest lipoproteins, are composed almost entirely of exogenous dietary triglyceride. In high concentrations, they cause turbidity in plasma. Chylomicrons are normally absent in the postabsorptive state. They seldom contribute significantly to hypertriglyceridemia unless serum triglyceride levels exceed 1000 mg/ml.
2. Very low-density lipoproteins (VLDL) are endogenously synthesized, triglyceride-rich lipoproteins composed of hepatic triglyceride (55–65%) and cholesterol (10–20%) combined with several protein subunits, the major components being apoproteins B and C. Only 5 to 10% of plasma cholesterol is normally found in the VLDL fraction. Unless chylomicrons are present, plasma triglycerides are highly correlated with VLDL levels.
3. Intermediate-density lipoproteins (IDL) are transitional lipoproteins resulting from the sequential delipidation of VLDL, with progressive triglyceride removal and loss of C apoproteins [9].
4. Low-density lipoproteins (LDL) are cholesterol-rich (45%) lipoproteins resulting from metabolism of VLDLs removed from plasma by binding to specific cellular receptors [12]. From 50 to 75% of plasma cholesterol is normally found in LDL. When triglyceride levels are

normal, total cholesterol levels usually provide a good measure of LDL levels.
5. High-density lipoproteins (HDL) are the smallest lipoproteins and are composed mainly of protein (45–50%). These are synthesized in the liver and function as a shuttle for cholesterol between the cells and the liver [28]. The fraction of total plasma cholesterol in the HDL fraction is somewhat sex dependent but approximates 25%.

The various protein constituents of lipoproteins are called *apoproteins*. These apoproteins serve structural as well as functional purposes and play a major role in determining the sites and rates of lipoprotein metabolism. Lipoprotein lipase is an enzyme found in close proximity to capillary endothelium of adipose and muscle tissue. This enzyme hydrolyzes triglycerides from chylomicrons and VLDLs to monoglycerides and fatty acids for storage in adipose cells.

CLINICAL CONSIDERATIONS
The finding of an elevated cholesterol or triglyceride level may be the incidental result of screening studies. However, in certain circumstances, these determinations should be made as part of a diagnostic evaluation in the asymptomatic patient:

1. Family history of premature cardiovascular disease
2. History of recurrent pancreatitis or abdominal pain
3. Presence of xanthoma or xanthelasma on physical examination
4. Lipemia retinalis or arcus juvenilis
5. Increased risk factors for coronary disease: abnormal glucose tolerance, increased uric acid, cigarette smoking, hypertension
6. Lipemic serum noted at phlebotomy
7. Family history of lipid disorders

The importance of characterizing the lipid disorders is apparent from numerous epidemiologic studies that have established a strong association between total cholesterol and ischemic cardiovascular disease [18,20,31]. In addition, eruptive xanthomas and pancreatitis may occur with marked triglyceride elevations. The predictive value of triglyceride elevations in the development of atherosclerotic vascular disease is less clear [5,19].

Fredrickson and Lees' original classification of hyperlipidemia based on elevations in the various classes of lipoproteins is still the major frame of reference for these diseases [10], but other classifications may also prove useful to the clinician. A more pathophysiologic approach is compared in Table 14-1 to the classic phenotypic and genetic classifications of hyperlipidemias. Secondary hyperlipoproteinemias are outlined in Table 14-2. Several points about these various classifications warrant

Table 14-1. Comparative Classifications of Hyperlipidemias

Physiologic Abnormality	Genetic Terminology	Lipoprotein Phenotype	Abnormal Lipoprotein
Abnormal LDL catabolism	Familial hyper- cholesterolemia Polygenic hyper- cholesterolemia	IIa	LDL
Increased endogenous triglyceride input	Familial hyper- triglyceridemia	IV	VLDL
Decreased triglyceride metabolism	Familial lipo- protein lipase deficiency C-II apoprotein deficiency	I	Chylomicrons
Mixed hyperlipidemia		V	Chylomicrons + VLDL
Abnormal remnant catabolism	Familial dysbeta- lipoproteinemia	III	β-VLDL
Combined hyperlipidemia	Familial multiple lipoprotein hyperlipidemia	IIa, IIb, IV, rarely V	LDL, VLDL

Table 14-2. Secondary Hyperlipidemias

Increased chylomicrons
  Dysglobulinemias
  Lupus erythematosus
Increased VLDL
  Diet
  Obesity
  Diabetes mellitus*
  Dysglobulinemia
  Uremia*
  Hypothyroidism*
  Nephrotic syndrome
  Drugs (estrogen, alcohol, glucocorticoids)*
Increased LDL
  Diet
  Hypothyroidism
  Dysglobulinemia
  Nephrotic syndrome
  Acute intermittent porphyria
  Obstructive liver disease

*May be associated with hyperchylomicronemia, particularly in combination with familial hyperlipidemia.

emphasis. (1) Most cases of hyperlipidemia are not readily subject to genetic classification. (2) Secondary hyperlipidemias are common and may present with lipid profiles consistent with lipoprotein or genetic classifications. (3) Significant elevations of triglycerides are often accompanied by some degree of cholesterol elevation since VLDL may contain 10 to 20% cholesterol.

The use of a pathophysiologic approach to hyperlipidemia allows inclusion of the classic hyperlipoproteinemia classification and recognition of genetic aspects of these disorders. In addition, such an approach provides a means of dealing with hyperlipidemic states, most of which are not due to definable genetic disorders, in a systematic fashion. In this framework, disorders include:

Abnormal LDL catabolism
Increased triglyceride input (endogenous hypertriglyceridemia)
Decreased triglyceride metabolism (exogenous hypertriglyceridemia)
Abnormal remnant lipoprotein metabolism (dysbetalipoproteinemia)
Combined hyperlipidemia

Abnormal Low-Density Lipoprotein Catabolism

Elevation of cholesterol levels in the presence of normal triglycerides is most often a result of a diet high in cholesterol or saturated fat or other secondary causes including hypothyroidism, the nephrotic syndrome, myeloma, porphyria, and obstructive liver disease. Diet has been established as a factor in cholesterol elevations. A net increase in the total cholesterol level in excess of 30% has been noted in normal and hyperlipidemic patients given a high-cholesterol diet, whereas a cholesterol-free diet resulted in comparable reductions to baseline values [7]. This observation is supported by the results using the American Heart Association (AHA) diet. The level of LDL cholesterol usually decreases by 10 to 15% when the diet is changed from the usual U.S. diet to the phase 1 AHA diet and decreases by 20 to 25% on the phase 2 diet [14]. Saturated fats have even stronger effects on plasma cholesterol than does dietary cholesterol [8,23].

The most clearly defined form of abnormal LDL metabolism is familial hypercholesterolemia (type IIa hyperlipoproteinemia). This is not, however, the most frequently encountered cause of elevated cholesterol levels. The homozygous form of this disorder is present in 1 in 1 million persons in the general population, whereas the heterozygous form accounts for only 1 in 25 of the estimated 5% of Americans with isolated elevation of cholesterol levels [17]. Familial hypercholesterolemia clearly documents the risk of elevated cholesterol levels. This disorder is inherited as an autosomal dominant trait and in the homozygous form is characterized by premature atherosclerosis, tendon xanthoma, and xanthelasma, with death usually occurring before age 30 due to cardiovascular complications. The heterozygous form is characterized by a lesser degree of hypercholesterolemia but an increased risk of atherosclerosis as compared to the unaffected population. Recent studies on homozygous forms have demonstrated deficiencies in LDL binding sites, whereas in the heterozygous form 50% reductions in receptors have been demonstrated [12]. Thus, the best-characterized hyperlipidemia clearly shows the risk of elevated cholesterol levels but accounts for a small proportion of clinical cases of isolated hypercholesterolemia.

Hypercholesterolemia may also present with increases of both LDL and VLDL in a combined hyperlipidemia (type IIb hyperlipoproteinemia). In fact, the estimated prevalence of this disorder (8%) is greater than that of isolated familial hypercholesterolemia (4%) in the hypercholesterolemic population. A polygenic form of hypercholesterolemia also exists; this disorder is not well defined.

Cholesterol levels greater than 350 mg/dl are most suggestive of heterozygous familial hypercholesterolemia. Xanthomas of the Achilles tendons occur in approximately half of these individuals after age 35 [14]. Xanthelasmas and corneal arcus may also be found in this population but are not specific for the presence of hyperlipidemia. Very high cholesterol levels may be found in the homozygous form of familial hypercholesterolemia, but the consequences of this disease (accelerated atherosclerosis) usually allow diagnosis at an early age. The adult with very high cholesterol levels in the absence of familial hypercholesterolemia probably has two disorders, such as combined hyperlipidemia and hypothyroidism or drug exposure.

Excess Endogenous Triglyceride Input
In some patients, hypertriglyceridemia is due to secondary causes of excess endogenous hypertriglyceridemia, manifested phenotypically as type IV hyperlipoproteinemia. Excess production of VLDL is commonly due to the high caloric intake associated with obesity. Potent stimuli of VLDL include carbohydrates and alcohol. Other causes of excess VLDL include the insulin-resistant state characteristic of obesity and secondary to estrogen or glucocorticoid therapy. Acromegaly and possibly uremia may be associated with this lipoprotein abnormality. Since VLDL contain some cholesterol, variable cholesterol elevations may be found. Sporadic and secondray hypertriglyceridemia account for approximately 4.5% of the population with triglycerides above the 95th percentile.

Monogenic familial hypertriglyceridemia, an autosomal dominant disorder with an estimated prevalence of 1 in 500 in the U.S. population, is included in this pathophysiologic category [5]. Most patients with this disorder manifest a type IV lipoprotein pattern. It is usually an asymptomatic condition. Xanthoma formation is rare, but hyperuricemia, impaired glucose tolerance, and pancreatitis are increased in frequency.

Hypertriglyceridemia is also seen in combined hyperlipidemia and may be aggravated by secondary factors (e.g., diabetes). Studies have suggested lesser abnormalities of apoprotein B and a lesser incidence of coronary artery disease in the familial form of hypertriglyceridemia as compared to that due to combined hyperlipidemia [16].

Decreased Triglyceride Catabolism

Removal of triglyceride from plasma VLDL and chylomicrons is accomplished by lipoprotein lipase. This enzyme, produced by fat cells, is insulin sensitive, enabling efficient clearing of dietary fat with meal-induced increases in insulin secretion. Chylomicronemia may be further categorized by the absence (type I hyperlipoproteinemia) or presence (type V hyperlipoproteinemia) of significant concurrent VLDL elevations. The latter presentation is seen more frequently and is most often due to the insulin-deficient state of uncontrolled diabetes mellitus. Hypothyroidism may be characterized by hypertriglyceridemia due to decreased lipoprotein lipase activity as well as abnormalities of cholesterol metabolism. Renal failure may also result in decreased adipose tissue activity of lipoprotein lipase.

Mixed hyperlipidemia (type V hyperlipoproteinemia) is characterized by markedly elevated triglycerides, both dietary chylomicrons and VLDL. In more severe forms, this disorder may present with lipemia retinalis, eruptive xanthomata, and bouts of pancreatitis. Such patients presumably have a combination of defects in triglyceride production and removal with major defects in lipoprotein lipase activity apparent in 5 to 10% of patients [17]. This disorder is not associated with a high incidence of pancreatitis unless other synergistic factors are present, such as estrogen, alcohol use, or diabetes mellitus in the setting of other hyperlipidemias such as familial hypertriglyceridemia or combined hyperlipidemia.

Lipoprotein lipase deficiency (type I hyperlipoproteinemia) may be inherited as a rare autosomal recessive condition presenting in childhood with eruptive xanthoma, hepatosplenomegaly, recurrent acute pancreatitis, and lipemia retinalis. Marked hyperchylomicronemia in this disorder is associated with recurrent pancreatitis and abdominal pain. A similar picture in adults is seen in the disorder characterized by autosomal recessive absence of the lipoprotein lipase activator, apoprotein C-II.

Abnormal Remnant Catabolism

Abnormal remnant catabolism is also known as *broad beta disease, dysbetalipoproteinemia,* or *type III hyperlipoproteinemia.* Familial dysbetalipoproteinemia occurs in about 1% of the population. However, not all affected individuals manifest hyperlipidemia. The presumed disorder involves a deficiency of one of the components of apoprotein E, with homozygotes having nearly total deficiency and heterozygotes having intermediate levels. Homozygotes do not have overt hyperlipidemia; they have a modest accumulation of remnant particles with low levels of LDL, presumably due to defective formation of LDL from VLDL. Homozygotes thus have low cholesterol and little or no elevation of triglycerides. The risk of developing atherosclerosis with this lipoprotein pattern is not known. The atherosclerotic risk for heterozygotes is also uncertain, although premature peripheral vascular disease has been suggested in some studies [15].

Hyperlipidemia and increased risk of atherosclerotic disease in individuals with dysbetalipoproteinemia are often due to the presence of another familial hyperlipidemia in individuals with abnormal apoprotein E. One of the characteristic features of dysbetalipoproteinemia is the presence of characteristic tuberous xanthomas over the elbows and knees or cutaneous xanthomas in the palmar and digital creases. The diagnosis of dysbetalipoproteinemia is based on an analysis of isoforms of apoprotein E separated by isoelectric focusing [15]. Such studies are indicated in patients with characteristic xanthomas as well as those with roughly comparable cholesterol and triglyceride levels.

Combined Hyperlipidemia

Combined hyperlipidemia (hypercholesterolemia and hypertriglyceridemia) has an estimated prevalence of 1 in 300. This disorder presents with variable lipid manifestations and complicates interpretation of the genetic origin of other disorders. Approximately one-third of patients have increased LDL alone, one-third have VLDL alone, and one-third have both. Environmental factors have some influence. Obese individuals tend to have VLDL elevations and thin individuals LDL elevations. This disorder can mimic other disorders on the basis of lipoprotein phenotypes. The diagnosis is dependent on the demonstration of increased VLDL, LDL, or both in approximately one-half of the first-degree relatives of a subject. Obviously, specific genetic diagnoses are not practical in most cases. This disorder may serve as the basis for more severe hyperlipidemic presentations when combined with secondary disorders such as estrogens, diabetes, and glucocorticoids (Table 14-2).

Marked Hypertriglyceridemia (Chylomicronemia Syndrome)

Plasma triglyceride levels in excess of 2000 mg/dl and associated with eruptive xanthomas, lipemia retinalis, and pancreatitis constitute the chylomicronemia syndrome [3]. This disorder is usually due to the interaction of one of the common familial forms of hypertriglyceridemia and an acquired form secondary to another disease, drug, or alcohol. The lipoprotein phenotype discussed previously is usually type V. Genetic abnormalities in lipoprotein lipase are rarely the cause of this syndrome.

DIAGNOSTIC METHODS
Refrigerated Plasma Test
For most hyperlipidemic states, quantitative determinations of cholesterol and triglycerides in the fasted state are adequate for diagnosis and classification. By merely refrigerating plasma obtained after an overnight fast of 10 to 12 hours, much valuable information may be obtained. Chylomicrons form a creamy layer at the top, whereas increased VLDL concentrations impart turbidity to the entire plasma, as do increased IDL characteristics of dysbetalipoproteinemia. High LDL and HDL do not produce turbidity; thus, patients with elevated concentrations of these cholesterol-carrying lipoproteins have clear plasma. It is best if patients are off any lipid-lowering agents or other drugs known to influence lipid levels (such as steroids or estrogens) for 1 month before baseline values are obtained. Myocardial infarction or severe stress may raise triglycerides and lower cholesterol significantly; thus, 4 to 8 weeks should intervene before studies are conducted.

Cholesterol
Plasma cholesterol levels are 3% lower than serum cholesterol measurements. Normal ranges for total cholesterol must be age and sex adjusted. Between ages 20 and 45 in men and 25 and 55 in women, both cholesterol and triglyceride levels rise. The 95th percentile for total cholesterol for men at age 25 is approximately 240 mg/dl; for women, it is 222 mg/dl. At age 55 the 95th percentile values are 276 and 300 mg/dl, respectively, reflecting the fact that serum lipid levels are higher in postmenopausal women.

Total cholesterol shows a high correlation with LDL cholesterol if triglycerides are not elevated. If triglycerides are increased as well, the contribution of VLDL to the total cholesterol may be estimated based on the observation that VLDL contain 1 gm of cholesterol for every 4 gm of triglyceride. In some circumstances, elevated HDL levels may also contribute to the total cholesterol measurement. These factors may be taken into account using the following formula to estimate LDL:

$$\text{LDL cholesterol} = \text{total cholesterol} - (\text{triglyceride}/5 + \text{HDL cholesterol})$$

The HDL cholesterol may be directly measured or estimated as 45 mg/dl in this formula. Quantitative HDL assays are now readily available in commercial laboratories. The above formula is not exact and is less useful if triglycerides are greater than 400 mg/ml or if dysbetalipoproteinemia is present. The 95th percentile values for LDL cholesterol at age 25 are 165 mg/dl in men and 150 mg/dl in women. At age 55, the values are 203 mg/dl for men and 213 mg/dl for women [14].

Triglycerides

Triglyceride measurements in the fasted patient normally assess the VLDL fraction. In the presence of chylomicronemia, triglyceride levels are usually quite elevated and VLDL levels cannot be readily determined. Chylomicrons are not present in the normal fasted state. Triglyceride levels, like cholesterol levels, are age and sex dependent. The 95th percentile values for men and women at age 25 are approximately 250 mg/dl and 145 mg/dl, respectively. At age 55 the values are 280 mg/dl for men and 260 mg/dl for women [14].

DISCUSSION

Hypercholesterolemia or hypertriglyceridemia should be confirmed by several determinations, with samples drawn after a 10- to 12-hour fast. If the problem appears to be persistent, a detailed history, particularly one dealing with alcohol intake and dietary patterns, is essential. At this point, one should also begin to consider the secondary causes of lipid disorders listed in Table 14-2. In the absence of obvious secondary disorders, familial forms of hyperlipidemia become more of a concern. A history of premature coronary artery disease or the presence of xanthomas certainly would support this suspicion. However, physical examination in hyperlipidemia is often totally unrevealing. If a patient has hypercholesterolemia, xanthelasma may be apparent. However, the corollary is not true—that is, the presence of xanthelasma does not mean that cholesterol levels are high. Patients with familial hypercholesterolemia may have xanthomas on the knuckles and tendons. Hypertriglyceridemia, on the other hand, must be severe to produce characteristic eruptive xanthomas over the knees, arms, and buttocks. Palmar and digital xanthomas are characteristic of dysbetalipoproteinemia.

Secondary hyperlipidemia affected largely by dietary factors accounts for most problems with hypercholesterolemia in the United States. Such hyperlipidemia is present even among children [6]. Most patients in the United States who have hyperlipidemia have plasma cholesterol levels ranging from 200 to 260 mg/dl, whereas in familial forms of hypercholesterolemia, levels of 350 mg/dl or more may be found. A serum cholesterol threshold level below which the development of atherosclerosis is minimized appears to be in the range of 150 to 180 mg/dl [20]. As noted, cholesterol levels above the 95th percentile for a given sex and age group are usually considered abnormal [18]. On a practical scale, a cholesterol level greater than 250 mg/dl requires further characterization as a possible lipid disorder. However, it should be borne in mind that there is no clear dividing line between a cholesterol level that increases the risk and one that does not. The prospective data of the Framingham study demonstrate that the risk of coronary artery disease in persons younger than 50 years of age is related to the total serum cholesterol level. Cholesterol is not a predictor of risk beyond age 65 [22].

Although persons with triglyceride elevations do on the average have a higher risk of coronary disease [19], the use of cholesterol, LDL, and HDL levels may better predict such risk. VLDL carry most triglyceride in the fasting state but also contain some cholesterol. The cholesterol associated with VLDL has not been shown to be an independent predictor of the risk of atherogenic disease. Triglycerides do, however, provide a reliable way to assess various hyperlipidemic states by using the refrigerated plasma test. A creamy layer indicating the presence of chylomicrons points toward the less common lipid disorders associated with abnormal VLDL catabolism. Turbidity throughout the plasma represents increased VLDL, most commonly due to endogenous hypertriglyceridemia. Clear plasma suggests normal triglyceride levels and selective LDL abnormalities.

As outlined in Figure 14-1, hyperlipidemic disorders may be largely investigated by using the refrigerated plasma test and measuring cholesterol and triglyceride levels after a 10- to 12-hour fast. In this sequence, the most straightforward diagnosis follows the finding of isolated hypercholesterolemia, evidenced by clear plasma and normal triglycerides. This points toward the diagnosis of familial hypercholesterolemia. Cholesterol levels are often in excess of 350 mg/dl in the heterozygous form. Levels are even higher in the homozygous state, but these patients usually present at a younger age with evidence of accelerated atherosclerosis. Most other patients have cholesterol levels less than 350 mg/dl and have less clearly defined reasons for these elevations. Hypothyroidism is a leading secondary cause of isolated cholesterol elevations. Diet, particularly one high in saturated fats, may also account for such intermediate cholesterol elevations.

When plasma is clear but triglycerides are modestly elevated, LDL cholesterol may be calculated. A calculated LDL of 200 mg/dl or more suggests predominant hypercholesterolemia as seen in familial hypercholesterolemia, whereas levels less than 200 mg/dl suggest that both LDL and VLDL are contributing to cholesterol elevation as may be found in combined hyperlipidemia, manifested in this instance by the IIb lipoprotein phenotype. The 200 mg/dl level is an arbitrary one, as 95th percentile LDL levels are lower in younger individuals.

In some instances, elevated HDL may contribute significantly to cholesterol elevations. In general, HDL levels correlate inversely with total cholesterol, as well as with the risk of atherosclerotic disease [20,21]. Measurement of HDL levels may enhance the predictive value of total cholesterol, particularly in subjects with modest hypercholesterolemia (240–300 mg/dl). High HDL levels in such instances may be somewhat reassuring. More severe hypercholesterolemia may warrant attempts at therapy regardless of the HDL levels [20].

When plasma is turbid after the overnight refrigerator test and cholesterol is normal, the presence of chylomicronemia serves to distinguish

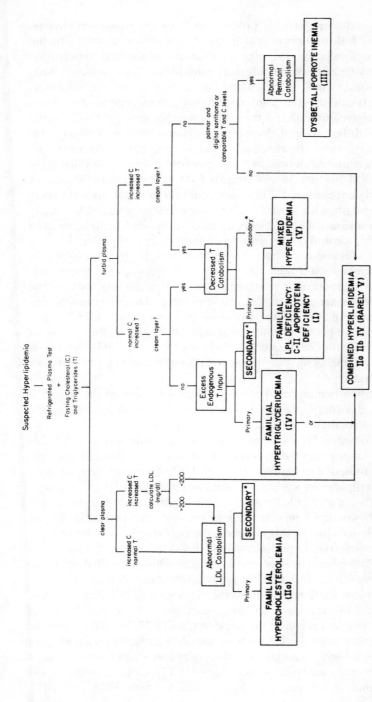

Figure 14-1. Diagnostic protocol: Suspected hyperlipidemia. LDL, low-density lipoprotein; LPL, lipoprotein lipase. *See Table 14-2 for causes.

excess endogenous triglyceride production from the exogenous hyperlipidemia that follows lipoprotein lipase deficiency or absence. In the
absence of chylomicrons, the primary disorder of familial hypertriglyceridemia may be considered. More common secondary causes include
high-carbohydrate diets, diabetes mellitus, estrogens, and other drugs.
Approximately one-third of combined hyperlipidemias present with isolated hypertriglyceridemia, so that this diagnosis may follow if family
studies show different lipid disorders. Chylomicronemia indicates inadequate triglyceride disposal and, as discussed earlier, is often associated with acquired deficiencies of lipoprotein lipase. Familial lipoprotein lipase deficiency in children or C-II apoprotein deficiency in
adults is rarely encountered. The more common disorder, mixed hyperlipidemia, presents with a type V lipoprotein phenotype and is usually
secondary to uncontrolled diabetes mellitus, dysglobulinemias, or drug
use (estrogens, alcohol) in the setting of another hyperlipidemia.

Significant elevations in both cholesterol and triglycerides without
chylomicronemia should raise the question of dysbetalipoproteinemia,
particularly if characteristic xanthomas are present and cholesterol and
triglyceride levels are approximately comparable. This diagnosis is confirmed by determination of the isoforms of apoprotein E [15]. Hyperlipidemia with dysbetalipoproteinemia usually occurs in the setting of
another lipid disorder such as combined hyperlipidemia, this latter condition again serving as the diagnostic term for abnormalities that are not
easily categorized.

The chylomicronemia syndrome may occur when any of the hypertri-
glyceridemic disorders in Figure 14-1 is combined with secondary disorders, such as diabetes mellitus, or with drug use.

Screening of adult family members should be considered in patients
suspected of having familial hypercholesterolemia, combined hyperlipidemia, or familial hypertriglyceridemia [26]. However, establishing
whether hyperlipidemia is genetic or acquired is often not possible unless
large kindreds are available for study. This is particularly true for familial combined hyperlipidemia, which may present with a type IIa, IIb, or
IV lipoprotein pattern. In this instance, the only way to establish a diagnosis is to demonstrate hyperlipidemia with various lipoprotein patterns
in relatives. The information gained from individual or familial lipid profiles may prove critical if significant lipid elevations are found. However,
in most instances moderate cholesterol elevations (250–300 mg/dl) are
encountered. The approach to these common nonfamilial forms of
hyperlipidemia is uncertain at the present time [2,27,30] and awaits the
results of further study [29]. Emphasis should be placed on identifying
those individuals with familial lipid disorders for which treatment programs are generally accepted as necessary [11,17]. Children with hypercholesterolemia should be carefully checked for both HDL and LDL

cholesterol since 20% will have elevated HDL and are at reduced risk for coronary disease [6,24].

REFERENCES

1. Ahrens, E. H. The management of hyperlipidemia: Whether, rather than how. *Ann. Intern. Med.* 85:87–93, 1976.
2. Ahrens, E. H. Dietary fats and coronary artery disease. Unfinished business. *Lancet* 2:1345–1348, 1979.
3. Brunzell, John D., and Bierman, E. L. Chylomicronemia syndrome. *Med. Clin. North Am.* 66:455–469, 1982.
4. Brunzell, J. D., Chait, A., and Bierman, E. L. Pathophysiology of lipoprotein transport. *Metabolism* 27:1109–1127, 1978.
5. Brunzell, J. D., et al. Myocardial infarction in the familial forms of hypertriglyceridemia. *Metabolism* 25:313–320, 1976.
6. Christensen, B., et al. Plasma cholesterol and triglyceride distributions in 13,665 children and adolescents. The prevalence study of the lipid research clinics program. *Pediatr. Res.* 14:94–202, 1980.
7. Connor, W. E., and Connor, S. L. The dietary treatment of hyperlipidemia. *Med. Clin. North Am.* 66:485–518, 1982.
8. Ehnholm, C., et al. Effect of diet on serum lipoproteins in a poulation with a high risk of coronary artery disease. *N. Engl. J. Med.* 307:850–855, 1982.
9. Fisher, W. R., and Truitt, D. H. The common hyperlipoproteinemias. An understanding of disease mechanisms and their control. *Ann. Intern. Med.* 85:497–508, 1976.
10. Fredrickson, D. S., and Lees, R. S. A system for phenotyping hyperlipoproteinemia. *Circulation* 31:321–327, 1965.
11. Glueck, C. J. Colestipol and probucol: Treatment of primary and familial hypercholesterolemia and amelioration of atherosclerosis. *Ann. Intern. Med.* 96:475–482, 1982.
12. Goldstein, J. L., and Brown, M. S. Familial hypercholesterolemia. A genetic regulatory defect in cholesterol metabolism. *Am. J. Med.* 58:147–150, 1975.
13. Gordon, T., et al. High density lipoprotein as a protective factor against coronary heart disease. The Framingham study. *Am. J. Med.* 62:707–713, 1977.
14. Havel, R. J. Approach to the patient with hyperlipidemia. *Med. Clin. North Am.* 66:319–335, 1982.
15. Havel, R. J. Familial dysbetalipoproteinemia. *Med. Clin. North Am.* 66:441–455, 1982.
16. Havel, R. J.: Treatment of hyperlipidemias: Where do we stand? *Am. J. Med.* 73:301–304, 1982.
17. Havel, R. J., and Kane, J. P. Therapy of hyperlipidemic states. *Ann. Rev. Med.* 33:417–433, 1982.
18. Heiss, G., et al. Lipoprotein-cholesterol distributions in selected North American populations: The Lipid Research Clinics Program Prevalence Study. *Circulation* 61:311–314, 1980.
19. Hulley, S. B., et al. Epidemiology as a guide to clinical decisions: The association between triglyceride and coronary heart disease. *N. Engl. J. Med.* 302:1383–1390, 1980.
20. Inkeles, S., and Eisenberg, D. Hyperlipidemia and coronary atherosclerosis: A review. *Medicine* 60:110–123, 1981.

21. Levy, R. I., and Rifkind, B. M. The structure, function, and metabolism of high-density lipoproteins: A status report. *Circulation* 62(Suppl. 5):4–8, 1980.
22. Kannel, W. B., et al. Cholesterol in the prediction of atherosclerotic disease: New perspectives based on the Framingham study. *Ann. Intern. Med.* 90:85–91, 1979.
23. Mistry, P., et al. Individual variation in the effects of dietary cholesterol on plasma lipoproteins and cellular cholesterol homeostasis in man. *J. Clin. Invest.* 67:493–502, 1981.
24. Morrison, J. A., et al. Lipids and lipoproteins in 927 school children, ages 6–17 years. *Pediatrics* 62:990–995, 1978.
25. Motulsky, A. G. The genetic hyperlipidemias. *N. Engl. J. Med.* 294:823–827, 1976.
26. Neill, C. A., Ose, L., and Kwiferovich, P. O., Jr. Hyperlipidemia: Clinical clues on the first two decades of life. *Johns Hopkins Med. J.* 140:171–176, 1977.
27. Oliver, M. F. Risks of correcting the risks of coronary disease and stroke with drugs. *N. Engl. J. Med.* 306:287–290, 1982.
28. Tall, A. R., and Small, D. M. Plasma high-density lipoproteins. *N. Engl. J. Med.* 299:1232–1236, 1978.
29. The Lipid Research Clinic Program. The coronary primary prevention trial: Design and implementation. *J. Chronic Dis.* 32:609–631, 1979.
30. The Pooling Project Research Group. Relationships of blood pressure, serum cholesterol, smoking habit, relative weight, and ECG abnormalities to incidence of major coronary events: Final report of the Pooling Project. *J. Chronic Dis.* 31:201–306, 1978.
31. Zampogua, A., Luria, M. H., and Munubens, S. T. Relationship between lipids and occlusive coronary artery disease. *Arch. Intern. Med.* 140:1067–1069, 1980.

15 Multiple Endocrine Neoplasia (MEN) Syndromes

T. Franklin Williams
William F. Streck

In the quarter century that spans their recognition, much has been learned about the syndromes of multiple endocrine neoplasia [23,27], commonly referred to as *MEN syndromes*. Knowledge has come from clinical and pathologic observations of the relatively frequent occurrence of certain endocrine abnormalities in both individuals and families. Recognition of these syndromes, particularly in their early stages, has also depended heavily on the development of laboratory methods for measuring the various hormones involved.

Two general MEN syndromes have come to be recognized. The MEN-I (Wermer's syndrome) consists typically of a combination of tumors or hyperplasia of the nonbeta islet cells of the pancreas, the parathyroids, and the anterior pituitary, with variable degrees of hyperfunction of these systems [40]. The MEN-IIa (Sipple's syndrome) consists typically of combinations of medullary thyroid carcinoma and pheochromocytoma with or without hyperfunction of the parathyroid glands [28]. A distinct subgroup of the MEN-II syndrome has been identified in which there is an association of multiple neuromas and a marfanoid habitus. This is now being referred to as the *MEN-IIb syndrome* [11]. Both MEN-I and MEN-IIa are inherited in an autosomal dominant fashion, usually with high penetrance, so that up to 50% of the members of affected families are likely to manifest the disease. Although the hereditary pattern of MEN-IIb is not entirely clear, familial forms do exist.

Because of both the potentially serious functional consequences and the risk of carcinoma, it is important to identify as early as possible, and treat appropriately, all affected members of such families. The usual components of the MEN syndromes are listed in Table 15-1.

These three syndromes have been related conceptually to the embryologic origin of their cell types in the neuroectoderm and possibly also the entoderm. More specifically, it is speculated that the cells that become involved in these tumors are of a common basic type, characterized as "amine precursor uptake and decarboxylation" (APUD) cells, that is, cells with the ability to take up the precursor amines and synthesize various peptide hormones [10,38]. Consistent with this theory is the fact that these tumors at times produce a number of ectopic hormones, including adrenocorticotropic hormone (ACTH), and that other tumors, probably derived from the same embryonic tissue, such as carcinoids and oat cell tumors of the lung, also produce a number of different ectopic peptide hormones.

Table 15-1. Multiple Endocrine Neoplasia Syndromes

Syndrome	Lesion	Incidence (%)
MEN-I		
Parathyroid	Hyperplasia or adenoma	80–90
Pancreas	Adenoma	75
Pituitary	Adenoma	60
MEN-IIa		
Thyroid	Medullary carcinoma	95–100
Adrenal	Pheochromocytoma	40–80
Parathyroid	Hyperplasia or adenoma	30–60
MEN-IIb		
Mucosal neuromas		100
Marfanoid habitus		100
Thyroid	Medullary carcinoma	80
Adrenal	Pheochromocytoma	30–60

CLINICAL CONSIDERATIONS
The three syndromes, although showing some overlap in the endocrine systems involved, are nevertheless completely distinct genetic and clinical entities.

Multiple Endocrine Neoplasia-I Syndrome
Parathyroid gland disease, usually due to hyperplasia or multiple adenomas, is the most frequently encountered component of the MEN-I syndrome, occurring in 80 to 90% of cases. Islet cell tumors occur in approximately 80% of cases; pituitary disease is somewhat less common, occurring in 60% of cases [3].

Although parathyroid disease is the most frequently encountered component of the MEN-I syndrome, it is also found in the general population, with an estimated incidence of approximately 27 per 100,000 [13]. The incidence of MEN syndromes in patients with hyperparathyroidism has been estimated by Mallette et al. [18], who found that 16% of 57 patients with primary hyperparathyroidism had the MEN-I syndrome. In another study by Jackson et al. in which first-degree relatives of 91 consecutive patients with parathyroid tumors were studied, 10 individuals (11%) were found whose other family members were affected. Of these 10 newly identified families, 5 had familial hyperparathyroidism, 3 had MEN-I, and 2 had MEN-IIa [15]. Multicentric origin is characteristic of the hyperparathyroid disease in MEN-I and MEN-IIa in 60 to 70% of cases [3,17]. This contrasts to an incidence of multicentric origin (hyperplasia or multiple adenomas) in 4 to 18% of the population with primary hyperparathyroidism [23,44]. In addition, patients with MEN-I tend to be younger, and their calcium levels may not be strikingly elevated [17].

Table 15-2. Relative Incidence of Manifestations of Zollinger-Ellison Syndrome

Manifestation	Incidence (%)
Ulcer pain	75–90
Bleeding	40
Diarrhea	30
Emesis	25
Bowel perforation	18
Radiographic changes (multiple small bowel ulcers)	60
Basal acid secretion, >15 mEq/hr	66
Basal/maximal acid production ratio, >0.6	75
Basal gastrin level, >400 pg/ml	70
Abnormal secretin stimulation	80–90

MEN-I may first be suspected when a patient has recurrent or intractable peptic ulcer disease. Further evaluation leads to findings of high gastric acid secretion and elevated serum gastrin levels. These findings, in combination with an islet cell tumor called *gastrinoma,* constitute the Zollinger-Ellison (ZE) syndrome [5,9,30]. The clinical features of the ZE syndrome are listed in Table 15-2.

The incidence of peptic ulcer disease has been estimated at 1.8 per 1000 patients in males, although some studies have shown that up to 10 to 12% of the population may have some history of peptic ulcer disease [33]. In contrast, the incidence of the ZE syndrome due to gastrin-secreting tumor is generally recognized as being less than 1% of patients with peptic ulcer disease. Thus, a patient presenting with peptic ulcer disease has a low probability of having a MEN syndrome and the ZE syndrome. Conversely, 15 to 26% of patients with the ZE syndrome have this as a subcomponent of the MEN-I syndrome [3,16]. In one study, 27% of 677 patients in a ZE syndrome registry were MEN patients [41]. Also of interest was the fact that a family history was present in only 6% prior to the diagnosis.

Although gastrin levels are typically elevated in the ZE syndrome, in some instances stimulation tests using calcium or secretin may be required to document significant hypersecretion of gastrin [8,14,16,19,20]. Radiologic findings, when present, are helpful in diagnosis. Thickened gastric folds or multiple ulcers are suggestive of the ZE syndrome [25].

Although gastrin-producing adenomas of non-beta, non-alpha cell origin are the most common pancreatic abnormalities in MEN-I, occasional beta cell insulin-producing tumors (insulinomas) and, rarely, alpha cell glucagon-producing tumors have been found [4,10]. Islet cell tumors of the pancreas are rare, with an estimated incidence of 1 per 100,000 per year [21]. Insulinomas are the second most commonly encountered islet cell tumor in the MEN syndrome. One study found that 4% of 951 cases of insulinomas were associated with the MEN-I syndrome [41]. Other tumors of the endocrine pancreas may also be found [10]. There are often multiple foci of the type of adenoma that is present in an individual patient. In those with islet cell tumors, watery diarrhea may be a significant symptom, and the evaluation of a patient with unexplained diarrhea should include consideration of both gastrinoma and the watery diarrhea-hypokalemia-achlorhydria (WDHA) syndrome [37].

Pituitary tumors, when they do occur, are often nonfunctioning and may produce only space-occupying signs. Occasionally, acromegaly or hyperprolactinemia may be found [24]. The incidence of MEN-I syndromes presenting with pituitary tumors is difficult to determine, possibly because the most common tumors found in the series of Ballard et al. [3] were nonfunctioning chromophobe adenomas (42%). These investigators did report that 55 of 85 MEN-I patients had pituitary lesions. Among the functioning tumors, 15 cases of acromegaly (27%) and 2 cases of Cushing's disease (3.6%) were included.

Adrenal cortical hyperplasia, multiple adenomas, and, rarely, adrenal cortical carcinoma have been reported, the overall incidence of adrenal gland involvement being 38% in one series [3]. The adrenal medulla has not been reported to be involved in the MEN-I syndrome, in clear contrast to the MEN-IIa syndrome. Similarly, thyroid medullary carcinoma has not been reported with the MEN-I syndrome. Other thyroid changes have occurred in association with this syndrome, including goiters, thyrotoxicosis, thyroiditis, and, rarely, thyroid carcinoma other than medullary. However, thyroid disease is so frequent in the general population that it is not clear that the incidence is any greater among members of families with MEN-I.

Other tumors described in members of these families have included carcinoid tumors, thymomas, schwannomas, and multiple lipomas [2,23,44]. Sometimes these other rarer tumors have been the first clue leading to the identification of families affected with MEN-I.

Once evidence for one or more types of neoplasia associated with MEN-I has been found, consideration should be given to the possibility of the other associated neoplastic changes, both in the individual patient and in all family members (parents, siblings, children) genetically at risk of having the syndrome.

Multiple Endocrine Neoplasia-IIa Syndrome

The discovery of the first person in a family with the MEN-IIa syndrome is often fortuitous, because tumors of the thyroid and adrenal medulla are often asymptomatic [29]. Medullary carcinoma of the thyroid (MCT) may be discovered at surgical exploration of an irregularly enlarged thyroid gland with or without regional lymph node enlargement and diagnosed on histological section. The pheochromocytomas characteristic of MEN-IIa may produce a hypertensive crisis for the first time during exploratory surgery of the thyroid gland.

MCT accounts for 7 to 12% of all thyroid malignancies [7,29]. This disorder occurs primarily in a sporadic fashion (75%), the remaining 25% presenting in a familial form of the MEN-II syndrome. As such, the presence of MCT has approximately a 25% chance of serving as an index case for an MEN syndrome on this statistical basis alone. Data similar to these have been found by Sizemore et al. [29] at the Mayo Clinic. In screening of the primary relatives of 36 patients with presumed sporadic cases of medullary carcinoma of the thyroid, 7 patients (19%) served as index cases to the familial disease. When MCT is encountered in the familial form, the natural history varies from family to family and also in individuals within a specific kindred. The sporadic form, unlike the familial form, is usually unilateral rather than multicentric and lacks the early phase of C-cell hyperplasia seen with the familial form.

The increased circulating levels of calcitonin that are characteristic of MCT usually produce no chemical or symptomatic changes. One of the few relatively common symptoms associated with this carcinoma is intractable diarrhea. Unfortunately, the diarrheal syndrome usually appears only after the carcinoma has metastasized.

A unique feature of MCT in the familial form is the established relationship between C-cell hyperplasia [43] and progression of the condition to frank malignancy. Calcitonin levels following stimulation provide a reliable tumor marker that may allow intervention prior to malignant progression in recognized cases. Since MCT in affected families is much more aggressive than usual thyroid malignancies, early diagnosis is essential.

Elevated calcitonin levels may be found in disorders other than MCT [7]. Ectopic calcitonin production has been found in carcinoid tumors, oat cell and islet cell carcinomas, and breast carcinoma. Calcitonin levels may also be elevated in renal disease, pregnancy, and hypergastrinemic states such as the ZE syndrome and pernicious anemia. In established cases of MCT, levels of calcitonin usually [32], although not always [36], show some correlation with tumor cell mass. In nonthyroid cancer, calcitonin levels may also be used as means of surveillance for tumor recurrence.

The incidence of pheochromocytoma is not known; it is estimated that between 0.5 and 0.7% of newly diagnosed hypertensive patients may harbor this tumor. Approximately 90% of patients with pheochromocytoma have sporadic disease (not associated with MEN). In these instances, tumors are unilateral in 80% of cases [23]. In contrast, the MEN-II syndrome is usually found in the remaining 10% of cases characterized by multicentric origin and bilateral disease. The incidence of pheochromocytoma in MEN-II varies from 13 to 21% in younger populations identified by screening to approximately 50% in older patients identified because of clinical evidence of MCT. It is also worth emphasizing that pheochromocytomas in MEN-II syndromes are often asymptomatic (8 of 17 cases in a Mayo Clinic series) yet lethal. Of 149 patients described in one literature review, 33 (22%) had deaths attributable to pheochromocytoma [6].

Hyperparathyroidism with hypercalcemia may occur as part of MEN-IIa, although less frequently than in MEN-I. As in MEN-I, multicentric foci are usually present, with hyperplasia of the parathyroid glands occurring in up to 80% of cases [29]. In at least a few instances, the hypercalcemia and elevated parathyroid hormone levels have returned to normal after removal of the pheochromocytomas [34]. Thus, it is speculated that in some instances the parathyroid abnormalities are secondary to the effects of either the calcitonin or the catecholamines.

Carcinoid tumors as well as tumors of the brain, including glioblastoma, glioma, and meningioma, have rarely been associated with MEN-IIa. As in MEN-I, once a person has been identified as having the pattern of MEN-IIa, it is essential that all genetically susceptible relatives be evaluated for the possibility of this syndrome. In fact, it is even more important in MEN-IIa because of the very frequent finding of asymptomatic early MCT in such relatives.

Multiple Endocrine Neoplasia-IIb Syndrome
The subgroup of persons with the MEN-IIb syndrome is clinically and genetically distinct [11]. These individuals have mucosal neuromas of the tongue, lips, conjunctiva, and occasionally elsewhere, hypertrophy of corneal nerves, and a habitus typical of Marfan's syndrome. The facial appearance is very characteristic, with broad lips, a flare to the alae, and laterally placed ears, such that it is said that even unrelated persons with this syndrome look like siblings. MCTs and pheochromocytomas are commonly found, but hyperparathyroidism is very rare in members of this subgroup. Although MEN-IIb is clearly familial, its precise genetic pattern is not yet defined. Sporadic cases occur with a frequency comparable to that of the familial form.

As the foregoing clinical considerations indicate, the initial symptom or clinical finding that may suggest one of the MEN syndromes can vary and thus lead to any one of many starting points for laboratory investigation. The basic requirements are these:

1. The ultimate establishment of the diagnosis of one of these syndromes depends on demonstrating excessive hormonal activity (or, rarely, a space-occupying, nonfunctioning tumor) of one or more of the endocrine systems typically involved.
2. Once such a finding has been made, it is essential to test for abnormalities of the other endocrine systems typically involved in the same syndrome.
3. Once an individual has been identified as having one of these syndromes, it is essential to test all family members at risk of having the same syndrome.

4. Involvement of all organ systems may not be present at a given time. Serial observation for other evolving components of a MEN syndrome may be required.

DIAGNOSTIC METHODS
Diagnostic tests for the MEN syndrome include:

Glucose and insulin levels (Chap. 16)
Skull x-ray (Chap. 2)
Serum calcium (Chap. 4)
Parathyroid hormone levels (Chap. 4)
Urinary catecholamines, vanillylmandelic acid, and metanephrines
   (Chap. 9)
Plasma catecholamines (Chap. 9)

Gastric Acidity
In persons with intractable or recurrent peptic ulcer disease, an important step is determination of the degree of gastric acidity in the basal state and the maximum acid secretion with stimulation. The standard test consists of gastric intubation in the overnight fasting subject, collection of basal samples every 15 minutes for 1 hour, administration of betazole (Histalog), 0.5 mg per kilogram of body weight, or pentagastrin, 6 μg per kilogram of body weight subcutaneously, and collection of four additional 15-minute samples. The total titratable acidity (titrated to pH 7.0) is measured and expressed as milliequivalents per hour.

Normal persons and most persons who have peptic ulcer disease not due to gastrin-secreting tumors have a basal acid secretion of less than 6 mEq/hr, and a ratio of basal/stimulated acid secretion of less than 0.6. Persons with gastrinomas have a higher basal acid secretion (most over 15 mEq/hr) and may have a basal/stimulated acid secretion ratio of more than 0.6 [8,42]. This latter low ratio has been questioned as a discriminatory tool and some believe it offers no advantage over the basal acid output alone [16].

Gastrin Levels
The normal range for fasting serum gastrin is variously reported as being up to 100 or 200 pg/ml. Most persons with gastrinomas will have higher values, but occasionally the fasting level has been reported to be as low as 75 pg/ml. Furthermore, elevated basal levels of serum gastrin in association with hyperacidity occur in three conditions other than gastrinomas, namely, antral G-cell hyperplasia, retained gastric antrum after previous gastric surgery, and gastric outlet obstruction and renal failure [16].

Persons with hypersecretion of gastric acid, as previously defined, or those with borderline values should have measurements of fasting levels of gastrin in the serum by radioimmunoassay techniques [20,30]. If the fasting gastrin level is elevated into the equivocally high range of 75 to 200 pg/ml or more, it should be followed by measurement of the gastrin response to secretin or calcium infusion.

Gastrin Stimulation Tests

SECRETIN STIMULATION TEST. The injection of secretin normally causes a fall in serum gastrin levels. In the ZE syndrome, a paradoxic stimulation of gastrin secretion takes place. This test is rapid and appears to give definitive results more often than the calcium infusion test. It consists of the intravenous injection of 2 units per kilogram of body weight of Secretin-Kabi as a bolus, with samples of blood for serum gastrin determinations at 0, 2, 5, 10, 15, and 30 minutes [20]. A rise of 200 pg/ml or more over basal levels of gastrin at 2, 5, or 10 minutes is considered to be diagnostic of gastrinoma [20]. These criteria apply when Secretin-Kabi (formerly GIH secretin) is used and will result in a rise in serum gastrin levels in 90% of patients with the ZE syndrome [16,20].

CALCIUM INFUSION TEST. The calcium infusion test consists of the intravenous administration of calcium as calcium gluconate, 4 mg per kilogram of body weight, over 3 hours. Blood samples are obtained for serum gastrin determinations at 0 time and at 30-minute intervals up to 3 hours. A change in serum gastrin of at least 395 pg/ml with stimulation is considered diagnostic, with an estimated 10% false-negative rate [8]. This test is more cumbersome than the secretin test and has more side effects. The secretin test using Secretin-Kabi is preferred [20].

Serum Calcitonin Levels

Serum calcitonin levels are determined through radioimmunoassay techniques that until recently have been available only in the research laboratories of the major investigators studying this entity [35]. Commercial laboratories are now offering this determination. Alternatively, one can usually obtain determinations through direct communication with the investigators in this field. Newer assays can detect levels as low as 25 pg/ml. In other assays, the normal range varies from less than 100 pg/ml up to 600 pg/ml. Familiarity with the assay used in studies of patients is required [2].

Calcitonin Stimulation Tests

PENTAGASTRIN STIMULATION. Pentagastrin injection is a quick procedure compared to the calcium infusion test, produces at least as many appropriately positive results, and causes fewer overall unpleasant symptoms.

It is reported that persons receiving pentagastrin injection almost always experience a brief feeling of tightness in the chest and faintness; however, no serious side effects have been reported. After a blood sample is drawn in the basal state, pentagastrin, 0.5 μg per kilogram of body weight, is administered as an intravenous bolus over a few seconds. Serum calcitonin determinations are done at 0, 1, 2, 4, 10, and 15 minutes [12,32].

CALCIUM INFUSION TESTS. Calcium infusion tests consist of administering 5 mg [32] to 15 mg [14] of calcium per kilogram of body weight over a 4-hour period, with determinations of serum calcitonin at 0, 3, and 4 hours. Since these large calcium loads can produce nausea and vomiting, short-form calcium infusion tests have also been advocated. In one test, 150 mg of calcium as calcium chloride is administered intravenously over 5 to 10 minutes. Serum calcitonin levels are measured at 0, 2, 5, 10, and 20 minutes [22]. A 1-minute infusion test has also been proposed, with the amount of calcium injected calculated to raise the serum calcium level 2 mg/dl using 20% of lean body weight as the volume of distribution of calcium [26].

A study comparing pentagastrin, short calcium infusion tests, and the combination of pentagastrin immediately after calcium administration in 1 minute as calcium gluconate, 2 mg per kilogram of body weight, concluded that the combined administration of pentagastrin and calcium gluconate constituted a more effective stimulus for calcitonin secretion than any of the tests used alone [39].

As noted, the limits of normal for basal serum calcitonin and the response to stimulation may vary somewhat from laboratory to laboratory [2]. Graze et al., in one of the largest reported series, give a normal basal range from undetectable to 0.38 ng/ml and after pentagastrin stimulation up to 0.63 ng/ml. They recommend that the serum calcitonin be considered abnormal when the basal level is above 0.40 ng/ml (400 pg/ml) and/ or the stimulated level after either pentagastrin or calcium infusion is above 0.58 ng/ml (580 pg/ml) [12].

DISCUSSION
Multiple Endocrine Neoplasia-I
The problem confronting the clinician becomes one of detecting the rare case of an MEN syndrome among a large number of endocrine tumors that appear sporadically with a varying incidence. In approaching the patient with one or more of these disorders, several guidelines may prove useful.

Family members of patients with MEN syndromes have a 50% chance of being affected. Manifestations of the MEN-I gene are usually apparent by age 20. Children of unaffected members of MEN families do not inherit the disease. So, an adult family member without disease would be expected to have normal children who would not require ongoing screening. In contrast, the children of an affected adult obviously require screening studies.

Yamaguchi et al. have divided the approach to patients with suspected MEN syndromes into three groups [44]. The first group is that of patients with a typical family history who present with two or more endocrine lesions. These persons obviously require evaluation. The second group includes family members who have a MEN-I type lesion. These again require complete evaluation for the full syndrome. Finally, the more difficult group is that composed of patients with sporadic endocrine lesions who have neither a family history nor any other disease belonging to a MEN-I syndrome. The tests available for screening the various syndromes are as follows [23]:

1. Calcium, phosphorous, and parathormone levels
2. Serum glucose after a 12-hour fast; serum insulin level if hypoglycemia occurs
3. Serum gastrin level and secretin stimulation test
4. Skull x-ray

These screening studies are obviously not applicable to every patient presenting with one of the sporadically occurring diseases of the MEN-I syndrome. For this reason, some guidelines are necessary.

Although hyperparathyroidism is the most common component of the MEN-I syndrome, all patients with evidence of primary hyperparathyroidism do not require screening for pituitary or pancreatic disease. In the presence of a history suggestive of clinical findings, screening may be performed. However, peptic ulcer disease is at least twice as common in patients with sporadic hyperparathyroidism [3], and in the absence of a suggestive history, the likelihood of the ZE syndrome or another pancreatic lesion is relatively small. Serum gastrin levels may also be elevated in hyperparathyroidism. However, the secretin test is normal, that is, gastrin levels decrease, in contrast to the paradoxic gastrin elevations found with gastrinomas. (Hypercalcemia may be characteristic of either the MEN-I or the MEN-II syndrome. In the MEN-I syndrome, hypercalcemia due to the WDHA syndrome has been shown to regress with treatment of this syndrome and presumably was not related to parathyroid disease [16]. Similarly, in the MEN-II syndrome, hypercalcemia due to pheochromocytoma has been reported [34]. Thus, in these two instances, it is important to treat one disease before treating the parathyroid disease.) The high incidence of multiple gland involvement in the parathyroid disease of both MEN syndromes should lead one to investigate for the possibility of either a MEN-I or MEN-II syndrome if such multiple gland involvement is found at surgery in the previously unsuspected patient.

Patients presenting with peptic ulcer disease do not require full screening studies for an MEN-I syndrome unless the ZE syndrome has been established. Conversely, all patients with the ZE syndrome should be evaluated for the MEN-I syndrome.

Persons symptomatic for peptic ulcer disease in whom suspicion of gastrinoma has been raised because of familial identification of MEN-I should be evaluated as outlined in Figure 15-1. A fasting serum gastrin level should be obtained in the hope of detecting gastrinomas before they have reached the clinically evident stage. The yield of positive results in asymptomatic family members has not yet been established in the MEN-I syndrome, but early screening has identified asymptomatic family members with ZE [23]. The finding of a clearly increased basal gastrin secretion that was further stimulated by secretin or calcium suggests the presence of a gastrinoma.

Although isolated insulinomas are encountered in most sporadic cases rather than the multicentric lesions characteristic of the MEN-I syndrome, this may not be easily established preoperatively. Since evidence of the MEN-I syndrome would alert the surgeon to possible multicentric disease, routine MEN-I screening is indicated if an adenoma is not localized preoperatively.

Inasmuch as endocrine tumors of the pancreas other than gastrin-producing tumors (e.g., insulinomas or glucagonomas) are less frequently found in association with MEN-I, further laboratory investigation for these possibilities appears justified only if clinical findings suggest their presence [4,10].

Evidence is also not yet available on which to base a decision about how often to repeat screening procedures for family members at risk of developing the MEN-I diseases. Since the risk of carcinoma is considerably lower in this syndrome than in MEN-II syndromes, a reasonable approach would be yearly reviews of any symptoms suggestive of any of the common elements of MEN-I and appropriate laboratory investigation of symptomatic persons. Yearly determination of fasting serum calcium and glucose combined with measurement of serum gastrin every 2 to 5 years in asymptomatic members of affected families appears reasonable.

Multiple Endocrine Neoplasia-IIa

Cases of MEN-IIa that are not clearly familial may be overlooked unless the association of certain disorders prompts further investigation. In regard to the MEN-II syndrome, the following screening studies have been proposed [23]:

1. Calcium level after fasting. If it is elevated, evaluation for hyperparathyroidism should be done.
2. Basal calcitonin level. If it is elevated, this is diagnostic of MCT in most instances. If it is normal, pentagastrin and/or calcium stimulation tests should be performed.

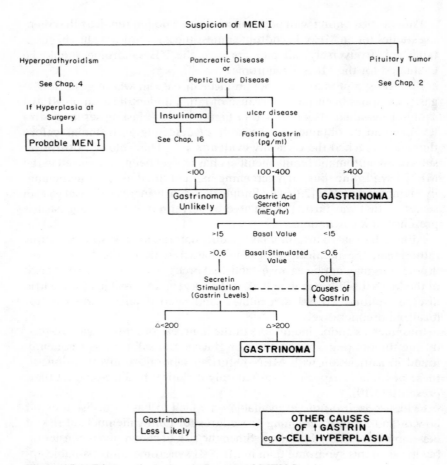

Figure 15-1. Diagnostic protocol: Suspected MEN-I.

3. Twenty-four-hour urine collections for metanephrines and/or determination of plasma catecholamine levels.

Using these screening tests, some general guidelines appear to be applicable (Fig. 15-2). All patients with pheochromocytomas, particularly those in whom the lesion is not clearly localized, should be screened for MCT. Conversely, all patients with MCT should be screened for pheochromocytoma. The presence of MCT defines a 25% chance of multicentric origin of the tumor characteristic of the MEN-IIa syndrome. For this reason, the simple presence of such a tumor should lead to evaluation for the syndrome. Since thyroid palpation or thyroid screening rarely distinguish MCT from other forms of thyroid enlargement, the possibility of encountering this disorder in an unsuspected fashion exists. In this instance, MCT that was previously unsuspected should be treated with full resection of the thyroid gland and subsequent screening for pheochromocytoma [29]. Investigation of children at risk for MCT in such families should begin at an early age, that is, ages 4 to 6, and should be repeated yearly. Based on experience to date, this approach offers a good prospect of identifying most of the persons at risk who are actually affected, before the age of 20 and at a time when the MCT is small and more likely to be completely removed, safely and prior to any metastases [12]. Also, in every family member at risk of MEN-IIa, there should be yearly laboratory determinations of urinary metanephrines, beginning at the same age, as screening for possible pheochromocytoma. At the Mayo Clinic, 19% of patients without family histories of MCT have been found to be index cases for the MEN-IIa syndrome [29].

The association of Cushing's syndrome with MCT and pheochromocytomas is frequent enough that laboratory screening for possible adrenal cortical hyperfunction should be carried out in all persons identified as having either of these tumors [31]. As noted before, in a number of such instances, Cushing's syndrome has been shown to be due to elevated circulating levels of ACTH, with disappearance of this syndrome following removal of the MCT or pheochromocytoma, thus establishing these tumors as the ectopic source of the ACTH.

Since MCT comprises a relatively small proportion of thyroid malignancies (which are not very common), routine calcitonin measurements are not indicated in the evaluation of all thyroid nodules. Patients with thyroid nodules and hypertension need not be screened for pheochromocytoma. The odds are not high that they will have the MCT of MEN-II, since this malignancy accounts for only 7 to 12% of thyroid malignancies, multicentric origin of MCT accounts for only 25% of the medullary carcinomas, and malignant nodules account for only 17% of solitary thyroid nodules [1].

Of all the components of the MEN syndromes, hyperparathyroidism is associated with both forms, although in a lesser incidence in the MEN-II syndrome. Hypertension is also present at a higher incidence in patients

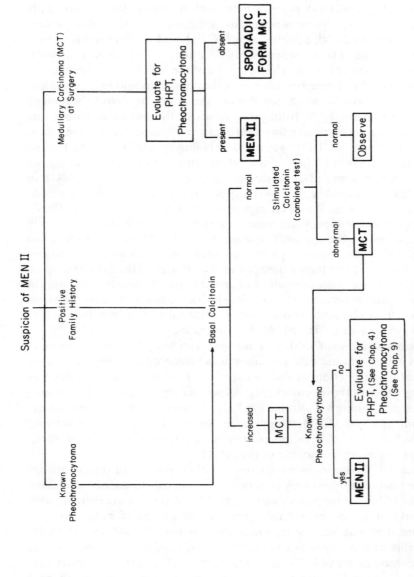

Figure 15-2. Diagnostic protocol: Suspected MEN-II. PHPT, primary hyperparathyroidism.

with hyperparathyroidism, so that the question of whether or not to study the patient for associated components of a MEN-II syndrome is fairly commonly encountered. This is heightened by the fact that the pheochromocytomas may often be asymptomatic in the patient with an MEN-II syndrome. In the patient with primary hyperparathyroidism who is not hypertensive and has no family history of MEN, it does not appear reasonable to recommend screening for pheochromocytoma. The broad experience with hyperparathyroidism has not been characterized by problems attendant to unsuspected pheochromocytoma at surgery, and the incidence of hyperparathyroidism as part of the MEN-II syndrome is not high. In contrast, a history suggestive of possible pheochromocytoma or more severe hypertension reasonably warrants screening studies before surgery.

It should be emphasized that, using the guidelines given, the discussion has focused on the asymptomatic patient without a family history. It cannot be emphasized too strongly that the patient who presents with an MEN syndrome or the family member of such a patient requires sequential evaluation for all components of the syndrome.

Multiple Endocrine Neoplasia-IIb
In persons suspected of having the MEN-IIb syndrome, laboratory investigation for hypercalcitoninemia should be conducted as described for MEN-IIa. In addition, there should be a careful search for pheochromocytomas, including radiographic procedures to identify possible adrenal masses even when catecholamine determinations have been normal.

Some mucosal neuromas have been shown on analysis after removal to contain large amounts of serotonin; however, this does not seem to result in a carcinoid-type syndrome, and a laboratory search for increased serotonin levels is probably not warranted. Hyperparathyroidism has been found only rarely in MEN-IIb. Serum calcium determination should be a sufficient preoperative screen. The parathyroid glands should be examined at the time of thyroid surgery in this syndrome, as well as MEN-IIa.

The genetic characteristics of this syndrome are much less consistent than those of the other two MEN syndromes; it is generally thought that the appearance of MEN-IIb represents a new mutation in most instances. The general appearance of persons with this syndrome is so characteristic that it serves well for initial screening of any other possible family members at risk. More elaborate laboratory investigation is not warranted in other family members of a person with this syndrome in the absence of the characteristic appearance.

REFERENCES
1. Ashcraft, M. W., and VanHerle, A. J. Management of thyroid nodules. 1. History and physical examination, blood tests, x-ray tests and ultrasonography. *Head Neck Surg.* 3:216–230, 1981.

2. Austin, L. A., and Heath, H., III. Calcitonin: Physiology and pathophysiology. *N. Engl. J. Med.* 304:269–279, 1981.
3. Ballard, H. S., Frame, B., and Hartsock, R. J. Familial multiple endocrine adenoma–peptic ulcer complex. *Medicine* 43:481–516, 1964.
4. Bloom, S. R., and Polak, J. M. Glucagonomas, lipomas and somatostatinomas. *Clin. Endocrinol. Metab.* 9:285–297, 1980.
5. Cameron, A. J., and Hoffman, H. N. Zollinger-Ellison syndrome: Clinical features and long-term follow-up. *Mayo Clin. Proc.* 49:44–51, 1974.
6. Carney, J. A., Sizemore, G. W., and Sheps, S. G. Adrenal medullary disease in multiple endocrine neoplasm, type 2. *Am. J. Clin. Pathol.* 66:279–290, 1976.
7. Deftos, L. J. Calcitonin in clinical medicine. *Adv. Intern. Med.* 23:159–193, 1978.
8. Deveney, C. W., et al. Use of calcium and secretin in the diagnosis of gastrinoma (Zollinger-Ellison syndrome). *Ann. Intern. Med.* 87:680–686, 1977.
9. Ellison, E. H., and Wilson, S. D. The Zollinger-Ellison syndrome: Re-appraisal and evaluation of 260 registered cases. *Ann. Surg.* 160:512–530, 1964.
10. Friesen, S. R. Tumors of the endocrine pancreas. *N. Engl. J. Med.* 306:580–590, 1982.
11. Gorlin, R. J., et al. Multiple mucosal neuromas, pheochromocytoma and medullary carcinoma of the thyroid—a syndrome. *Cancer* 22:293–299, 1968.
12. Graze, K., et al. Natural history of familial medullary thyroid carcinoma: Effect of a program for early diagnosis. *N. Engl. J. Med.* 299:980–985, 1978.
13. Heath, H. H., Hodgson, S. F., and Kennedy, M. A. Primary hyperparathyroidism: Incidence, morbidity and potential economic impact in a community. *N. Engl. J. Med.* 302:189–193, 1980.
14. Hennessey, J. F., et al. A comparison of pentagastrin injection and calcium infusion as provocative agents for the detection of medullary carcinoma of the thyroid. *J. Clin. Endocrinol. Metab.* 39:487–495, 1974.
15. Jackson, C. E., Frame, F., and Block, M. A. Prevalence of Endocrine Neoplasia Syndromes in Genetic Studies of Parathyroid Tumors. In J. J. Mulvihill, R. W. Miller, and J. F. Fraumeni, Jr. (Eds.), *Genetics of Human Cancer*. New York: Raven Press, 1977. Pp. 205–208.
16. Jensen, R. T., et al. Zollinger-Ellison syndrome. Current concepts and management. *Ann. Intern. Med.* 98:59–75, 1983.
17. Lamers, C. B., and Froeling, P. G. Clinical significance of hyperparathyroidism in familial multiple endocrine adenomatosis type 1 (MEA I). *Am. J. Med.* 66:422–424, 1979.
18. Mallette, L. E., et al. Primary hyperparathyroidism: Clinical and biochemical features. *Medicine* 53:127–146, 1974.
19. McGuigan, J. E. The Zollinger-Ellison Syndrome. In M. H. Sleisenger and J. S. Fordtran (Eds.), *Gastrointestinal Disease*. Philadelphia: Saunders, 1978. Pp. 860–868.
20. McGuigan, J. E., and Wolfe, M. M. Secretin injection test in the diagnosis of gastrinoma. *Gastroenterology* 79:1324–1331, 1980.
21. Murlow, R. E., and Connelly, R. R. Epidemiology of pancreatic cancer in Connecticut. *Gastroenterology* 55:667–686, 1978.
22. Parthemore, J. G., et al. A short calcium infusion in the diagnosis of medullary carcinoma of the thyroid. *J. Clin. Endocrinol. Metab.* 39:108–111, 1974.
23. Pont, A. Multiple endocrine neoplasia syndromes. *West. J. Med.* 132:301–313, 1980.

24. Prosser, P. R., Karam, J. H., and Townsend, J. J. Prolactin secreting pituitary adenomas in multiple endocrine adenomatosis type I. *Ann. Intern. Med.* 91:41–44, 1979.
25. Regan, P. T., and Malagelada, J. R. A reappraisal of clinical, roentgenographic, and endoscopic features of the Zollinger-Ellison syndrome. *Mayo Clin. Proc.* 53:19–23, 1978.
26. Rude, R. K., and Singer, F. R. Comparison of serum calcitonin levels after a 1 minute calcium injection and after pentagastrin injection in the diagnosis of medullary thyroid carcinoma. *J. Clin. Endocrinol. Metab.* 44:980–983, 1977.
27. Schimke, R. N. Multiple endocrine adenomatosis syndromes. *Adv. Intern. Med.* 21:249–265, 1976.
28. Sipple, J. H. The association of pheochromocytoma with carcinoma of the thyroid gland. *Am. J. Med.* 32:163–166, 1961.
29. Sizemore, G. W., Heath, H., III, and Carney, J. A. Multiple endocrine neoplasia type 2. *Clin. Endocrinol. Metab.* 8:299–315, 1979.
30. Stadil, F., and Stage, J. G. The Zollinger-Ellison syndrome. *Clin. Endocrinol. Metab.* 8:433–446, 1979.
31. Steiner, A. L., Goodman, A. D., and Powers, S. R. Study of a kindred with pheochromocytoma, medullary thyroid carcinoma, hyperparathyroidism, and Cushing's disease: Multiple endocrine neoplasia, type 2. *Medicine* 47:379–409, 1968.
32. Stepemas, A., Samaan, N., and Hill, C. S., Jr. Medullary thyroid carcinoma—importance of serial calcitonin measurements. *Cancer* 43:825–837, 1979.
33. Sturdevant, R. A. L., and Walsh, J. H. Duodenal Ulcer. In M. H. Sleisenger and J. S. Fordtran (Eds.), *Gastrointestinal Disease*. Philadelphia: Saunders, 1978. P. 841.
34. Swinton, N. W., Jr., Clerkin, E. P., and Flint, L. D. Hypercalcemia and familial pheochromocytoma—correction after adrenalectomy. *Ann. Intern. Med.* 76:455–457, 1972.
35. Tashjian, A. H., Jr., et al. Immunoassay of human calcitonin: Clinical measurement, relation to serum calcium and studies in patients with medullary carcinoma. *N. Engl. J. Med.* 283:890–895, 1970.
36. Trump, D. L., Mendelsohn, G., and Baylin, S. B. Discordance between plasma calcitonin and tumor mass in medullary thyroid carcinoma. *N. Engl. J. Med.* 301:253–256, 1979.
37. Verner, J. V., Jr., Morrison, A. B. Islet cell tumor and a syndrome of refractory watery diarrhea and hypokalemia. *Am. J. Med.* 25:374–380, 1958.
38. Weichert, R. F. The neural ectodermal origin of the peptide-secreting endocrine glands: A unifying concept for the etiology of multiple endocrine adenomatosis and the inappropriate secretion of peptide hormones by nonendocrine tumors. *Am. J. Med.* 49:232–241, 1970.
39. Wells, S. A., et al. Provocative agents and the diagnosis of medullary carcinoma of the thyroid gland. *Ann. Surg.* 188:139–141, 1978.
40. Wermer, P. Genetic aspects of adenomatosis of endocrine glands. *Am. J. Med.* 16:363–370, 1954.
41. Wilson, S. D. Ulcerogenic Tumors of the Pancreas: The Zollinger-Ellison Syndrome. In L. C. Carey (Ed.), *The Pancreas*. St. Louis: Mosby, 1973. Pp. 295–318.
42. Winship, D. H., and Ellison, E. H. Variability of gastric secretion in patients with and without the Zollinger-Ellison syndrome. *Lancet* 1:1128–1130, 1967.

43. Wolfe, H. J., et al. C-cell hyperplasia preceding medullary thyroid carcinoma. *N. Engl. J. Med.* 289:437–441, 1973.
44. Yamaguchi, K., Kamoya, T., and Abe, K. Multiple endocrine neoplasia type I. *Clin. Endocrinol. Metab.* 9:261–284, 1980.

16   Hypoglycemia

Dean H. Lockwood
Zachary R. Freedman

In normal humans, the level of plasma glucose is tightly controlled, rarely varying by more than 40 to 50 mg/dl throughout a 24-hour period. This aspect of glucose homeostasis is a consequence of the interplay of a number of hormones, enzymes, and substrates in several organs, most prominently the liver and muscle. An imbalance between glucose utilization and glucose ingestion and/or hepatic glucose production can cause either hyperglycemia (i.e., diabetes mellitus) or hypoglycemia. With regard to hypoglycemia, the physician must search for those factors that cause either excessive glucose utilization or reduced hepatic glucose production.

Several major underlying diseases or disorders are manifested as hypoglycemia. Unfortunately, the signs and symptoms of hypoglycemia can be mild or severe, diffuse or specific, and can mimic either organic or functional disorders. This diversity, coupled with the lack of complete agreement among physicians concerning the diagnosis of hypoglycemia, has probably been responsible for the recent tendency to label many conditions as hypoglycemia. This overdiagnosis of hypoglycemia is especially prevalent among lay people who are frequently exposed to television programs and magazine articles about hypoglycemia. More often than not, these are based on personal experiences rather than clinical studies. There are clinical studies, however, that allow us to define hypoglycemia and to approach the differential diagnosis in a logical manner.

CLINICAL CONSIDERATIONS

The majority of the signs and symptoms of hypoglycemia are a consequence of either an excessive adrenergic response, provoked by decreased glucose levels, or an impairment of the nervous system that usually requires an adequate supply of glucose for normal function. The symptoms associated with increased catecholamine release include palpitations, sweating, tremor, anxiety, acral and perioral numbness, and hunger. Symptoms of neuroglycopenia include hypothermia, headache, confusion, fatigue, motor incoordination, amnesia, and, if severe enough, loss of consciousness, seizures, and coma. When the occurrence of hypoglycemic symptoms is compared to antecedent food intake, two major forms of hypoglycemia can be defined—postprandial and fasting.

Postprandial hypoglycemia is the more prevalent form and classically occurs as a transient event during the transition from the fed to the fasted (postabsorptive) state. With this type of hypoglycemia, the plasma glucose has usually declined to low levels rapidly, provoking a brisk adrenergic response and the attendant symptoms. In contrast, during fasting hypoglycemia, the onset is more gradual, and one is apt to see the neuroglycopenic symptoms predominate. Although these are important differential points elicited by a careful medical history, it must also be realized that any combination of symptoms can occur in either type of hypoglycemia. In addition, it should be appreciated that whereas post-prandial hypoglycemia is invariably provoked by food ingestion, fasting hypoglycemia may occur not only in the early morning but occasionally between meals as well.

As indicated earlier, there is no universal agreement concerning the biochemical definition of hypoglycemia. The problem arises from studies of plasma and blood glucose in normal subjects during oral glucose tolerance tests (OGTTs) and during fasting [24]. The results of these studies indicate that during a 72-hour fast, the plasma glucose can decline dramatically, especially in young women, without accompanying symptoms [23]. In this situation, plasma glucose values as low as 25 to 30 mg/dl have been observed. Studies during an oral glucose tolerance test reveal that plasma glucose levels of less than 55 mg/dl are seen in approximately 25% of asymptomatic normal subjects, but this percentage decreases to less than 10% when the cutoff is reduced to 50 mg/dl. Furthermore, studies of insulin-induced hypoglycemia in normal subjects indicate that the greatest release of counterregulatory hormones (growth hormone, cortisol, glucagon, and catecholamines) usually occurs when the plasma glucose concentration is less than 50 mg/dl [3,13]. In contrast, similar studies in diabetics with persistent hyperglycemia reveal that rapidly lowering the plasma glucose level can result in the release of these hormones at a considerably higher threshold than that found in normal humans [4,22]. Taken together, these studies provide a reasonable rationale for arbitrarily defining fasting or postprandial hypoglycemia as a plasma glucose value of 50 mg/dl or less. Clearly, one must recognize that in fasting normal women one may encounter hypoglycemic values in the absence of symptoms, and in type I diabetics one may encounter symptoms in the absence of true hypoglycemia. Thus, in the approach to hypoglycemia, it is of paramount importance to attempt to correlate symptoms with biochemical verification and the relief of these symptoms with carbohydrate ingestion.

Fasting Hypoglycemia

In normal humans, starvation per se does not result in hypoglycemia. The normal adaptive processes that maintain glucose production and plasma glucose levels greater than 50 mg/dl include a fall in plasma insulin levels, a rise in the counterregulatory hormones (growth hormone, cortisol, glucagon, and epinephrine), and an increase in liver glycogenolysis and gluconeogenesis [26]. Hypoglycemia in adults occurs because

Table 16-1. Fasting Hypoglycemia in Adults

Increased glucose utilization
  Endogenous insulin (insulinoma, sulfonylurea)
  Extrapancreatic tumor
  Exogenous insulin (factitious)
  Autoimmune insulin syndrome (spontaneous insulin antibodies)
Underproduction of glucose
  Hypoadrenalism
  Hypopituitarism or isolated ACTH deficiency
  Severe liver disease
  Alcohol

of excessive glucose utilization or deficient glucose production (see Table 16-1).

Patients of all ages may be diagnosed with an insulinoma, but the peak years are between 40 and 70 years of age. Symptoms may be present for days to years, with a mean duration of 32½ months [6,28]. Although symptoms of hypoglycemia typically occur in the fasting state, patients can also have symptoms postprandially since a well-differentiated tumor may secrete insulin after glucose administration.

The extrapancreatic tumors associated with fasting hypoglycemia include mesenchymal tumors found in the retroperitoneal space or thorax, hepatomas, and adrenocortical adenomas. Unlike insulinomas, most of the tumors are large, with symptoms and signs caused by a space-occupying mass. Thoracic tumors produce dyspnea, cough, and chest pain, whereas abdominal tumors present as palpable masses or fullness.

It is often difficult to rule out factitious hypoglycemia as the result of either exogenous insulin administration or ingestion of oral hypoglycemic agents. Surreptitious insulin administration is often seen in young women, nurses, and others associated with the medical profession [7,27]. The findings include a large and absolute elevation in the serum insulin concentration associated with low connecting peptide (C-peptide) and proinsulin immunoreactivity. In the nondiabetic, the finding of positive insulin antibodies further strengthens the likelihood of exogenous insulin administration. Factitious hypoglycemia secondary to sulfonylurea use may mimic the clinical signs and symptoms of insulinoma and may be precipitated by concomitant use of sulfonamides or phenylbutazone, which displace insulin from binding sites on plasma proteins. Hypoglycemia secondary to oral hypoglycemic agents may also be found in the clinical setting of alcohol use, reduced food intake, and liver or renal disease [8,9]. More prevalent in insulin-treated diabetics is the occurrence of asymptomatic nocturnal hypoglycemia. The hypoglycemia may be prolonged and is associated with high doses of intermediate acting insulin [12].

In the past few years, a rare syndrome of severe fasting or postprandial hypoglycemia has been detected in individuals who have insulin binding antibodies in serum but no history of exogenous insulin administration. It is thought that hypoglycemia in the fasting state may result from dissociation of insulin from insulin-antibody complexes, resulting in excessive intact insulin [14].

Except for extrapancreatic tumor, the cause of fasting hypoglycemia in patients with appropriately suppressed serum insulin is glucose underproduction. Since glucocorticoids are required for optimal gluconeogenesis, adrenal insufficiency resulting from either Addison's disease, isolated adrenocorticotropic hormone (ACTH) deficiency, or hypopituitarism may lead to fasting hypoglycemia. Treatment with exogenous glucocorticoids will prevent hypoglycemia. Although uncommon, severe liver disease (more than 80% parenchymal destruction) can lead to profound and prolonged fasting hypoglycemia. This is usually the result of fulminant hepatitis, metastatic infiltration, or drug toxins. In malnourished chronic alcoholics who lack sufficient glycogen stores, the metabolism of alcohol leads to the accumulation of reduced nicotinamide adenine dinucleotide (NADH) and inhibition of gluconeogenesis, with resulting hypoglycemia.

Postprandial Hypoglycemia
Postprandial hypoglycemia can usually be diagnosed following a careful medical evaluation and a 5-hour OGTT. The major difficulty for the physician is the judgment concerning the correlation between the symptoms and the corresponding plasma glucose level. Many patients mistakenly believe that they have hypoglycemia, and unfortunately, there are physicians who believe that postprandial hypoglycemia is a rare condition. Obviously, the correct answer lies somewhere between these two extremes. A better understanding of the various forms of postprandial hypoglycemia should provide the physician with a better basis for making the correct diagnosis.

Alimentary Hypoglycemia
Alimentary hypoglycemia, which is usually seen 1 to 3 hours after glucose ingestion (Fig. 16-1), occurs most frequently in patients who have a history of upper gastrointestinal surgery. Procedures associated with alimentary hypoglycemia include vagotomy, gastrectomy, gastrojejunostomy, and pyloroplasty. With the altered gastrointestinal physiology, there is a rapid gastric emptying leading to augmented glucose absorption, hyperglycemia, and excessive insulin secretion. The combination of a heightened but shortened glucose absorption phase and hyperinsulinemia can lead to subsequent hypoglycemia. Sometimes blood sampling every 15 minutes during the first 1 to 2 hours of an OGTT is required to document the hyperglycemia peak. Biochemical

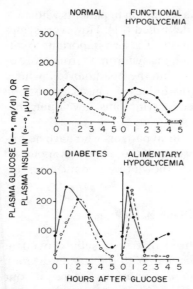

Figure 16-1. Comparison of glucose and insulin levels during a 5-hour oral glucose tolerance test.

evidence for postprandial hypoglycemia is common in patients who have had the types of procedures previously described [21]. However, symptomatic hypoglycemia is much less common. It is also important to differentiate the signs and symptoms of "dumping syndrome" from those of hypoglycemia. Dumping usually occurs within the first hour following a meal and is characterized by epigastric fullness, nausea, peristaltic rushes, and weakness, with hypoglycemia symptoms developing between 1 and 3 hours.

Alimentary hypoglycemia may also occur in patients who have no history of gastrointestinal surgery. At least some of these patients appear to have enhanced gastric emptying for either known (e.g., peptic ulcer disease) or unknown reasons.

Hypoglycemia Associated with Type II Diabetes Mellitus or Impaired Glucose Tolerance

For over 50 years, it has been recognized that noninsulin-dependent diabetics can have episodes of hypoglycemia. With the standardization of the OGTT and the advent of the radioimmunoassay for insulin, our understanding of this form of postprandial hypoglycemia has been partially increased.

As shown in Figure 16-1, virtually all these patients have a normal fasting plasma glucose level. In fact, a fasting plasma glucose above 130 mg/dl virtually rules out the possibility of this form of postprandial hypoglycemia [29]. During the first 2 hours of the OGTT, the criteria is met for impaired glucose tolerance and sometimes for type II diabetes mellitus (see Chap. 1). Characteristically, between 3 and 5 hours after glucose ingestion, the plasma glucose rapidly falls and reaches its nadir. Compared to normals, there is delayed initial insulin secretion and later hyperinsulinemia presumably due to the initial and persistent hyperglycemia. Of interest, however, is the demonstration that there are no differences in the insulin secretory responses between diabetics who develop hypoglycemia and those who do not [16]. This observation suggests that factors other than abnormal insulin secretion contribute to the development of hypoglycemia. Typically, these patients have mild episodes of adrenergic symptomatology, but occasional cases of severe neuroglycopenia have also been reported. Whether most patients later develop more severe glucose intolerance with fasting hyperglycemia, thereby eliminating their transient episodes of hypoglycemia, requires further longitudinal studies.

Functional Postprandial Hypoglycemia

The syndrome of functional postprandial hypoglycemia has also been labeled *idiopathic* or *reactive hypoglycemia,* emphasizing our lack of understanding of the etiology of this condition. As shown in Figure 16-1, transient hypoglycemia usually develops between the second and fifth hours during an OGTT or after a meal. Unlike the other two types of postprandial hypoglycemia, antecedent hyperglycemia does not occur. The early portion of the glucose curve is either normal or in some cases nearly horizontal, indicating little deviation from the fasting condition. Studies in a large number of patients indicate that neither hyperinsulinemia nor inappropriate insulin secretion is a prominent etiologic factor in this syndrome. However, some patients have delayed insulin secretion. Perhaps the most common features of this syndrome are that it occurs in young women and is associated with abnormal psychodynamics. Psychologic testing shows that these patients' personality profiles are frequently characterized by hypersomatization and hypochondriac complaints [18]. Along with symptoms of increased adrenergic activity, they may also complain of problems associated with increased vagal activity, including nausea, vomiting, indigestion, and irritable colon. Clearly, this form of hypoglycemia is likely to be most difficult to document if the physician requires a close correlation between hypoglycemia and symptomatology.

It should be recognized that certain states of hormone deficiency can cause postprandial hypoglycemia, although fasting hypoglycemia is the rule. In adults, hormonal deficiencies likely to cause postprandial hypoglycemia include hypothyroidism and hypoadrenocorticism.

DIAGNOSTIC METHODS
Fasting Insulin/Glucose Determinations
Hyperinsulinism is clearly demonstrated in nonobese individuals when their fasting insulin levels are greater than 24 μU/ml. Also, normal values for fasting insulin may be inappropriately elevated for the prevailing blood glucose. When fasting glucose levels are less than 50 mg/dl, plasma insulin will fall to less than 10 μU/ml [9]. When plasma glucose levels are less than 40 mg/dl, insulin values should be less than 5 μU/ml. Furthermore, the ratio of insulin to glucose (I : G) normally decreases with serial observation during fasting. Increasing ratios or ratios greater than 0.3 are suspicious for hyperinsulinism, and values greater than 0.4 indicate an insulinoma [23].

Oral Glucose Tolerance Test
The OGTT has no place in the evaluation of suspected fasting hypoglycemia. It may prove useful in assessing postprandial hypoglycemia if extended to 4 to 5 hours (see Fig. 16-1). Preparation of the patient and proper administration of the test are explained in Chapter 1.

Proinsulin (Percentage of Immunoreactive Insulin) and Connecting Peptide
Normal plasma contains a small amount of proinsulin, the single-chain precursor of insulin (proinsulin = C-peptide + insulin) [8,25]. Insulinomas generally secrete increased amounts of proinsulin into the cir-

culation [1,30]. Normally, proinsulin constitutes less than 22% of the total immunoreactive insulin. In over 85% of patients with islet cell tumors the proinsulin percentage exceeds 25% [8]. The higher the percentage of proinsulin, the more undifferentiated the tumor.

The radioimmunoassay of the C-peptide helps to distinguish endogenous from exogenous hyperinsulinism [7,27]. C-peptide is secreted in equal molar concentrations with insulin [25]. It is not present in measurable quantities in exogenous hyperinsulinism. Thus, a high C-peptide level implies endogenous insulin secretion, whereas a low C-peptide level suggests an exogenous source for the elevated plasma insulin level. The most useful application of the C-peptide measurement has been in diabetic patients who may have circulating antibodies that will interfere with the radioimmunoassay for insulin. Unfortunately, assays currently can be found only in research institutions and are unavailable to most commercial laboratories.

Species of Insulin
In patients with hypoglycemia and hyperinsulinemia, the use of species-specific human antiserum may help resolve the origin of the insulin–insulinoma (human insulin) versus factitious (beef or pork insulin, etc.) [2a]. However, the restricted availability of the antisera will limit its use to the most difficult diagnoses.

Insulin Antibodies
The presence of insulin antibodies in plasma can suggest either preexisting insulin administration or, rarely, a syndrome associated with spontaneously occurring insulin antibodies. The presence or absence of insulin antibodies can be determined by several commercial laboratories.

Plasma Sulfonylureas and Urinary Metabolites
Detection of sulfonylureas in plasma or metabolites in urine will diagnose drug-induced hyperinsulinism. Chlorpropamide's high protein binding and long life enhance its toxic risk. Sulfonylurea-induced fasting hypoglycemia can masquerade as an insulinoma; thus, this diagnosis must always be considered [8,9]. The current availability of a plasma or urine assay, in our experience, is best referred to the drug manufacturer.

Suppression Tests
In a patient with asymptomatic fasting hypoglycemia or inconstant or borderline hyperinsulinism, suppression tests have been useful in differentiating autonomous insulin-producing cells from islet tissue under normal physiologic control. These tests primarily involve exogenous insulin infusion with measurement of endogenous C-peptide and proinsulin [25,30]. In patients with insulinomas, the autonomous production of C-peptide and proinsulin is not completely suppressed by exogenous in-

sulin. However, in several patients with insulinomas, near-normal suppression of C-peptide has been reported. The additional measurement of plasma human proinsulin has produced a more reliable discrimination between patients with insulinomas and normals [30].

Provocative Testing

The OGTT has no place in the evaluation of suspected fasting hypoglycemia. Other provocative tests used to discriminate patients with insulinomas from normals are less sensitive than the I : G ratio, C-peptide, proinsulin level, or suppression test. Tests commonly used include tolbutamide [28], leucine [10], and glucagon [20]. Utilizing plasma insulin criteria, 80% of patients with insulinomas had abnormal tolbutamide tests, 74% had abnormal leucine tests, and 58% had abnormal glucagon tests [8]. In the last few years, a calcium infusion test has been reported to distinguish normals from patients with insulinoma [11]. In patients with insulinoma, calcium infusion stimulates insulin secretion. However, a recent report documents the fact that in many patients with islet cell tumors there is no stimulation of insulin secretion after calcium infusion [5]. Since all tests have false-negative responses, provocative tests are rarely employed for diagnostic purposes.

Localization of Insulinomas

Once the biochemical diagnosis of an insulinoma has been made, the preferred mode of treatment is surgical extirpation of the tumor [6]. Localization of the tumor greatly increases the chance of a successful first operation. However, the tumors are small; 65% are less than 1.5 cm in diameter and 40% are less than 1 cm in diameter. Over 10% of the tumors are multiple [6]. Due to the smallness of the tumors, current ultrasound and computed tomography (CT) scanning techniques have not been helpful in preoperative localization [6,8]. In most series 50 to 75% of tumors can be localized by pancreatic arteriography [6,8]. There have been false-positive localizations using arteriography but, in general, this technique is safe and helpful when used in conjunction with magnification, stereoscopy, and subtraction techniques. More recently, percutaneous transhepatic catheterization of the splenic and portal veins with selective blood sampling for insulin levels has been used to determine the site of the tumor [17]. This technique has not received widespread use and has been restricted to large medical centers.

DISCUSSION

Fasting Hypoglycemia

In patients with suspected fasting hypoglycemia, the first step is to obtain a 12-hour overnight fasting blood glucose determination and a simultaneous insulin value (Fig. 16-2). Patients strongly suspected of harboring an insulinoma or reporting severe symptoms should be hospitalized. In patients with milder symptoms, outpatient evaluation can proceed in the physician's office. It is prudent to request a spouse or friend to transport and accompany the patient to the laboratory or office when obtaining the fasting plasma glucose and insulin determinations.

If the plasma glucose is low (less than 50 mg/dl), the laboratory should proceed to analyze the simultaneously collected serum or plasma insulin. If after a 12-hour overnight fast hypoglycemia has not ensued, further fasting may induce symptomatic hypoglycemia. Serial plasma glucose and insulin determinations are obtained with constant patient observation by a physician or nurse. An unattended patient may lapse into unconsciousness or convulsions, especially if the initial plasma glucose is low normal. Insertion of a heparin lock or intravenous catheter with saline infusion prior to prolonging the fast will allow prompt glucose infusion if severe hypoglycemia ensues. Almost 80 to 85% of patients with an insulinoma will experience hypoglycemia merely by prolonging the fast to midday [6,8].

If hypoglycemia has not developed by late in the day, a decision to hospitalize the patient for prolonged fasting must be made. The prolonged fast must be supervised to prevent surreptitious food ingestion. In addition, daily urine samples should be tested for ketones to ensure maintenance of the fasting state. If symptomatic hypoglycemia has not resulted after 72 hours of fasting plus 15 minutes of vigorous exercise, further fasting will not be helpful. This occurs in approximately 5% of patients with proven insulinoma and may reflect an insulin-resistant state secondary to the chronic hyperinsulinism [2]. Normoglycemia associated with appropriately suppressed insulin values warrants no further evaluation. In patients who develop hypoglycemia after a period of fasting, the simultaneously obtained insulin value will determine further diagnostic evaluation (see Figs. 16-2 and 16-3). The critical observation required is the ratio of insulin to glucose rather than the absolute level of either. An I : G ratio of more than 0.3 is strongly suggestive of insulinoma, particularly if the ratio tends to increase throughout the course of a fast. Hyperinsulinism associated with hypoglycemia may be absolute or too high for the prevailing blood glucose. In the insulinoma patient, both C-peptide immunoreactivity and proinsulin are elevated. Over 95% of patients can be detected by prolonged fasting plus exercise, the majority within a 12- to 16-hour fast.

In the diabetic with fasting hypoglycemia, the diagnosis of insulinoma is made more difficult due to the presence of insulin binding antibodies. In this situation, measurement of free C-peptide and proinsulin is mandatory. In patients in whom the diagnosis is in question, provocative testing and/or suppression tests may be helpful. Since insulinomas may be a

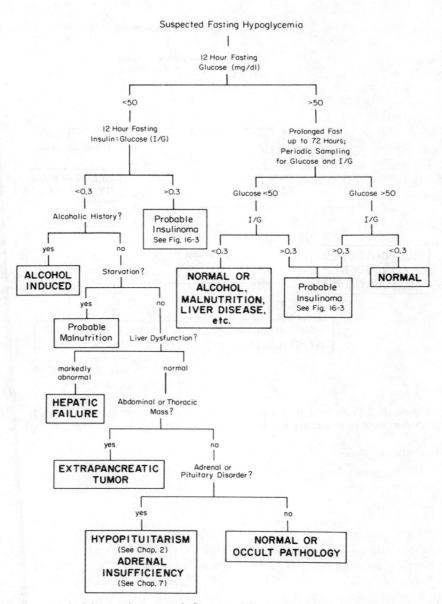

Figure 16-2. Diagnostic protocol: Suspected fasting hypoglycemia.

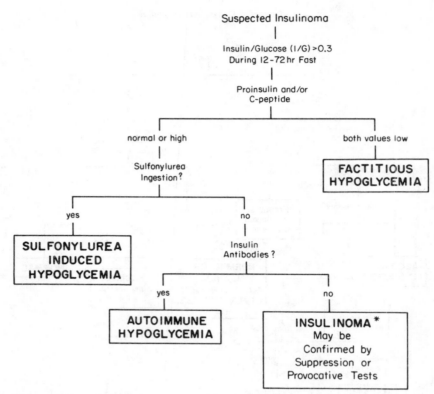

Figure 16-3. Diagnostic protocol: Suspected insulinoma (suggestive history).
*Attempts at preoperative localization indicated (i.e., CT scan, angiography).

feature of multiple endocrine neoplasia type I (MEN-I) (10% are patients with insulinoma), evaluation for parathyroid, pituitary, and adrenocortical hyperfunction is appropriate.

Other conditions with an elevated I : G ratio (>0.3) include factitious insulin administration, use of oral agents, and a rare autoimmune syndrome. In fasting hypoglycemia and hyperinsulinemia secondary to surreptitious insulin administration, the findings include a large and absolute elevation in the serum insulin concentration associated with low C-peptide and proinsulin immunoreactivity. Detection may also be aided by examining the plasma insulin with species-specific human antiserum. In the nondiabetic, the finding of positive insulin antibodies further strengthens the likelihood of exogenous insulin administration. Both immunoreactive insulin and C-peptide may be elevated in hypoglycemia secondary to oral agent use, mimicking an insulinoma. However, a normal I : G ratio may be seen with hypoglycemia due to the ability of oral agents to potentiate insulin action. A distinguishing feature is the presence of sulfonylureas or metabolites in blood and/or urine. A characteristic that distinguishes patients with the insulin autoimmune syndrome from nondiabetic patients with insulinoma is the presence of circulating insulin antibodies in the former and its absence in the latter. In the insulin autoimmune syndrome, C-peptide levels may be elevated. This is in contradistinction to patients with factitious hypoglycemia, who lack measurable C-peptide or proinsulin.

When the fasting I : G ratio is less than 0.3 [23], hypoglycemia due to causes other than insulinoma should be considered. These include adrenal hypofunction or hypopituitarism including isolated ACTH deficiency, severe liver disease, alcohol ingestion, and increased utilization of glucose from an extrapancreatic tumor. The appropriate diagnostic work-up includes the evaluation of adrenal and pituitary function, as outlined in Chapters 2 and 7; liver function testing, including a prothrombin time; and a careful abdominal and chest examination. If these tests are normal, then a more extensive search for an extrapancreatic tumor should be performed. Patients with extrapancreatic tumors may contain in their serum a nonsuppressible insulin-like activity that is soluble in acid ethanol (NSILA-s) [15,19]. This is a heterogeneous group of peptide molecules with insulin-like activity that is not suppressed by an excess of insulin antibodies. The peptides comprising NSILA-s include insulin-like growth factors IGF-1 and IGF-2. IGF-1 is identical to somatomedin-C. These molecules have insulin-like activity as well as growth-promoting effects.

Postprandial Hypoglycemia
Since postprandial hypoglycemia does not become apparent during fasting but is provoked by food ingestion, a careful dietary history usually

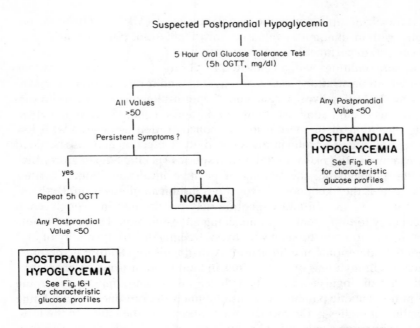

Figure 16-4. Diagnostic protocol: Suspected postprandial hypogycemia.

reveals that large meals high in carbohydrate are most frequently associated with subsequent hypoglycemic symptoms. This observation has led physicians to use the OGTT for diagnostic purposes. This test is employed with the knowledge that ingestion of pure glucose does not mimic a normal meal and that the reproducibility of the test can be variable. Clinical experience has shown that symptoms can occur as early as 1 hour and as late as 4 to 5 hours after a meal. Appropriately, the standard OGTT, when used for evaluation of postprandial hypoglycemia, is extended from 2 to 5 hours (Fig. 16-4).

Sampling procedures are usually as follows: (1) before and every half hour after ingestion of 75 gm of glucose for 5 hours and (2) any time the patient experiences symptoms during the testing period.

As discussed previously, the medical history may prompt the physician to determine plasma glucose levels every 15 minutes during the initial hour or two of testing. Postprandial hypoglycemia, if present, can usually be classified into one of three forms depending on the history and pattern of glucose response during the tolerance test: (1) alimentary hypoglycemia, (2) hypoglycemia associated with type II diabetes mellitus or impaired glucose tolerance, and (3) functional (idiopathic, reactive) hypoglycemia. The typical plasma glucose pattern and the representative insulin response for each condition are illustrated in Figure 16-1. It is evident that simultaneous measurements of insulin values are not useful in making the appropriate laboratory diagnosis and thus should not be employed in the usual approach to this problem. Finally, it must be appreciated that the 5-hour OGTT may not elicit hypoglycemia on every occasion. If there is a high index of suspicion, repeated testing may be indicated. In this regard, we have found on occasion that reproduction of hypoglycemic symptoms can be accomplished only by ingestion of certain foods. The physician may want to re-create this situation in the office in order to obtain a specimen for plasma glucose when symptoms occur.

REFERENCES

1. Alsever, R., et al. Insulinoma with low circulating insulin levels. The diagnostic value of proinsulin measurements. *Ann. Intern. Med.* 82:347–350, 1975.
2. Barr, R., et al. Insulin receptors in patients with insulinomas: Changes in receptor affinity and concentration. *J. Clin. Endocrinol. Metab.* 44:1210–1213, 1977.
2a. Bauman, W. A., and Yallow, R. S. Differential diagnosis between endogenous and exogenous insulin induced refractory hyperglycemia in a non-diabetic patient. *N. Engl. J. Med.* 303:198–199, 1980.
3. DeFronzo, R., et al. A test of the hypothesis that the rate of fall in glucose concentration triggers counterregulatory hormonal responses in man. *Diabetes* 26:445–452, 1977.

4. DeFronzo, R., Hendler, R., and Christensen, N. Stimulation of counter-regulatory hormonal responses in diabetic man by a fall in glucose concentration. *Diabetes* 29:125–131, 1980.
5. DePalo, C., et al. Lack of effect of calcium infusion on blood glucose in plasma insulin levels in patients with insulinoma. *J. Clin. Endocrinol. Metab.* 52:804–806, 1981.
6. Editorial. Diagnosis and treatment of insulin secreting tumors. *Lancet* 1:22–23, 1980.
7. Editorial. Factitious hypoglycemia. *Lancet* 1:1293–1294, 1978.
8. Fajans, S., and Floyd, J. Diagnosis in the medical management of insulinomas. *Ann. Rev. Med.* 30:313–328, 1979.
9. Felig, P. Disorders of Carbohydrate Metabolism. In P. Bondy and R. Rosenberg (Eds.), *Metabolic Control and Disease*. Philadelphia: Saunders, 1980.
10. Floyd, J., et al. Plasma insulin in organic hyperinsulinism: Comparative effects of tolbutamide, leucine and glucose. *J. Clin. Endocrinol. Metab.* 24:747–760, 1964.
11. Gaeke, R., et al. Insulin and proinsulin released during calcium infusion in a patient with islet cell tumor. *Metabolism* 24:1029–1034, 1975.
12. Gale, E., and Tattersall, R. Unrecognized nocturnal hypoglycemia in insulin treated diabetics. *Lancet* 1:1049–1052, 1979.
13. Garber, A., et al. The role of adrenergic mechanisms in the substrate and hormonal response to insulin-induced hypoglycemia in man. *J. Clin. Invest.* 58:7–15, 1976.
14. Goldman, J., et al. Characterization of circulating insulin and proinsulin binding antibodies in autoimmune hypoglycemia. *J. Clin. Invest.* 63:1050–1059, 1979.
15. Gordon, P., et al. Hypoglycemia associated with non-islet cell tumor and insulin-like growth factors. *N. Engl. J. Med.* 305:1452–1455, 1981.
16. Hofeldt, F. D., et al. Are abnormalities in insulin secretion responsible for reactive hypoglycemia? *Diabetes* 23:589–596, 1974.
17. Ingemansson, S., et al. Islet cell hyperplasia localized by pancreatic vein catheterization in insulin radioimmunoassay. *Am. J. Surg.* 133:643–645, 1977.
18. Johnson, D. D., et al. Reactive hypoglycemia. *J.A.M.A.* 243:1151–1155, 1980.
19. Kahn, R. The riddle of tumour hypoglycemia revisited. *Clin. Endocrinol. Metab.* 9:335–360, 1980.
20. Kumar, D., Mehtalea, J., and Miller, V. Diagnostic use of glucagon-induced insulin response: Studies in patients with insulinoma or other hypoglycemic conditions. *Ann. Intern. Med.* 80:697–701, 1974.
21. Leichter, S. B., and Permutt, M. A. Effect of adrenergic agents on postgastrectomy hypoglycemia. *Diabetes* 24:1005–1010, 1975.
22. Lilavivathana, U., et al. Counterregulatory hormonal responses to rapid glucose lowering in diabetic man. *Diabetes* 28:873–877, 1979.
23. Merimee, T., and Tyson, J. Hypoglycemia in man: Pathogenic and physiologic variants. *Diabetes* 26:161–165, 1977.
24. Permutt, M. A. Postprandial hypoglycemia. *Diabetes* 25:719–733, 1976.
25. Rubenstein, A., Kuzuya, H., and Horowitz, D. Clinical significance of circulating C-peptide in diabetes mellitus in hypoglycemic disorders. *Arch. Intern. Med.* 137:625–632, 1977.
26. Saudek, C., and Felig, P. Metabolic events of starvation. *Am. J. Med.* 60:117–126, 1976.

27. Scarlett, J., et al. Factitious hypoglycemia. *N. Engl. J. Med.* 297:1029–1032, 1977.
28. Service, J., et al. Insulinoma. *Mayo Clin. Proc.* 51:417–429, 1976.
29. Seltzer, H. S., Fajans, S. S., and Conn, J. W. Spontaneous hypoglycemia as an early manifestation of diabetes mellitus. *Diabetes* 5:437–441, 1956.
30. Turner, R. C., and Heding, L. G. Plasma proinsulin, C-peptide, and insulin in diagnostic suppression tests for insulinoma. *Diabetalogia* 13:571–577, 1977.

17 Interference in Endocrine Testing

Lewis B. Morrow

Final endocrine diagnosis is dependent on laboratory tests for confirmation of clinical impressions. Most laboratories now have the capability to perform the great majority of tests enumerated in earlier chapters. Generally, the laboratory procedures are sensitive, specific, and highly reproducible. In spite of this precision, however, diagnostic errors occur because of the ability of many drugs and metabolic conditions to interfere with the assessment of hormone concentrations. This chapter reviews some of these considerations in endocrine testing.

The endocrine system maintains homeostasis through feedback mechanisms. This has two implications. First, it is frequently necessary to measure both limbs of this system. For example, a low thyroxine (T_4) level may be found in association with either an elevated thyroid-stimulating hormone (TSH) level, suggesting primary failure of the thyroid gland, or with a low TSH level, compatible with hypothalamic-pituitary disease. A high serum calcium level with an elevated parathyroid hormone level is seen in primary or tertiary hyperparathyroidism, but depressed parathyroid hormone (PTH) levels in that setting suggest other diagnostic possibilities ranging from malignancy to sarcoid. Similar parallels are seen with adrenocorticotropic hormone (ACTH) and cortisol, renin-aldosterone, sodium, and others. Drugs may interfere with either limb of the loop. Evaluation of endocrine testing depends on an understanding of the feedback control and on the understanding that certain drugs may influence one part of the loop, with effects apparent elsewhere.

Second, since the endocrine system generally responds promptly to changes, many tests must be conducted under standardized conditions. Activity and stress are stimuli for cortisol and growth hormone (GH) release and alter insulin secretion. In addition to these rapid fluctuations, some systems change cyclically depending on the time of day (cortisol, PTH, testosterone) or month (follicle-stimulating hormone/luteinizing hormone [FSH : LH], estrogen in women). Aging can profoundly alter other tests, such as adrenal androgen steroidogenesis and gonadotropin production and response to thyrotropin-releasing hormone (TRH). A correct interpretation of endocrine tests requires an appreciation of the normal hormonal cyclic responses and the effects of age, activity, associated diseases, and nutritional status on hormone production.

DISEASE STATES THAT ALTER TESTING

A comprehensive review of diseases that alter tests is available [8], as is an integrated review of specific problems incurred by metabolic, endocrine, or drug influences on pituitary testing [3]. In this section, attention will focus on endocrine tests in liver disease, renal disease, pregnancy, anorexia nervosa, and obesity.

Liver Disease

Hepatic disease may alter endocrine tests by influencing the production of certain proteins or by changing the clearance rate of hormones. The liver synthesizes angiotensin precursors and the carrier proteins for cortisol (transcortin), thyroid hormone (thyroid binding globulin [TBG]), testosterone, and estrogen (sex hormone binding globulin). Significant changes can occur in plasma levels of these proteins with liver disease. Inflammatory diseases such as acute viral hepatitis, and possibly primary biliary cirrhosis and chronic active hepatitis, may be associated with increased T_4 levels due to transudation or augmented synthesis of hepatic TBG. In contrast, alcoholic cirrhosis is characterized by normal to low T_4 and TBG concentrations, reflecting impaired globulin production [18].

Cortisol is metabolized in the liver by conjugation with glucuronide. In cirrhosis this metabolism is impaired. Although free cortisol levels remain unchanged, the urinary 17-hydrosteroids are low and the normal diurnal variation in plasma cortisol is blunted by the prolonged half-life of steroids.

Renal Disease

The endocrine changes associated with renal disease have been recently reviewed and include alterations in several of the endocrine tests [6,7]. Glucose intolerance is frequently identified. Fasting blood sugars may be normal, but basal insulin levels are increased. Uremia also probably impairs the early phase of insulin release. Basal GH levels are elevated in uremia, and in some individuals a paradoxic increase in GH following intravenous glucose administration as well as an exaggerated response to an insulin challenge is seen. These findings may be explained in part by a prolonged metabolic clearance rate of GH. Prolactin levels may also be increased and suppress poorly with levodopa (L-dopa) in these patients. Testosterone levels are depressed in men and luteinizing hormone (LH) levels may be increased.

The influence of uremia on thyroid function testing is variable, but nearly all parameters are affected. The half-lives of T_4 and triiodothyronine (T_3) are prolonged, but serum T_4 and T_3 levels are usually depressed. The free T_4 levels are frequently normal. The TSH values are usually normal and these patients are generally euthyroid. Since many of the physical findings in uremia tend to mimic those of hypothyroidism, special care is required in the laboratory evaluation of thyroid function. The ^{131}I uptake is unreliable and is usually found to show low 2- or 6-hour uptake values and elevated 24-hour values.

PTH is uniformly elevated in normal physiologic compensation for the impaired calcium absorption and increased tissue calcium deposition associated with the progressive deterioration in renal function.

Plasma cortisol levels are generally normal, although significant elevations have been reported. Furthermore, the standard 1-mg overnight dexamethasone test may fail to suppress cortisol levels adequately [16].

Pregnancy

Many of the endocrine changes associated with pregnancy can be attributed directly to the effects of high levels of estrogens and progesterone. Other differences from the nonpregnant state are noted that may be related to the interaction of the maternal and fetal endocrine systems or to hypothalamic-pituitary modulations occurring in pregnancy [9].

Cortisol levels increase from the second month until term. The circadian rhythm is normal, but the afternoon plasma cortisol level is higher than that seen with estrogen therapy alone. Free plasma cortisol concentrations are increased, and the urinary free cortisol may rise above normal: Urinary 17-hydroxycorticosteroids (17-OHCS) are normal.

Plasma renin, angiotensin II, and aldosterone levels are increased in pregnancy. Interestingly, the aldosterone secretion rate falls precipitously in severe toxemia.

Insulin levels rise progressively during pregnancy, probably because of contrainsulin factors such as increased free cortisol, rising placental lactogen, and the anti-insulin properties of the placenta itself. Basal glucagon levels are normal, but the insulin/glucagon ratio is increased so that generally blood sugar is maintained in the normal range.

GH has been difficult to assess during pregnancy because its immunologic similarity to human placental lactogen makes radioimmunoassay (RIA) measurements difficult. Recently, more specific antibodies have been developed, and GH dynamics show normal basal values with arginine hyperresponsiveness during the first two trimesters. A profound GH suppression occurs during the third trimester and persists into the postpartum period. This has been attributed to hypothalamic-pituitary suppression of GH release by placental lactogen in association with increased free cortisol.

Prolactin increases during pregnancy, and values above normal are seen as early as the first trimester.

Total calcium and phosphorus fall with pregnancy, with the lowest values seen at 28 to 32 weeks. Ionized calcium remains normal. PTH rises significantly during the third trimester, especially at term. These alterations in calcium and PTH metabolism are not seen with estrogen treatment.

Anorexia Nervosa and Obesity

Anorexia nervosa is frequently confused with hypopituitarism, although the clinical presentation is characteristically distinctive. Amenorrhea is common. Serum gonadotropins may be normal, although urinary gonadotropins are low, as is estradiol. Prolactin is usually normal and the FSH : LH response to luteinizing hormone-releasing hormone (LHRH) is variable, although some studies suggest a delayed responsiveness. GH is usually elevated, which is a valuable diagnostic indicator since patients with hypopituitarism have low, nonresponsive levels [15]. The T_3 values are low [5], as in other acutely starved patients. The morning cortisol is higher than in controls, but the circadian rhythm is normal. There is a prolongation of the cortisol half-life that accounts in part for the low to normal 17-OH and a urinary free cortisol that is normal but increased above control values [1,2].

In the infant, emotional deprivation may produce an endocrine picture, including growth failure, that is difficult to differentiate from that of hypopituitarism.

Obesity also alters endocrine tests. The GH response to insulin is diminished, and there is increased estrogen production, decreased serum testosterone, and augmented insulin secretion. The presumed mechanism for this insulin resistance is a reduction in peripheral insulin receptors that can produce an overtly diabetic glucose tolerance test. Weight loss may lead to normal carbohydrate handling.

DRUG INTERFERENCE

A complete listing of all drugs that are capable of altering endocrine tests is beyond the scope of this chapter. Several excellent reviews are available [4,10,20]. When an unexpected result is obtained, drug interference must be the first consideration. Some medications and hormones are unique in their ability to influence endocrine tests by a variety of in vivo mechanisms. The following discussion provides examples of the kinds of alterations that can be produced.

Phenytoin

Phenytoin interferes with several endocrine tests [11]. Total T_4 values may be falsely low since phenytoin is bound to TBG, displacing T_4 from its usual binding sites. Phenytoin also accelerates the urinary and fecal excretion of T_4, so that free T_4 values may also be low. T_4 conversion to T_3 is probably enhanced to explain this phenomenon. The patients remain euthyroid, as demonstrated by normal TSH values.

Phenytoin accelerates the metabolism of glucocorticoids. Thus, the overnight 1-mg dexamethasone test may fail to show cortisol suppression even in individuals with an intact pituitary-adrenal axis. The rapid disposal of dexamethasone results in the delivery of a suboptimal dose. With chronic administration, plasma cortisol levels are normal, although urinary 17-OHCS and 17-ketosteroids (17-KS) are slightly depressed due to changes in the hepatic metabolism of steroids. The metyrapone test is unreliable in a patient who is taking Dilantin.

PTH levels are also increased by phenytoin. The putative mechanism is through hepatic interference with vitamin D metabolism, which results in vitamin D deficiency, osteomalacia with slightly depressed serum calcium levels, and secondary hyperparathyroidism.

Psychotropic Drugs

Many psychotropic drugs, neuroleptics, and antipsychotics have antidopaminergic properties that produce prolactin elevation and hyperresponsiveness to stimuli through inhibition of prolactin-inhibiting factor [13]. Administration of the phenothiazines, chlorpromazine, trifluoperazine, fluphenazine, butaperazine, perphenazine, and thiethylperazine all result in prolactin secretion. The effects of the phenothiazines on GH are variable. Some studies show a decreased basal GH level with a poor response to hypoglycemia, but others have less consistently demonstrated GH hyperresponsiveness. The nonphenothiazines such as haloperidol, primozide, thiothixene, molindone, and loxapine have similar effects on prolactin.

Estrogens

Estrogens stimulate hepatic synthesis of TBG, so that total T_4 levels are elevated. Since total TBG is increased, there is a proportionate increase in unbound binding sites as well, which lowers the T_3 resin uptake test. Neither the T_4 nor the T_3 resin uptake test accurately reflects thyroid function in a patient on estrogen therapy. Estrogens also increase transcortin and may lead to an elevation in plasma cortisol. The standard overnight 1-mg dexamethasone suppression test may consistently give values greater than 5 μg/dl because of this increase in carrier protein.

Angiotensin levels are also affected by estrogen administration through a similar mechanism, making evaluation of renovascular hypertension confusing at times. Estrogens augment basal GH levels and the GH response to insulin and arginine. This does not lead to diagnostic errors, however, since these infusion tests are employed to assess GH deficiency. Male subjects are occasionally pretreated with estrogens to take advantage of this property. Although other perturbations such as an increase in prolactin (PRL) or gonadotropin suppression are well known, they rarely cause problems in interpretation. Hyperresponsiveness to TRH has also been reported.

Cortisol

The adrenal glucocorticoids, whether given exogenously or produced in excess endogenously, alter many parameters of endocrine testing. GH responses are blunted and suppressed entirely at high doses of steroids [14]. Prolactin, TSH, and, of course, ACTH responses to stimulation tests are similarly affected. A direct effect of glucocorticoids on the thyroid is observed, with decreased T_4 serum levels. With acutely administered pharmacologic doses of steroids, T_3 levels are also suppressed. All these effects can be attributed to a suppressive effect on both pituitary TSH and the thyroid gland. The LH response to LHRH may also be inhibited.

Thyroid Hormone
Thyroid hormone at physiologic replacement concentrations has no effect on endocrine testing except that the TSH response to TRH is blunted. When T_3 alone is administered, a euthyroid state can be achieved with very low T_4 levels. Thyroid hormone preparations containing a mixture of T_3 and T_4 may give confusing test results because of the rapid absorption and metabolism of T_3. Generally, the use of these mixed preparations is discouraged because of the variability in serum concentrations of T_3. At supraphysiologic levels of T_4, either endogenously or exogenously produced, the GH response to insulin is blunted and the prolactin response to stimulation is decreased. Because of increased catabolism, the adrenal steroid production rate is increased and urinary 17-OHCS and 17-KS are elevated despite normal plasma cortisol levels. LH and FSH may be elevated.

In hypothyroidism, prolactin levels tend to rise above the normal limits. Because of slow catabolism of adrenal steroids, 17-OHCS and 17-KS levels in the urine are low, but plasma cortisol is maintained in the normal range. However, the diurnal variation is blunted, with afternoon cortisol levels being slightly higher.

Antihypertensive Drugs
Antihypertensives may also alter endocrine tests. Galactorrhea and elevated prolactin levels can be produced by reserpine and methyldopa, and the GH response to hypoglycemia is blunted by reserpine. For the clinician, the most common problem associated with these drugs is interference with the evaluation of the patient with suspected pheochromocytoma. A number of methods are currently available for the estimation of catecholamine secretion, and the degree of drug interference depends on the method used [12]. Alpha-methyldopa (Aldomet) and madelamine, as well as some nosedrops and bronchodilators, react in urinary catecholamine assays to give falsely elevated results. Exogenous catecholamines in bananas and other fruits produce minor elevations in urinary free catecholamines, but these are usually not significant. However, to avoid confusion, these dietary sources of catecholamines should be avoided before testing. Forty-eight hours off these drugs and on a restricted diet is sufficient. Hypoglycemia and exercise can lead to physiologic increases in catecholamines. Emotional stress can result in minor elevations that do not, however, produce abnormal values.

A variety of methods are available for the vanillylmandelic acid (VMA) assay. Methyldopa and monoamine oxidase inhibitors tend to suppress VMA secretion and increase total metanephrines. However, these compounds usually do not depress the VMA to normal levels in patients with pheochromocytoma. Salicylates interfere with the two-dimensional paper chromatography assay. The colorimetric methods for VMA assay that rely on the diazotized p-nitroaniline reaction have been largely replaced because of errors induced by dietary ingredients such as coffee, tea, chocolate, bananas, cheese, and vanilla.

Metanephrines are considered to be the best screening test for pheochromocytoma. Renografin, however, may alter the spectrophotometric assay, and at least 1 week should be allowed following administration before the urine is collected. Reserpine, guanethidine, antihistamines, chlorothiazides, and spironolactone do not interfere and need not be withdrawn. As in all urine tests, incompleteness of the urine collection frequently leads to erroneous conclusions. The sample must be collected in acid to ensure that the pH remains below 3.

Miscellaneous Drugs
Other drugs that may influence endocrine testing include the oral hypoglycemics, the sulfonylureas, which may inhibit thyroid hormone formation, with a resultant fall in T_4, and elevation in TSH. T_4 is also, in part, depressed by binding of the sulfonylureas to TBG with displacement of T_4 from their binding sites. Salicylates lower the circulating T_4, probably by displacing T_4 from TBG; the ^{131}I uptake is suppressed, although this result is not fully explained. Antihistamines and phenylbutazone also reduce ^{131}I uptake. Lithium is goitrogenic and may result in hypothyroidism, as well as a type of nephrogenic diabetes insipidus and changes in the renin-angiotensin system [19].

Spironolactone is effective in the treatment of hypertension because of its aldosterone antagonistic properties. One of the side effects of this drug is an acceleration in the peripheral conversion of testosterone to estrogens [17]. Testosterone levels in men receiving this drug may fall to clearly abnormal levels. LH secretion tends to be elevated. Since gynecomastia and decreased libido are seen in these patients, an adequate endocrine evaluation requires that spironolactone be discontinued before studies are ordered.

In summary, many drugs and metabolic alterations must be considered in the interpretation of endocrine tests. These factors may give inappropriate results through (1) direct interference in the assay itself, (2) changes in the sensitivity of the pituitary or target endocrine gland, (3) altered metabolism of the hormone measured or the stimuli administered, (4) fluctuations in binding properties, or (5) perturbations in the

Table 17-1. Selected Tests Used to Evaluate Thyroid Function

Test	Site Tested	Increase	Decrease
TRH infusion	Hypothalamus	Estrogens	Aspirin
TSH	Pituitary	Sulfonylureas	Glucocorticoids
^{131}I uptake	Thyroid gland	Iodine deficient	Phenylbutazone
T_4		Estrogens	Prednisone
T_3		After ^{131}I treatment	Starvation
T_3 resin uptake		Androgens	Estrogens
Free T_4		Heparin	Phenytoin

feedback mechanism. As an example, Table 17-1 shows some of the tests used to evaluate thyroid function. Each test may be influenced by a variety of drugs or pathologic conditions, although only one example of each is shown. Appreciation of these limitations of laboratory testing is crucial for proper patient management.

REFERENCES

1. Boyar, R. M., et al. Cortisol secretion and metabolism in anorexia nervosa. *N. Engl. J. Med.* 296:190–193, 1977.
2. Casper, R. C., Chatterton, R. T., Jr., and Davis, J. M. Alterations in serum cortisol and its binding characteristics in anorexia nervosa. *J. Clin. Endocrinol. Metab.* 49:406–411, 1979.
3. Cohen, K. L. Metabolic, endocrine and drug interference with pituitary function tests: A review. *Metabolism* 28:1165–1177, 1977.
4. Constantino, N. V., and Kabat, H. F. Drug induced modifications of laboratory test values. *Am. J. Hosp. Pharm.* 30:24–71, 1973.
5. Croxson, M. S., and Ibbertson, H. R. Low serum triiodothyronine and hypothyroidism in anorexia nervosa. *J. Clin. Endocrinol. Metab.* 44:167–174, 1977.
6. Emmanouel, D. S., Lindbreimer, M. D., and Keitz, A. I. Pathogenesis of endocrine abnormalities in uremia. *Endocrine Rev.* 1:28–45, 1980.
7. Feldman, H. A., and Singer, I. Endocrinology and metabolism in uremia and dialysis: A clinical review. *Medicine* 54:345–376, 1975.
8. Friedman, R. B., et al. Effects of disease on clinical laboratory tests. *Clin. Chem.* 26(4):ID–476D, 1980.
9. Fuchs, F., and Klopper, A. *Endocrinology of Pregnancy* (2nd ed.). New York: Harper & Row, 1977.
10. Galen, R. S. The effects of drugs on laboratory tests. *Orthop. Clin. North Am.* 10:465–494, 1979.
11. Gharib, H., and Munoz, J. M. Endocrine manifestations of diphenylhydantoin therapy. *Metabolism* 23:515–524, 1974.
12. Gitlow, S. E., Mendlowitz, M., and Bertaini, L. M. Biochemical techniques for detecting and establishing the presence of pheochromocytoma. *Am. J. Cardiol.* 26:270–279, 1970.
13. Gruen, P. H. The prolactin response in clinical psychiatry. *Med. Clin. North Am.* 2:409–424, 1978.

14. Hartog, M., Gaayar, M. A., and Fraser, R. Effect of corticosteroids on serum growth hormone. *Lancet* 2:376–378, 1964.
15. Mecklenberg, R. S., et al. Hypothalamic function in patients with anorexia nervosa. *Medicine* 53:147–159, 1974.
16. McDonald, W. B., et al. Adrenocorticotropin-cortisol axis abnormalities in hemodialysis patients. *J. Clin. Endocrinol. Metab.* 48:92–95, 1979.
17. Rose, L. I., Underwood, R. H., and Newmark, S. R. Pathophysiology of spironolactone induced gynecomastia. *Ann. Intern. Med.* 87:398–403, 1977.
18. Schussler, G. C., Schaffner, F., and Korn, F. Increased serum thyroid hormone binding and decreased free hormone in chronic active liver disease. *N. Engl. J. Med.* 299:510–515, 1978.
19. Transbol, I., et al. Endocrine effects of lithium. *Acta Endocrinol.* 88:619–624, 1978.
20. Young, D. S., Pesanter, L. C., and Gibberman, V. Effects of drugs on clinical laboratory tests. *Clin. Chem.* 21:1D–432D, 1975.

Index

Acne, in Cushing's syndrome, 143, 144
Acromegaly
  clinical considerations, 33–35
  diagnostic methods, 35–37
  discussion, 37–39
  in MEN-I syndrome, 264
  pituitary tumors and, 18
ACTH, 15
  and aldosterone regulation, 173
  APUD cell synthesis of, 261
  disordered regulation, 125
  ectopic production, 143, 145, 146
    and amenorrhea, 199
    dexamethasone suppression test in, 153
  exogenous. *See also* ACTH stimulation tests
    and Cushing's syndrome, 143
    and hirsutism, 209
  and hirsutism, 209, 210, 211–212
  intracranial pressure and, 16
ACTH levels
  in adrenal insufficiency, 126, 133
  assays
    in adrenal insufficiency, 133
    in Cushing's syndrome, 149
    in hypopituitarism, 24, 26
  in Cushing's syndrome
    assays, 149
    diagnosis, 152, 153, 154–155
    dexamethasone suppression test and, 153, 214
  glucocorticoid administration and, 127–128, 143
  and hypoglycemia, 281, 282, 291
ACTH stimulation tests
  in adrenal insufficiency, 129–131
    diagnosis, 127
    urinary metabolites, 133–135
  adrenal vein sampling during, 181–182, 185
  in Cushing's syndrome, 150
  exogenous cortisol and, 301–302
  in hirsutism, 214
  in hyponatremia, 123
  in hypopituitarism, 25
Addison's disease, 125
  ACTH measurements in, 23
  clinical considerations, 126–127
  and hypoglycemia, 282

  and short stature, 40
Adolescence
  goiter in, 71
  puberty. *See* Puberty
Adrenal disorders. *See also specific disorders*
  aldosteronism. *See* Aldosteronism, primary
  hypercortisolism. *See* Cushing's syndrome
  hypoadrenalism. *See* Adrenal insufficiency
  MEN syndromes, MEN-IIa, 273
  and reproductive disorders
    female, 143, 144, 145, 196, 199, 205, 207
    male, 240, 242, 243
Adrenal hyperplasia
  adrenal scintiscan with, 182, 185, 187
  bilateral. *See* Cushing's disease
  congenital, 194
    amenorrhea with, 192
    diagnosis, 202, 203
    and hirsutism, 209, 210, 211–212, 216, 217, 218
    and hypogonadism, male, 240
    and gynecomastia and feminization, 227
  idiopathic, 180, 181, 182, 185, 186
  MEN syndromes, MEN-I, 264
  nodular, 143, 145, 149, 155
  and primary aldosteronism, 175–178, 184–188
Adrenal insufficiency
  acromegaly and, 34
  clinical considerations, 125–128
  diagnostic methods, 128–134
  diluting capacity assessment in, 118
  discussion, 134–139
  and hypercalcemia, 82
  and hypoglycemia, 41, 281, 282, 285, 289, 295
  secondary, 127–128, 137–139
Adrenal scintiscan, 150, 182, 185, 187
Adrenal steroids, exogenous thyroid hormone and, 302
Adrenal tumors
  ACTH levels in, 154
  and Cushing's syndrome, 145

307

Adrenal tumors—*Continued*
  dexamethasone suppression tests
    in, 153, 155
  and hirsutism, 212
  and hypoglycemia, 281
  MEN syndromes, 262, 264
  metapyrone test in, 149–150
  and reproductive disorders, male,
    240, 242
Adrenal venography, 182, 185, 186,
  187
Adrenalectomy, 126
alpha-Adrenergic blocking test, 164–
  165
Albumin. *See* Proteins, serum
Alcohol
  and dexamethasone suppression
    test, 155
  and gynecomastia, 228
  and hyperlipidemias, 249, 253, 258
  and hypocalcemia, 102
  and hypoglycemia, 281, 282, 289,
    291
  and reproductive disorders, male,
    225, 228, 239
  and vasopressin release, 108
Aldactone. *See* Spironolactone
Aldosterone
  ACTH stimulation test and, 127
  adenomas producing, 176, 177, 180,
    181, 182, 185, 186
  assays, 180
  cortisol ratios, 181, 182
  excretion and secretion measure-
    ments, 180, 184, 185
  excretion rate, 183
  plasma levels, 180, 184, 185, 186,
    187
  pregnancy and, 299
  spironolactone and, 303
Aldosteronism, primary, 120, 173–174
  clinical considerations, 174–178
  diagnostic methods, 178–182
  discussion, 182–187
Aldosteronism, secondary, 173–174,
  177
Alimentary hypoglycemia. *See* Hypoglycemia
Alkaline phosphatase, 88
Alkalosis
  in Cushing's syndrome, 143, 145
  in primary aldosteronism, 174,
    175
Alpha-adrenergic blocking test, 164–
  165

5-Alpha-reductase deficiency, 234
Amenorrhea
  anorexia nervosa and, 299
  clinical considerations
    primary disorders, 191–195
    secondary disorders, 195–200
  Cushing's syndrome and, 18, 143,
    144, 145
  diagnostic methods, 201–202
  diagnostic protocols, 203, 205
  discussion, 202–207
  hypopituitarism and, 25, 28
  oral contraceptives and, 28
  ovarian disease and, 211
Amine precursor uptake and decar-
    boxylation cells, 261
Amino acid metabolism, disorders of,
    40
Anabolic steroids, and hirsutism, 209
Androgen insensitivity, 192, 194, 207,
    226, 235, 239, 242
Androgens. *See also* Testosterone
  and amenorrhea, 192, 204
  congenital adrenal hyperplasia and,
    194
  in Cushing's syndrome, 143
  enzymatic abnormalities, 234, 243
  and hirsutism, 210, 211, 216, 217,
    218
  hypopituitarism and, 25
  in male hypogonadism, 225
  ovarian tumors producing, 199
  urinary metabolites, 134. *See also*
    17-Ketosteroids
Androstenedione, 210, 215, 217
Angiography, 21
  in hypercalcemia, 88
  in pheochromocytoma, 169
Angiotensin
  liver disease and, 298
  pregnancy and, 299
Anorchia, 225, 233, 242
Anorexia nervosa, 20
  and amenorrhea, 192, 193, 196, 197
  endocrine test interference, 299–
    300
  and euthyroid sick syndrome, 57
  growth hormone in, 36
Antacids, and hypercalcemia, 82
Antibodies. *See also* Autoimmune dis-
    orders; Globulins
  insulin-binding, 281, 282, 286, 288
  thyroid-stimulating, 54, 65
Antibody tests, in thyroid disorders,
    61, 65–66, 73

Antidiuretic hormone. *See* Arginine
    vasopressin; Diabetes insipidus
    and SIADH
Antihistamines, 303, 304
Antihypertensives
    assay interference by, 169, 301,
        302–303
    and gonadal function, male, 233
Apomorphine test, 44
Apoproteins, 247, 248, 252–253, 258
Arcus juvenilis, 248
Arginine provocative test, 44, 301
Arginine vasopressin
    assays, 117
    deficiencies, 109–111
    excess of, 111–114
    and free water clearance, 118
    Pitressin infusion, 114, 116, 119
    in polyuria, 120
    saline infusion test and, 116–117
Arsenic, 233
Arteriography
    adrenal, 150
    pancreatic, 287
    in pheochromocytoma, 166, 168
Aspirin, 233
Atherosclerosis. *See also* Cardiovas-
    cular disorders
    acromegaly and, 34–35
    hyperlipidemias and, 248, 251, 253
Autoimmune disorders. *See also* Anti-
    bodies; Globulins
    and adrenal insufficiency, 126, 127
    insulin antibodies, 281, 282, 286,
        288, 291
    and premature menopause, 198–199
    thyroid, 58, 65–66, 73

Baroreceptors, 108
Barr body, 201, 241
Benzamides, 27, 28
Betazole, 267–268
Bicarbonate, in primary aldosteron-
    ism, 174, 175
Biopsy, thyroid, 73, 75, 76
Birth control pills. *See* Oral contracep-
    tives
Birth weight, 41
Bisulfan, 233
Blood pressure. *See also* Hyperten-
    sion
    AVP deficiency and, 110
    pheochromocytoma and, 159, 160
Blood volume, and vasopressin re-
    lease, 108

Body size
    males, 235
    short stature, 39–48
Bone(s). *See also* Skeletal disorders
    in acromegaly, 34
    calcium metabolism, 98
    in Cushing's syndrome, 144
    in short stature, 40, 42
    and vitamin D metabolism, 81–82
Bone scans, in hypercalcemia, 88, 89,
    90
Broad beta disease, 252–253
Bromocryptine, 32, 34
Buccal smears
    in growth retardation, 45
    in reproductive disorders
        female, 201, 205
        male, 236
BUN
    in osmolality determination, 114,
        115
    in short stature, 42
    in SIADH, 121
Butyrophenones, 27, 28

Calcitonin
    assays, 268
    and hypocalcemia, 99, 102
    MEN syndromes
        MEN-IIa, 271, 273, 274
        MEN-IIb, 275
    stimulation tests, 268–269
Calcium infusion tests, 268, 269
    in hypoglycemia, 287
    in MEN syndromes, 268, 269–271
Calcium levels. *See also* Hypercalce-
    mia; Hypocalcemia
    laboratory determinations, 85, 86
    in MEN syndromes
        MEN-I, 270
        MEN-IIa, 271
        MEN-IIb, 275
    phenytoin and, 301
    pregnancy and, 299
    serum proteins and, 85, 90, 97, 103
Calculi, 83
Carbamazepine, 108, 112, 113
Carcinoid, 261
    and dexamethasone suppression
        tests, 155
    MEN syndromes, 264, 266
Cardiovascular disorders, 174
    acromegaly and, 34–35
    and catecholamine assays, 167, 169
    diluting capacity assessment in, 118

Cardiovascular disorders—*Continued*
  hyperlipidemias and, 248, 249, 252,
    255, 256, 259
  and hyponatremia, 112, 122
  pheochromocytoma and, 159, 160,
    161
  primary aldosteronism and, 175
  and short stature, 40
Carotid angiography, 21
Carpal tunnel syndrome, acromegaly
    and, 34
Carrier proteins. *See* Proteins, serum
Catecholamines. *See also* Pheochro-
    mocytoma
  assays
    interference with, 165, 301, 302
    in pheochromocytoma, 162–164,
      167, 168, 169
  hypoglycemia and, 279
  in MEN-IIa syndrome, 273
Catheterization
  neck, 88–89, 93
  splenic and portal veins, 287
C-cell hyperplasia, 265
Celiac disease, and short stature, 42
Central nervous system disorders. *See
    also* Hypothalamic disorders;
    Pituitary disorders
  and adrenal insufficiency, 127
  and amenorrhea, 192, 193, 196, 197,
    204
  and growth retardation, 47
  and male hypogonadism, 229
  MEN-IIa syndrome, 266
  and short stature, 40, 41
  and SIADH, 112, 113
Central nervous system symptoms.
    See also Seizures
  in diabetes insipidus, 110
  in hypoglycemia, 288
  with pheochromocytoma, 160
Chemotherapy, and gonadal function
  female, 196, 199
  male, 233
Children. *See* Pediatric patients
Chlorambucil, 233
Chloride
  in hypercalcemia, 86, 93
  in hyperparathyroidism, 89
Chlorpromazine, 22, 27, 29
Chlorpropamide, 108, 112, 113, 286
Cholelithiasis, with pheochromocy-
    toma, 160
Cholesterol, 247. *See also* Hyperlipid-
    emias; Lipoproteins

assays, 254
  in broad beta disease, 253
  diet and, 255, 256
  in differential diagnosis, 256, 257
  LDL catabolism abnormalities,
    250–251
  radioiodinated, adrenal scans with,
    150, 182, 187
  in VLDL, 250, 251
Chromosomal disorders. *See also*
    Genetic factors
  and reproductive disorders
    female, 192–193, 204, 205, 206
    male, 227, 229, 232, 241, 242
  and short stature, 40, 42
Chromosome analysis. *See* Karyotyp-
    ing
Chvostek's sign, 99
Chylomicronemia, 253
  differential diagnosis, 256, 257, 258
  in lipoprotein lipase deficiency, 252
  triglycerides in, 255
  VLDL elevations and, 252
Chylomicrons, 247, 248, 249
Cimetidine, 227, 233
Cirrhosis. *See* Liver disease
Cisternography, metrizamide, 21
Clinitest, 5, 10
Clofibrate, 108, 112, 113
Clomiphene stimulation test
  and gonadotropin secretion, 23,
    223
  in reproductive disorders
    female, 202, 203, 204
    male, 228, 237, 240, 241
Clonidine suppression test, in pheo-
    chromocytoma, 165–166
Colchicine, and gonadal function,
    male, 233
Computed tomography
  adrenal, 150
    in adrenal insufficiency, 135
    in Cushing's syndrome, 150
    in primary aldosteronism, 180–
      181
  in growth retardation, 47
  in hypopituitarism, 21, 24, 26, 31
  insulinoma localization, 287
  in pheochromocytoma, 166, 168
Congenital disorders. *See also* Chro-
    mosomal disorders; Genetic
    factors
  adrenal hyperplasia. *See* Adrenal
    hyperplasia, congenital
  anorchia, 233, 242

and male hypogonadism, 225
and short stature, 40
Connecting peptide. *See* C-peptide
Contraceptives, oral. *See* Oral contra-
    ceptives
Corneal arcus, 251
Corticosteroids
    and amenorrhea, 199
    in Cushing's syndrome, 145
Corticotropin-releasing factor, 15
Cortisol, 134
    ACTH stimulation tests and, 129,
        130–131, 134–139
    in adrenal insufficiency, 126, 127,
        133–134
    aldosterone ratios, 181, 182
    in amenorrhea, 204
    anorexia nervosa and, 300
    assays
        in adrenal insufficiency, 128–
            129
        in Cushing's syndrome, 147, 151,
            213
        interfering factors, 301–302
    dexamethasone suppression test
        and, 147, 151, 154–155
    fasting and, 280
    and hyponatremia, 113
    in hypopituitarism, 24, 25
    in insulin tolerance test, 131
    kidney disease and, 298–299
    liver disease and, 298
    metapyrone and, 149
    phenytoin and, 300
    pregnancy and, 299
    urinary free
        in adrenal insufficiency, 133–134
        in Cushing's syndrome, 147, 151,
            213
Cortisol suppression test, phenytoin
    and, 300
Cortisone, 134
    and calcium levels, 88
    exogenous, and adrenal insufficien-
        cy, 128
Cosyntropin test, 129–130, 135, 136,
    139
C-peptide, 12
    assays, 285–286
    factitious insulin use and, 281
    in hypoglycemia, fasting, 288, 291
    suppression of, 286–287
Creatinine, 147. *See also* Kidney func-
    tion
    in short stature, 42

with urinary steroid assay, 134
Cushing's disease
    with amenorrhea, 18, 199
    defined, 143
    and dexamethasone suppression
        test, 155
    and hirsutism, 213
    in MEN-I syndrome, 264
    pituitary tumors and, 18
Cushing's syndrome
    amenorrhea in, 18
    clinical considerations, 143–145
    defined, 143
    diagnostic methods, 145–150
        etiology, determination of, 148–
            150
        screening tests, 146–148
        supplemental studies, 150
    discussion, 150–156
    and hirsutism, 211, 217, 218
    in MEN-IIa syndrome, 273
    and Nelson's syndrome, 17
    and short stature, 40
Cyclic AMP
    assays, 86–87
    in hypercalcemia, 83, 85, 92–93
    in hyperparathyroidism, 89, 90
    PTH infusion and, 101, 102–103,
        105
Cyclophosphamide, 232
Cyproheptadine, 144

Dehydration, AVP deficiency and,
    110
Dehydration test, 115–116, 120,
    121
Dehydroepiandrosterone, 210, 211.
    See also Androgens
    in Cushing's syndrome, 150, 152,
        154
    in hirsutism, 215, 218
Demethylchlortetracycline, 111
11-Deoxycortisol, 133, 134
Depression
    and dexamethasone suppresion
        test, 155
    growth hormone in, 36
    hypocalcemia and, 99
Desoxycorticosterone, in Cushing's
    syndrome, ectopic ACTH and,
        145
Development, sexual differentiation,
    223–224
Developmental abnormalities. *See*
    Gonadal dysgenesis

Dexamethasone
  with ACTH stimulation tests, 130
  exogenous, and adrenal insuffi-
    ciency, 128
  in glucocorticoid-responsive hyper-
    aldosteronism, 184, 185
  in hirsutism, 219
Dexamethasone suppression tests
  in congenital adrenal hyperplasia,
    212
  in Cushing's syndrome
    atypical responses, causes of, 155
    diagnostic, 148–149
    in diagnostic protocols, 150–155
    nodular hyperplasia and, 145
    screening, 146–148
  exogenous estrogens and, 302
  in hirsutism, 214, 217, 218–219
  kidney disease and, 299
  phenytoin and, 300
DHEA. See Dehydroepiandrosterone
Diabetes insipidus, 41
  with growth retardation, 47
  lithium and, 303
  nephrogenic, 110–111
  neurogenic, 109–110
  pituitary tumors and, 16, 17–18
Diabetes insipidus and SIADH, 107–
    109
  clinical considerations
    AVP deficiencies, 109–111
    AVP excess, 111–114
  diagnostic methods
    AVP levels, 117
    dehydration test, 115–116
    diluting capacity assessment,
      117–118
    free water clearance, 118
    hypertonic saline infusion, 116–
      117
    osmolality determinations, 114,
      115
  discussion, 118–123
    hyponatremia, 121–123
    polyuria and hypernatremia, 118–
      121
Diabetes mellitus
  with adrenal insufficiency, primary,
    126
  clinical considerations, 1–4
  with delayed puberty, 230
  diagnostic methods, 4–8
    special categories, 6–8
    tests, 4–6

  discussion, 8–12
    insulin, proinsulin, and C-pep-
      tide, 11–12
    laboratory tests, 9–12
  and hyperlipidemias
    combined, 253
    hypertriglyceridemia, 258
    secondary, 249
  hypoglycemia with, 284
  and osmotic diuresis, 109
  and reproductive disorders, male,
    225, 293
  and short stature, 40
  with Turner's syndrome, 193
Diagnostic protocols
  acromegaly, 38
  adrenal insufficiency, 136, 138
  aldosteronism, primary
    laboratory evaluation, 177
    localization, 185
  amenorrhea
    primary, 205
    secondary, 203
  Cushing's syndrome, 151, 152
  diabetes mellitus, 7
  hirsutism, 217
  hypercalcemia, 90
  hyperlipidemia, 257
  hypocalcemia, 104
  hypoglycemia
    fasting, 289
    insulinoma, 290
    postprandial, 292
  hypogonadism, male, 239, 240, 242
  MEN syndromes
    MEN-I, 272
    MEN-II, 274
  pheochromocytoma, 168
  pituitary disorders
    acromegaly, 38
    hyperprolactemia, 31
    hypopituitarism, 26
    short stature, 46
  thyroid disorders
    hyperthyroidism, 68
    hypothyroidism, 70
    solitary nodule, 75
  water conservation disorders
    hyponatremia, 122
    polyuria, 120
Diastix, 10
Diazoxide, and hirsutism, 209
Diet. See also Nutrition
  in aldosteronism, 176

and hyperlipidemias
    cholesterol levels, 250, 255
    hypertriglyceridemia, 258
    secondary, 249
and hypocalcemia, 99, 104
and hypoglycemia, 281, 291–293
salt depletion, 179–180, 184
Diethylstilbestrol, and gonadal function, male, 233
Digitalis, and gynecomastia and feminization, 227
Dihydrotestosterone
    enzymatic abnormalities, 234
    in male sexual development, 223
Dilantin
    and gonadal function, male, 233
    and hirsutism, 209
    and hypocalcemia, 99, 102
Diluting capacity assessment, 117–118
Diuretics, 89
    and hypercalcemia, 82, 84
    and hypocalcemia, 100
    and hyponatremia, 112, 121, 122
    and polyuria, 119
    for volume depletion, 184
Diurnal rhythms, cortisol levels, 134–135, 148, 154–155
L-Dopa
    and growth hormone secretion, 21
    kidney disease and, 298
L-Dopa test
    in acromegaly, 36, 37, 38
    in short stature, 44
Dopamine, 15
    agonists
        and pituitary adenomas, 33
        TRH responses, 36
    antagonists of, 22, 27, 28
    and prolactin, 27, 29–30
Drugs
    and catecholamine assays, 163, 165, 169
    in chylomicronemia syndrome, 253
    and dexamethasone suppresion test, 155
    and diabetes insipidus, 110
    dopamine antagonists, 22, 27, 28
    endocrine test interference
        antihypertensives, 302–303
        cortisol, 301–302
        estrogens, 301
        miscellaneous, 303–304
        phenytoin, 300, 301
        psychotropic drugs, 301

thyroid hormone, 302
and glucose tolerance, 3
and gynecomastia and feminization, 227
and hirsutism, 209
and hypercalcemia, 82, 84, 87, 89
and hyperglycemia, 286
and hyperlipidemias, 251
    combined, 253
    hypertriglyceridemia, 258
    secondary, 249
and hyperprolactinemia, 31
and hypocalcemia, 99, 102, 104
and hypoglycemia, 282
hypoglycemics, oral, 281, 291, 303
and hyponatremia, 112, 113
and reproductive disorders
    female, 192, 196, 198
    male, 225–228, 232, 233
and vasopressin release, 108
and water conservation, 111
Ductal obstruction, and male infertility, 231–232
Dumping syndrome, 284
Dwarfism, pituitary, 225
Dysbetalipoproteinemia, 252–255
Dysglobinemias, 249

Ectopic ACTH syndrome, 145, 146, 153
    and amenorrhea, 199
    defined, 143
    and hirsutism, 218
Ectopic PTH syndrome, 90, 92
Edema, 173–174
    in Cushing's syndrome, 143, 144, 145
    hyponatremia and, 122
Elderly
    goiter in, 71
    hyperthyroidism in, 54
Electrolytes. See also specific ions
    in primary aldosteronism, 172–173, 174, 176, 177
    in short stature, 42
Empty sella syndrome, 19, 225. See also Sella turcica
Endocrine disorders
    and amenorrhea, 196, 197–198
    and delayed puberty, 230
    and hypercalcemia, 82
    and short stature, 40
Endorphins, 15
Epinephrine, fasting and, 280

Epiphyses, in short stature, 40
Estradiol
    anorexia nervosa and, 300
    and reproductive disorders, male,
        243
Estrogen levels
    hypopituitarism and, 25
    liver disease and, 298
    in reproductive disorders
        female, 201
        male, 235, 236
Estrogen-progesterone test, in amen-
    orrhea, 200
Estrogens
    in Cushing's syndrome, 143
    exogenous. See also Oral contra-
        ceptives
        and ACTH stimulation tests, 130
        and amenorrhea, 196
        and dexamethasone suppression
            test, 155
        endocrine test interference, 155,
            301
        and gynecomastia and feminiza-
            tion, 227
        and hyperlipidemias, 249, 251,
            253, 258
        and thyroid function, 55
    obesity and, 300
    in reproductive disorders, male,
        223, 235
    in testicular feminization, 235
    tumors secreting, 242
Estrogen suppression test, in hirsut-
    ism, 217, 218
Eunuchoid habitus, 235, 238
Euthyroid sick syndrome, 24–25,
    57–58
Exercise
    and amenorrhea, 192, 193, 196–197
    and catecholamines, 302
    and growth hormone secretion, 21,
        43
Exophthalmos, 53, 68
Extracellular fluid volume
    assessment of, in polyuria, 119
    and AVP release, 108
    hyponatremia and, 112
    in SIADH, 121

Failure to thrive, 40, 41
Familial hypocalciuric hypercalcemia,
    82, 85
Family history. See also Genetic fac-
    tors

hyperlipidemia diagnosis, 248, 258
thyroid carcinoma, 76, 77
Fasting hypoglycemia. See Hypo-
    glycemia
Febrile illness, and male infertility,
    226, 232
Feminization. See also Androgen in-
    sensitivity
    defined, 226–227
    in hypogonadism, 230
Fertile eunuch syndrome, 225
Fluorescent Y test, 201, 205, 236
Follicle-stimulating hormone. See also
    Gonadotropins
    alpha subunit, 18
    and oligospermia, 231
Fractures, and hypercalcemia, 82
Framingham study, 255
Free water clearance, 118, 121
Fröhlich's syndrome, 225
Furosemide, volume depletion with,
    184

Galactorrhea, 28, 30
Gastrinomas, 263, 272
    diagnosis, 272
    gastrin levels with, 267–268
    screening for, in MEN syndromes,
        270, 272
Genetic factors
    in amenorrhea, 206
    in androgen insensitivity syndrome,
        235
    in diabetes, 1, 2, 3, 8–9
    in hirsutism, 209
    in hypercalcemia, 82, 85
    in hyperlipidemias, 248–251
        diagnosis, 255–258
        screening, 248, 258
        secondary, 250
    in MEN syndromes, 261
        MEN-I, 264
        MEN-IIa, 264, 266
        MEN-IIb, 266
    in rickets, vitamin D-resistant, 102
    in short stature, 40
    in thyroid cancer, 76, 77
Genitourinary tract
    developmental abnormalities. See
        Gonadal dysgenesis
    infections, 225
Gestational diabetes, 3, 7–8
Gilbert-Dreyfus syndrome, 234
Globulins. See also Antibodies
    dysglobulinemias, 249

hormone-binding, liver disease and,
    298
testosterone-binding, 228
thyroid-stimulating, 54–55, 66
thyroxine-binding, 55, 61, 63–64,
    68, 69–70, 298, 300, 301
Glomerular filtration rate. *See* Kidney
    function
Glucagon, fasting and, 280
Glucagon infusion test
in hypoglycemia, 287
in short stature, 44
Glucagonomas, 271. *See also* Pancre-
    atic tumors
Glucocorticoid-remediable hyper-
    aldosteronism
clinical considerations, 176, 178
diagnostic tests, 180, 181, 182
differential diagnosis, 184–187
Glucocorticoids. *See also* Dexameth-
    asone; Prednisone
and adrenal insufficiency, 125, 127–
    128, 137–139
and Cushing's syndrome, 143
and hyperlipidemias
    combined, 253
    secondary, 249
and hypoglycemia, 282
and hyponatremia, 112, 123
in hypopituitarism, 25
phenytoin and, 300
and short stature, 41
suppression by. *See also* Dexameth-
    asone suppression tests
of hypercalcemia, 88
of hypothalamic-pituitary axis,
    127–128
and VLDL excess, 251
withdrawal of, 138, 139
Gluconeogenesis, inhibition of, 281,
    282
Glucopeptides, pituitary tumors and,
    18
Glucose
deficient production, 281, 282
exogenous, and GH levels, 298
Glucose:insulin ratio, in hypoglyce-
    mia, 288, 289
Glucose levels. *See also* Hypoglycemia
assays
    in diabetes diagnosis, 4, 5, 7
    in diabetes management, 9–11
    in hypoglycemia, 285
fasting
    in diabetes mellitus, 4

in fasting hypoglycemia, 287–288,
    289
hyperglycemia
and osmotic diuresis, 120
pheochromocytoma and, 160
and pseudohypernatremia, 112
and pseudohyponatremia, 114
in hypoglycemia, 280
in MEN-I syndrome, 270
in osmolality determination, 114,
    115
with pheochromocytoma, 160
in polyuria diagnosis, 120
and pseudohypernatremia, 112
Glucose tolerance
abnormalities
    hypoglycemia associated with,
        284
    types of, 2, 3–4
acromegaly and, 35
in Cushing's syndrome, 144
in hyperlipidemias, 248, 251
Glucose tolerance tests
in acromegaly, 36
in diabetes, 4–6, 7, 8
in hypoglycemia, 280, 282, 284–285
    glucose vs. insulin levels, 283
    postprandial, 292, 293
Glycogen storage diseases, and short
    stature, 40
Glycosuria, 5, 8, 9–10
Glycosylated hemoglobin, 9, 11–12
Goiter, 68
clinical considerations, 71–72
diagnostic methods, 72–73
discussion, 73–74
in Graves' disease, 69
lithium and, 303
in MEN syndromes, 264
thyroid scans in, 67
thyrotrope cell hyperplasia and, 19
toxic multinodular, 54
Gonadal dysgenesis
female, 192–193, 195, 198, 205,
    206–207
male, 231–232, 234. *See also* Hypo-
    gonadism and infertility, male
in short stature, 45, 46
Gonadal function. *See also* Amen-
    orrhea; Hypogonadism and in-
    fertility, male
acromegaly and, 34
with adrenal insufficiency, primary,
    126
in Cushing's syndrome, 143, 144, 145

Gonadal function—*Continued*
  prolactin and, 33
  tests of, with insulin tolerance test,
    132
Gonadotropin-releasing hormone
  in hypopituitarism, 22
  with insulin tolerance test, 132, 135
  stimulation test
    interference with, 300, 302
    in reproductive disorders, 202,
      203, 237
Gonadotropins. *See also* Follicle-
    stimulating hormone; Luteiniz-
    ing hormone
  androgens and, 223, 224
  anorexia nervosa and, 299–300
  assays
    in amenorrhea, 201
    interference with, 302, 303
    in male hypogonadism, 236
  CNS tumors and, 127
  deficiency of, 193
  exogenous thyroid hormone and,
    302
  and gynecomastia and feminization,
    227
  in hirsutism, 211, 212, 215, 217, 218
  human chorionic. *See* Human chori-
    onic gonadotropin
  in males, 236
  in pituitary hormone failure, 41
  pituitary tumors and, 18
  prolactin and, 33
  in reproductive disorders, female,
    198, 201, 203, 204, 205
  in reproductive disorders, male, 227
    androgen enzymatic defects, 234,
      235
    diagnosis, 238–242
    hypogonadism, 229
  stimulation tests
    in amenorrhea, 201, 203, 204
    in hypopituitarism, 22–23
Granulomatous disease
  and hypercalcemia, 82, 84, 85
  and male hypogonadism, 225
Graves' disease, 58, 68
  clinical considerations, 53–55
  diagnosis of, 69
  LATS in, 65
  with primary adrenal failure, 126
Growth factors, insulin-like, 291
Growth hormone, 15–16
  acromegaly, 33–39

anorexia nervosa and, 300
assay, 43
and delayed puberty, 230
exogenous thyroid hormone and,
  302
fasting and, 280
in hypopituitarism, 21, 25, 26, 27
with insulin tolerance test, 135
kidney disease and, 298
obesity and, 300
pituitary tumors and, 16, 17, 18
pregnancy and, 299
provocative tests, 43–45
psychotropics and, 301
radioreceptor assay, 45
receptor deficiency, 47
secretion rate estimation, 45
short stature, 39–48
Gynecomastia, 242, 243
  in alcoholism, 228
  defined, 226
  in hypogonadism, 230
  spironolactone and, 303

Hair, body
  gonadotropin deficiency and, 25
  hirsutism. *See* Hirsutism
Haloperidol, 27
Hand-Schuller-Christian syndrome.
    See Histiocytosis
Hashimoto's thyroiditis, 58–59
  antibody test in, 66
  with primary adrenal failure, 126
  TSH levels in, 64
  Turner's syndrome and, 193
Headache, pheochromocytoma and,
  160
Heart disease. *See* Cardiovascular dis-
    orders
Heat
  and euthyroid sick syndrome, 57
  and infertility, male, 226
  intolerance of, in acromegaly, 34
Hematocrit, in short stature, 42
Hemochromatosis, and hypopituitar-
    ism, 17, 20
Hemoglobin, glycosylated, 9, 11–12
Hepatosplenomegaly, in lipoprotein
    lipase deficiency, 252
Hereditary factors. *See* Genetic fac-
    tors
Hermaphroditism, 192, 194–195
  and amenorrhea, 205, 207
  androgen abnormalities, 234, 235

Hirsutism
  with amenorrhea, 202, 204, 206
  clinical considerations, 209–213
  in Cushing's syndrome, 143, 144
  diagnostic methods, 213–215
  discussion, 215–219
  idiopathic, 211, 217, 218
Histalog, 267
Histiocytosis
  and growth retardation, 47
  and hypopituitarism, 17, 20
  and short stature, 40
Histocompatability antigens, in dia-
    betes mellitus, 1
Human chorionic gonadotropin
  alpha subunit, 18
  and gynecomastia and feminization,
    227
  in males, 236
  in reproductive disorders
    female, 203
    male, 227, 228, 237, 242, 243
  stimulation test, 237
  tumors secreting, 242
Human placental lactogen, 299
H-Y antigen
  in amenorrhea, 201–202
  in reproductive disorders, male, 237
Hydrocortisone, and calcium levels,
    88
17-Hydroxycorticosteroids
  ACTH stimulation tests, 131
  in adrenal insufficiency, 134
  anorexia nervosa and, 300
  dexamethasone suppression test
    and, 147–155
  glucocorticoids and, 139
  in hirsutism, 213, 217
  phenytoin and, 300
  pregnancy and, 299
  in reproductive disorders, male, 237
Hydroxylase deficiencies, 194
  and amenorrhea, 205
  in hirsutism, 211–212, 213
17-Hydroxyprogesterone, in hirsut-
    ism, 211, 212, 219
17-Hydroxysteroids
  in amenorrhea, 207
  exogenous thyroid hormone and,
    302
  liver disease and, 298
  in primary aldosteronism, 175
Hyperaldosteronism, 120. See also
    Aldosteronism, primary

glucocorticoid remediable, 176,
    178, 184–187
  idiopathic, 175–178, 180, 181, 182,
    184–188
Hypercalcemia, 81–82
  clinical considerations, 82–85
  diagnostic methods, 85–89
  discussion, 89–93
  MEN syndromes, MEN-I, 270
  and water conservation, 110, 111
Hypercholesterolemia, in children,
    258–259
Hypercortisolism. See Cushing's syn-
    drome
Hyperglycemia. See Glucose levels
Hyperkalemia. See Potassium levels
Hyperlipidemias, 247–248
  clinical considerations
    chylomicronemia, 253
    combined, 253
    LDL catabolism abnormalities,
      250–251
    remnant catabolism abnormal-
      ities, 252–253
    secondary, 249
    triglyceride catabolism defects,
      252
    triglycerides, endogenous input,
      251–252
  combined, 251, 252, 253
  diagnostic methods, 254–255
  discussion, 255–259
  and osmolality, 115
  and pseudohypernatremia, 112
  and pseudohyponatremia, 113–114
  and short stature, 40
Hyperlipoproteinemia, type III, 252–
    253
Hypernatremia
  AVP deficiency and, 110
  diagnosis, 118–121
Hyperparathyroidism
  acromegaly and, 35
  and hypercalcemia, 82
  MEN syndromes, 262
    MEN-I, 270, 272
    MEN-IIa, 266, 273, 274, 275
    MEN-IIb, 275
  normocalcemic, 83
  phenytoin and, 301
  primary, diagnosis, 89–91
Hyperprolactinemia
  acromegaly and, 35
  clinical considerations, 27–29

Hyperprolactinemia—*Continued*
  diagnostic methods, 29–30
  discussion, 30–33
  in MEN-I syndrome, 264
  pituitary tumors and, 18
  and reproductive disorders
    female, 193, 197–198, 200–204
    male, 225, 229, 236, 238–241
  secondary, 31
Hyperproteinemia. *See* Proteins,
    serum
Hypertension
  acromegaly and, 34–35
  in Cushing's syndrome, 144
  with hypercalcemia, 83
  with hyperlipidemia, 248
  in MEN syndromes, 273, 275
  pheochromocytoma and, 159, 160,
    161
  plasma renin in, 179
  in primary aldosteronism, 174–177
Hyperthyroidism, 68
  clinical considerations, 53–55
  diagnosis of, 69
  diagnostic methods, 59–67
    thyroid scans, 67
    TRH assay in, 64–65
  diagnostic protocol, 68
  Hashimoto's thyroiditis and, 58
  and hypercalcemia, 82
  and male infertility, 232
Hypertriglyceridemia, 251–252, 253
  and cardiovascular disease, 256
  xanthomas in, 255
Hypoadrenalism. *See* Adrenal insuf-
    ficiency
Hypocalcemia
  clinical considerations, 97–103
    other disorders, 102
    PTH disorders, 100–101
    vitamin D disorders, 101–102
  diagnostic methods, 102–103
  discussion, 103–105
Hypocalciuric hypercalcemia, famil-
    ial, 85
Hypoglycemia
  and catecholamine assays, 169, 302
  clinical considerations
    alimentary, 282, 284
    diabetes-associated, 284
    fasting, 280–282
    postprandial, 282
  cortisol response to, in Cushing's
    syndrome, 146, 148

diagnostic methods, 285–287
discussion
  fasting, 287–289, 291
  postprandial, 291–293
growth hormone deficiency and, 41
insulin, 27
nocturnal, 281
and vasopressin release, 108
Hypogonadism and infertility, male,
    223–224
  clinical considerations, 224–235
    causes, 226, 227–229
    gynecomastia and feminization,
      230
    hormonal factors, 234–235
    infertility, 231–233
    pubertal failure, 229–230
  diagnostic measures, 235–237
  discussion, 237–243
  pituitary hormones and, 16, 25, 34
Hyponatremia, 121–123
  in adrenal insufficiency, 126
  and catecholamines, 164
  clinical conditions with, 112
  SIADH, 111–114
  signs and symptoms, 111
Hypoparathyroidism. *See also* Para-
    thyroid hormone
  with adrenal insufficiency, primary,
    126
  hypocalcemia with, 99, 100–101
  MEN-IIa syndrome, 274
Hypophysitis, and hypothyroidism, 57
Hypopituitarism
  and adrenal insufficiency, insulin
    tolerance test in, 132
  anorexia nervosa and, 299
  clinical considerations
    empty sella syndrome, 19
    postpartum pituitary necrosis,
      19–20
    tumors, 16–19
  diagnostic flow sheet, 26
  diagnostic methods, 20–23
    endocrine evaluation, 21–23
    neuroradiologic evaluations, 21
  discussion, 24–27
  growth hormone deficiency in, 41
  and hypoglycemia, 281, 289, 291
  and hypothyroidism, 57
  and short stature, 40
Hypotension, AVP deficiency and,
    110
Hypothalamic disorders. *See also*

Central nervous system disorders
and adrenal insufficiency, 127
and hypopituitarism, 17, 18, 20
and hypothyroidism, 57
prolactin secretion in, 24
and reproductive disorders
female, 193, 197
male, 225, 238–241
TSH levels in, 71
and water conservation disorders, 109, 110
Hypothalamic-pituitary-adrenal axis. *See also* Pituitary disorders
in adrenal insufficiency, 137–139
suppression of, 125, 127–128
Hypothalamic-pituitary-gonadal axis
in amenorrhea, 199
in male infertility, 232
Hypothalamic-releasing hormone, 25
Hypothalamus
and ACTH secretion, 144
dopamine depletion, 27
Hypothyroidism
acromegaly and, 34
with adrenal insufficiency, 127
cholesterol levels in, 250
clinical considerations, 55–58
and delayed puberty, 230
diagnosis of, 69
diagnostic methods, 59–67
TRH assay, 64
triiodothyronine, 67
diagnostic protocol, 70
diluting capacity assessment in, 118
and galactorrhea, 28
growth hormone therapy and, 48
and hyperlipidemias, 249, 251
and hypoglycemia, 285
and hyponatremia, 112, 113
in hypopituitarism, 25
hypothalamic, 70
lithium and, 304
pituitary, 70
with primary adrenal failure, 126
radioiodine therapy and, 56
and short stature, 40, 41
thyrotrope cell hyperplasia and, 19

Immobilization, and hypercalcemia, 82, 84, 85
Immotile cilia syndrome, and infertility, male, 226, 232
Immunoglobulins. *See* Antibodies; Autoimmune disorders; Globulins
Immunologic infertility, male, 226
Impotence, 232
in Cushing's syndrome, 143, 144
defined, 225–226
Infants. *See also* Pediatric patients
emotional deprivation, 300
growth disorders, 40, 41
Infections
and diabetes mellitus, 1
and hypercalcemia, 82, 84, 85
and hypopituitarism, 17
and infertility, male, 225, 226, 231–232
and short stature, 40
Infertility
female. *See* Amenorrhea
male, 225, 231–233, 239
Inhibin, 223–224
Insulin
antibodies, 281, 282, 286, 288, 291
assays, in hypoglycemia, 285, 286
autoimmune syndrome, 291
circulating, 12
factitious administration, 281, 291
fasting and, 280
vs. glucose, in GTT, 283
in hypoglycemia, fasting, 287–288, 289
immunoreactive, 285–286, 291
and nocturnal hypoglycemia, 281
obesity and, 300
pregnancy and, 299
Insulin:glucose ratios, in hypoglycemia, 288, 289
Insulin hypoglycemia
clinical considerations, 281–282
and prolactin levels, 22, 27
Insulin resistance, and VLDL excess, 251
Insulin tolerance test, 43
in adrenal insufficiency, 131–132, 135, 136, 137
in Cushing's syndrome, 146, 148
exogenous hormones and, 301, 302
and growth hormone secretion, 43–44
Insulinomas
calcium infusion tests in, 287
C-peptide and proinsulin in, 286–287
diagnosis, 288, 289, 291
diagnostic protocol, 290

Insulinomas—*Continued*
  and hypoglycemia, 281
  localization of, 287
  MEN syndromes, MEN-I, 263–264,
    271
Intrauterine growth retardation, 40,
    41
Intravenous pyelography, in pheo-
    chromocytoma, 166
Iodine
  organic, and thyrotoxicosis, 55
  radioactive. *See* Radioiodine
Islet cell tumors, acromegaly and, 35
Isolated LH deficiency, 225

Kallman's syndrome, 193, 225
Karyotyping
  females, 201, 205, 206
  males, 232, 236, 242, 243
Ketoacidosis, and euthyroid sick syn-
    drome, 57
17-Ketogenic steroids
  defined, 134
  in hirsutism, 213
17-Ketosteroids
  in adrenal insufficiency, 134
  assay interference
    exogenous thyroid hormone and,
      302
    phenytoin and, 300, 301
  in Cushing's syndrome, 154
  in hirsutism, 211, 213, 217, 218, 219
  in primary aldosteronism, 175
  in reproductive disorders
    female, 204, 207
    male, 237, 242, 243
Kidney disease, 174
  cholesterol levels in, 250
  endocrine test interference, 298–
    299
  growth hormone in, 36
  and hypercalcemia, 83
  and hyperlipidemias, 249, 250, 251
  and hypocalcemia, 99, 101, 103,
    104, 105
  hyponatremia with, 112
  and polyuria, 119
  with primary aldosteronism, 174,
    175
  and prolactin levels, 28
  and reproductive disorders, male,
    225, 228, 239
  and short stature, 40, 42
  and VLDL excess, 251

Kidney function. *See also* Creatinine
  and euthyroid sick syndrome, 57
  hypocalciuric hypercalcemia, 82, 85
  phosphorus regulation, assays of,
    87–88
  in primary aldosteronism, 173
  and SIADH, 113
  and water conservation disorders,
    109, 110–111
Klinefelter's syndrome, 242
  and gynecomastia and feminization,
    227
  and male hypogonadism, 225, 241

Laboratory. *See also specific disorders
    and tests*
  in diagnostic protocols. *See* Diag-
    nostic protocols
  interference in endocrine testing
    disease states, 297–300
    drugs, 300–304
Lactotrope hyperplasia, 18
Laron dwarfism, 40, 46, 47
LATS. *See* Long-acting thyroid-stimu-
    lating globulin
Laurence-Moon-Biedl syndrome, 225,
    229
Leucine infusion test, in hypoglyce-
    mia, 287
Levodopa. *See* L-Dopa
Leydig cells
  failure of, 224, 239
  and hormone secretion, 223, 224
  in male hypogonadism, 228, 238
Libido, in Cushing's syndrome, 143
Lipemia, 248
Lipemia retinalis, 248, 252, 253
Lipidoses. *See* Hyperlipidemias
Lipids, in osmolality determination,
    115
Lipomas, 264
Lipoprotein lipase, 248
  deficiencies of, 252, 258
  in differential diagnosis, 257
Lipoproteins
  high-density
    defined, 248
    in differential diagnosis, 256, 257
  intermediate density, 247, 254
  low-density
    abnormal catabolism, 250–251
    in broad beta disease, 253
    defined, 247–248
    in differential diagnosis, 256, 257

in hyperlipidemias, 249, 253
total cholesterol and, 254
very low density
    cholesterol in, 250
    cholesterol contribution to, 254
    and chylomicronemia, 252, 255
    in combined hyperlipidemia, 251, 253
    defined, 247
    in differential diagnosis, 256, 257
    excess production of, 251–252
    and plasma turbidity, 254
    in secondary hyperlipidemia, 249
Lithium
    goitrogenicity, 303
    and hypercalcemia, 82
    and water conservation, 108, 110, 111
Liver disease, 174
    endocrine test interference, 298
    and euthyroid sick syndrome, 57
    growth hormone in, 36
    and gynecomastia and feminization, 227
    and hyperlipidemia, secondary, 249
    and hypocalcemia, 99, 101, 104, 105
    and hypoglycemia, 281, 282, 289, 291
    hyponatremia with, 112
    and prolactin levels, 28
    and reproductive disorders, male, 227, 239
    and short stature, 40, 42
Liver function
    exogenous estrogens and, 301
    phenytoin and, 300, 301
Long-acting thyroid-stimulating globulin, 54, 65–66
Lubs syndrome, 234, 235
Lupus erythematosus, and hyperlipidemias, 249
Luteinizing hormone. See also Gonadotropins
    in fertile eunuch syndrome, 225
    in males, 236
    spironolactone and, 303
Luteinizing hormone-releasing hormone. See also Gonadotropin-releasing hormone
    in amenorrhea, 203, 204
    anorexia nervosa and, 300
    cortisol and, 301
Lymphoma, 90

Magnesium deficiency, and hypocalcemia, 99, 102, 103, 104
Malabsorption
    and hypocalcemia, 99, 102, 105
    and short stature, 40, 42
Malignancy. See also Metastatic disease; Tumors; specific tumor sites
    and hypercalcemia, 82, 83–89
    thyroid, 72–73, 74–76
Malnutrition. See Nutrition
Marfanoid habitus, 262, 266
Marijuana, and gonadal function, male, 233
Mass lesions
    and pituitary hormone secretion, 16
    and short stature, 41
Maturation, delayed, 229–230. See also Puberty
Medullary carcinoma of thyroid. See Thyroid tumors
Menopause
    and lipids, 254
    premature, 198–199
Menses. See also Amenorrhea
    in Cushing's syndrome, 143, 144
    hypopituitarism and, 25
MEN syndromes. See Multiple endocrine neoplasia syndromes
Metabolic alkalosis, in primary aldosteronism, 174, 175
Metabolic disorders. See Systemic disorders
Metanephrines, 303
    in MEN-IIa syndrome, 273
    in pheochromocytoma, 162–163, 167, 168, 169
Metapyrone test
    ACTH stimulation test and, 25
    in adrenal insufficiency, 129, 132–133, 137
    in Cushing's syndrome, 149–150
Metastatic disease
    growth hormone in, 36
    hypercalcemia in, 90
    and hypoglycemia, 282
    and hypopituitarism, 17
Methadone, 233
Methotrexate, 233
Methyldopa, 27, 28, 303
Metoclopramide, 27
    and PRL secretion, 22
    and prolactin levels, 27, 28

Metrizamide cisternography, in pituitary tumors, 21
Mineralocorticoid escape, 173. *See also* Aldosteronism, primary
Mineralocorticoids, in Cushing's syndrome, 143
Minoxidil, and hirsutism, 209
Mithramycin, and hypocalcemia, 99
Monoamine oxidase, 162
Monoamine oxidase inhibitors, 303
    and catecholamine assays, 163
    and gonadal function, male, 233
Mosaicism
    in females, 192–193, 205, 206
    in males, 241, 242
Mucosal neuromas, 262, 275
Mullerian regression factor, 223
Multinodular goiter. *See* Goiter
Multiple endocrine neoplasia (MEN) syndromes, 261–262
    acromegaly in, 35
    clinical considerations
        MEN-I, 262–264
        MEN-IIa, 264–266
        MEN-IIb, 266–267
    diagnostic methods, 267–269
    discussion
        MEN-I, 269–271
        MEN-IIa, 271–275
        MEN-IIb, 275
    and hypercalcemia, 82, 83, 84
    insulinomas, 291
    pheochromocytoma in, 161, 162, 169
    thyroid carcinoma, 76
Murphy-Patte method, 59
Myeloma, 90
Myocardial infarction
    and euthyroid sick syndrome, 57
    and glucose tolerance, 3
Myopathy, acromegaly and, 35
Myotonia dystrophica, 225

Needle biopsy, thyroid, 73, 75, 76
Nelson's syndrome, 17, 23
Neonatal hyperthyroidism, 65
Neonatal hypocalcemia, 99, 102
Nephrotic syndrome. *See* Kidney disease
Neuroglycopenia, 284
Neurohypothalamic control, of ACTH secretion, 144
Neurologic abnormalities. *See also* Central nervous system symptoms

acromegaly and, 35
in hypercalcemia, 83
in hypocalcemia, 99, 100
in hypoglycemia, 279, 288
in hyponatremia, 111
in hypopituitarism, 26
and impotence, 226
in pheochromocytoma, 160
pituitary disorders and, 23, 35, 41
Neuromas, mucosal, 262, 275
Neurophysin, 228
Neuroradiology. *See* Radiology
Nitrofurantoin, 233
Nodular adrenal hyperplasia. *See* Adrenal hyperplasia, nodular
Nodules, thyroid, 55
    clinical considerations, 71–72
    diagnostic methods, 72–73
    discussion, 74–76
    radioactive iodine uptake in, 66, 67
Nonsuppressible insulin-like activity, 291
Noonan's syndrome, 229, 255
Nutrition. *See also* Diet
    in aldosteronism, 176
    and amenorrhea, 196, 197
    and euthyroid sick syndrome, 57
    and growth abnormalities, 42
    and gynecomastia, 227
    and hypocalcemia, 102
    and hypoglycemia, 289
    Vitamin D deficiency, 101

Obesity
    in Cushing's syndrome, 143, 144
    endocrine test interference, 300
    and hyperlipidemia, secondary, 249
    hypothyroidism and, 41
    LHRH in, 202, 203
    morbid, 240
    VLDL excess in, 251
Oligomenorrhea, hypopituitarism and, 25
Oligospermia
    in Cushing's syndrome, 143
    idiopathic, 231, 238, 239, 240
    and infertility, male, 226
Oral contraceptives
    and amenorrhea, 196, 197
    and cortisol levels, 155
    in hirsutism, 218
    and hyperprolactinemia, 27, 28
Oral hypoglycemics
    and hypoglycemia, 281, 291
    test interference by, 303

Orchitis, and male infertility, 233
Osmolality
    assays, 114, 115
    AVP and, 107–108
    in diabetes insipidus, 120, 121
    polydipsia and, 111
    in SIADH, 121
    water load and, 118
Osmolarity, AVP deficiency and, 110
Osmoreceptors, 107–108
Osmotic diuresis, 109, 110, 119, 120
Osteomalacia, phenytoin and, 301
Osteopenia, in Cushing's syndrome,
        144
Ovaries
    polycystic disease
        and amenorrhea, 192, 195–196
        diagnosis, 202, 203
        and hirsutism, 209–212, 216–219
    premature menopause, 198–199
    prolactin and, 33
    resistant ovary syndrome, 194
    tumors, 199

Padre-Willi syndrome, 229
Paget's disease, and hypercalcemia,
        82, 85
Pancreatic tumors, MEN syndromes,
        262, 263–264, 271
Pancreatitis
    with hypercalcemia, 83
    with hyperlipidemias, 248, 251,
        252, 253
    with hypocalcemia, 99, 103
    with hyponatremia, 112
Panhypopituitarism, 112, 113
Parathyroid hormone. See also Hyper-
        parathyroidism; Hypoparathy-
        roidism
    assays, 86, 89, 90
    and calcium regulation, 81–82, 97,
        98
    ectopic secretion, 90, 92
    in familial hypercalciuric hyper-
        calcemia, 85
    and hypercalcemia, 82, 85
    and hypocalcemia, 99
    kidney disease and, 298–299
Parathyroid hormone infusion test, in
        hypocalcemia, 102–103, 105
Parathyroid hyperplasia, 83
Parathyroid tumors, MEN syn-
        dromes, 262
Pediatric patients
    diabetes mellitus in, 6, 7, 8

growth disorders, 40, 41, 300
growth hormone secretion in, 21
hyperlipidemias in, 258–259
MEN-I syndrome, 269–270
neonatal hyperthyroidism, 65
neonatal hypocalcemia, 99, 102
pheochromocytoma in, 160, 161
Pendred's syndrome, goiter and, 71
Pentagastrin stimulation tests, in
        MEN syndromes, MEN-IIa,
        271
Pentolium suppression test, 166
Peptic ulcer disease
    with hypercalcemia, 83
    in MEN-I syndrome, 263, 267, 270,
        271, 272
Perchlorate washout test, 61, 66–67
Phenothiazines
    and amenorrhea, 196
    and prolactin levels, 27, 28, 31
Phentolamine adrenergic blocking
        test, 164–165, 167
Phenylbutazone, 303, 304
Phenytoin, endocrine test interference
        by, 155, 300, 301
Pheochromocytomas
    antihypertensive drugs in, 302
    assay interference, 302–303
    clinical considerations, 159–162
    diagnostic methods, 162–165
    discussion, 166–169
    MEN syndromes, 262
        MEN-I, 270
        MEN-IIa, 265–266, 273, 274
        MEN-IIb, 266, 274
Phosphate, exogenous, and hypocal-
        cemia, 99
Phosphorus levels
    assays
        in hypercalcemia, 85, 86, 89, 93
        in hypocalcemia, 102, 104, 105
        and renal regulation, 87–88
    in MEN-I syndrome, 270
    in mineral homeostasis, 98
    parathyroid hormone and, 97, 103,
        105
    pregnancy and, 299
    and vitamin D metabolism, 81
Pigmentation
    in adrenal insufficiency, 125–128
    in Cushing's syndrome, 144, 145
Pitressin infusion, 114, 116, 119
Pituitary disorders, 15–16. See also
        specific disorders
    acromegaly, 33–39

Pituitary disorders—*Continued*
  and adrenal insufficiency, 127
    evaluation, 137, 138
    insulin tolerance test in, 132
  and gynecomastia and feminization,
    227
  and hirsutism, 212
  hyperprolactinemia, 27–33
  hypoglycemia with, 281, 289, 291
  hypopituitarism, 16–27
  and hypothyroidism, 57
  and reproductive disorders
    female, 192, 193, 199
    male, 225, 227, 228–229, 238–241
  short stature, 39–48
  thyrotropin-releasing hormone
    assay in, 64
  and water conservation disorders,
    109, 110
Pituitary dwarfism, 225
Pituitary failure, and male hypogonadism, 225
Pituitary suppression
  in congenital adrenal hyperplasia,
    212
  glucocorticoid, 137–139. *See also*
    Dexamethasone suppression
    tests
Pituitary tumors, 16–19
  and amenorrhea, 197–198, 204
  and Cushing's syndrome, 145
  growth hormone secretion, 33–35
  MEN syndromes, 262, 264, 272
  and prolactin levels, 28, 29–33
Placental lactogen, 299
Pneumoencephalography, 21
Polycystic ovarian disease. *See* Ovaries
Polydipsia, 109, 110, 111, 116, 120,
  121, 122
Polytomography, of sella turcica, 21,
  24, 30, 31, 32
Polyuria
  AVP deficiencies and, 109
  in Cushing's syndrome, 144
  diagnosis, 118–121
Porphyria, and hyperlipidemia, secondary, 249
Porter-Silber chromogens, 134
Postpartum necrosis, and hypopituita-
  rism, 17, 19–20
Potassium levels
  in adrenal insufficiency, 126
  in Cushing's syndrome, 143, 144, 145

  in hyponatremia, 122
  in primary aldosteronism, 174–177,
    183–184
  and water conservation, 110, 111
Prader-Willi syndrome, 225
Prednisone. *See also* Glucocorticoids
  and adrenal insufficiency, 127–128
  and calcium levels, 88
Pregnanetriol, 134
  in hirsutism, 214, 217
  in reproductive disorders
    female, 204, 207
    male, 237
Pregnancy
  and diabetes, 3, 7–8
  endocrine test interference, 299
  goiter in, 71
  Graves' disease in, 65
  and hypocalcemia, 100
  luteoma of, 219
  molar, 54
  postpartum necrosis, 17, 19–20
  postpartum pituitary hemorrhage,
    127
  sellar enlargement in, 18
  thyroid function in, 55
Primary aldosteronism. *See* Aldosteronism, primary
Progesterone test, in amenorrhea, 200
Progestins
  in amenorrhea, 207
  in hirsutism, 209, 211–212, 219
Proinsulin
  assays
    in diabetes, 12
    in hypoglycemia, 285–286
  factitious insulin use and, 281
  in hypoglycemia, 288
  suppression of, 286–287
Prolactin, 15–16
  acromegaly and, 35
  and amenorrhea, 197–198
  assays
    exogenous hormones and, 301,
      302
    in hyperprolactinemia, 29, 31
    in hypopituitarism, 22, 26
  hyperprolactinemia, 27–33
  in males, 236
  in MEN-I syndrome, 264
  pituitary tumors and, 16, 17, 18
  pregnancy and, 299
  psychotropics and, 301
Prolactin-inhibiting factor, 15

Propranolol, 44
Propylthiouracil, 67
Protein-bound iodine, 60
Proteins, serum
    and calcium levels, 103
    and cortisol levels, 155
    estrogens and, 301
    liver disease and, 298
Pseudohermaphroditism, 225, 234
Pseudohyperparathyroidism, 90, 92,
    101, 105
Pseudohyponatremia, 112, 113
Pseudohypoparathyroidism
    and hypocalcemia, 99, 101, 104, 105
    and short stature, 40
Pseudo-pseudohypoparathyroidism,
    40, 101
Pseudo-Turner's syndrome, 225
Psychological factors
    emotional deprivation, 300
    and impotence, 226
Psychosocial dwarfism, 40, 42
Psychotropic drugs, endocrine test
    interference, 301
Pubertal failure, male, 229–230
Puberty. See also Amenorrhea
    delayed
        female, 192, 206
        male, 225, 239, 240
    delayed maturation, 229–230
    precocious
        hypothyroidism and, 28
        and short stature, 40
Pulmonary disease
    and ectopic ACTH, 146
    and short stature, 40
    and SIADH, 112, 113

Radiation
    and hypopituitarism, 17
    and hypothyroidism, 57
    and parathyroid function, 103
    and reproductive disorders
        female, 196, 199
        male, 225
    and thyroid nodules, 76
Radioiodine, 61. See also Thyroid
    scans
    adrenal scans, 150, 182, 185, 187
    drugs interfering with uptake, 304
    and hypothyroidism, 56
    and parathyroid function, 103
    thyroid nodule uptake, 66, 67, 76

Radioisotope studies. See Scintig-
    raphy
Radiologic dyes
    endocrine test interference by, 163,
        303
    and thyrotoxicosis, 55
Radiology
    in acromegaly, 37, 38
    in adrenal insufficiency, 135
    in Cushing's syndrome, 150, 154
    in hypercalcemia, 88
    in pheochromocytoma, 166, 168,
        169
    in pituitary tumors, 21
    in short stature, 42
Radioreceptor assay, prolactin, 29
5-alpha-Reductase deficiency, 234
Refrigerated plasma test, 256, 257
Reidel's thyroiditis, 59
Reifenstein syndrome, 234, 235
Remnant catabolism abnormalities,
    249, 252–253
Renin
    in aldosterone-producing adenoma,
        176, 177
    aldosterone ratio, 186
    low-sodium diet and, 184
    pregnancy and, 299
    in primary aldosteronism, 174, 175,
        177, 179–180, 183, 184–187
Renin-aldosterone system, in adrenal
    insufficiency, 126
Renin-angiotensin system, and vaso-
    pressin release, 108
Renografin, 163, 303
Reproductive axis. See Amenorrhea;
    Gonadal function; Hypogonad-
    ism
Reserpine, and prolactin levels, 27, 28
Resistant ovary syndrome, 192, 194
Retina
    lipemia and, 248, 252, 253
    pheochromocytoma and, 160
    in primary aldosteronism, 174,
        175
Rickets
    and hypocalcemia, 99, 101, 104
    and short stature, 40
Rosewater syndrome, 234

Salicylates, 303, 304
Saline infusion test, in primary aldo-
    steronism, 183–184

Sarcoidosis, and hypopituitarism, 20
Schwannomas, 264
Scintigraphy
    adrenal, 150, 182, 185, 187
    bone, 88, 89, 90
    thyroid, 61, 66, 67, 69, 76, 304. *See also* Radioiodine; Thyroid scans
Secretin, 268
Seizures. *See also* Central nervous system symptoms
    with hypocalcemia, 99, 100
    hyponatremia and, 111
Sella turcica, 16–19, 21, 24, 30, 31, 32
Semen analysis, 235, 238, 239, 240
Seminiferous tubule failure, 233
Serotonin, in mucosal neuromas, 275
Sertoli cell factor, 223–224
Sertoli cell only syndrome, 225, 232–233, 241
Sex hormones. *See also* Androgens; Estrogens; *specific hormones*
    in amenorrhea, 202, 204, 205, 206
    androgen defects, 234–235
    enzymatic abnormalities, 234
    and hirsutism, 209
    in hypopituitarism, 26
Sexual development. *See also* Amenorrhea; Gonadal dysgenesis; Puberty
    androgen enzymatic defects, 234
    differentiation, 223–224
Sheehan's syndrome, 17, 19–20
Short stature
    clinical considerations, 39–42
    diagnostic evaluation, 42–45
    discussion, 45–48
SIADH, 111–114. *See also* Diabetes insipidus and SIADH
    clinical considerations, 111–114
    diagnosis, 121–123
    diagnostic criteria, 113
    diagnostic methods, 114–119
    etiologies, 113
Sipple's syndrome. *See* Multiple endocrine neoplasia (MEN) syndromes
Skeletal disorders. *See also* Bone(s)
    with hypercalcemia, 83
    and short stature, 40, 42
Sleep, and growth hormone secretion, 43
Sodium. *See also* Aldosteronism, primary; Arginine vasopressin;

Diabetes insipidus and SIADH; Hypernatremia; Hyponatremia
    in adrenal insufficiency, 126
    in primary aldosteronism, 174–177, 183
Soft tissue, in acromegaly, 34
Somatomedin
    in acromegaly, 36–37, 38
    glucocorticoids and, 41
    growth hormone and, 47, 48
    insulin-like growth factors, 291
    in Laron dwarfism, 47
    liver disease and, 42
    measurement of, 45
Somatostatin, 15, 48
Spironolactone, 303, 304
    and ACTH stimulation tests, 130
    and dexamethasone suppression test, 155
    and gonadal function, male, 233
    and gynecomastia and feminization, 227
    renin ratios, 176
    therapeutic trial, 182, 184–187
Starvation, 227. *See also* Nutrition
Stein-Leventhal criteria, 211
Steroids. *See specific hormones*
Stones, 83
Stress
    and amenorrhea, 196
    and catecholamines, 165, 302
Sulfonamides, 281, 303
Sulfonylureas, 281, 286
Suppressive therapy, with thyroid nodules, 76
Surgery
    in acromegaly, 39
    and amenorrhea, 196
    and euthyroid sick syndrome, 57
    in gonadal dysgenesis, female, 206–207
    and hyperprolactinemia, 27
    and hypoparathyroidism, 100
    and hypopituitarism, 17, 20
    and impotence, 226
    and male hypogonadism, 225
    in pheochromocytoma, 169
    for pituitary adenomas, 32–33
    in primary aldosteronism, 175
    thyroid resection, 56
Sweating, acromegaly and, 34
Systemic disorders. *See also* Cardiovascular disorders; Infections;

Pulmonary disease
and hyperlipidemia, 249
and male infertility, 226, 228, 232, 233
and short stature, 40, 41–42

T3. *See* Thyroid function tests; Triiodothyronine
T4. *See* Thyroid function tests; Thyroxine
Technetium, in thyroid scans, 67
Tes-Tape, 10
Testes, formation, 223–224
Testicular failure, 241, 242. *See also* Hypogonadism and infertility, male
and gynecomastia and feminization, 227
and male infertility, 232–233
Testicular feminization, 192, 194, 207, 226, 235, 239, 242
Testicular size, 25, 235. *See also* Hypogonadism and infertility, male
Testosterone. *See also* Androgens; Sex hormones
assays, 236
and clomiphene stimulation tests, 241
in diagnosis, 239, 240
enzymatic abnormalities, 234
and gonadal function, male, 233
and gynecomastia and feminization, 227
in hirsutism, 210, 211, 214–215, 217
liver disease and, 298
in male sexual development, 223
normal levels, 238
obesity and, 300
in seminiferous tubule failure, 233
spironolactone and, 303
Testosterone-binding globulin, 228
Tetany, with hypocalcemia, 99, 100
Thiazides, 89, 113
Thymomas, MEN syndromes, 264
Thyroid carcinoma. *See* Thyroid tumors
Thyroid disorders. *See also specific disorders*
with adrenal insufficiency, 126, 127
and amenorrhea, 196, 199–200
glucose tolerance tests in, 5
goiters and nodules
clinical considerations, 71–72

diagnostic methods, 72–73
discussion, 73–77
and hypercalcemia, 82
and hyperlipidemia, 249, 251
hyperthyroidism, hypothyroidism, and thyroiditis
clinical considerations, 53–59
diagnostic methods, 59–67
discussion, 67–71
hyponatremia with, 112
MEN syndromes, MEN-I, 264
and short stature, 40
Thyroid function
acromegaly and, 34
with thyroid nodules, 74
Thyroid function tests, 59–67
assay interference, 60
anorexia nervosa and, 300
drugs, 303, 304
exogenous cortisol and, 302
kidney disease and, 298
phenytoin and, 300
propylthiouracil and, 67
factors affecting, 60
in growth hormone therapy, 48
in hyperthyroidism, 54, 55
in hypopituitarism, 24–25
with insulin tolerance test, 132
in short stature, 42
with thyroid nodules, 74
Thyroid hormones. *See also* Thyroid function tests; *specific hormones*
exogenous, assay interference by, 302
in hyperthyroidism, 54, 55
liver disease and, 298
Thyroid scans, 67. *See also* Radioiodine
in goiter, 73
interfering factors, 304
with thyroid nodules, 66, 67, 74, 76
in thyroiditis, 69
Thyroid tumors, medullary carcinoma, 262
in MEN-IIa syndrome, 264–265, 273, 274
in MEN-IIb syndrome, 266
pheochromocytoma with, 162
Thyroiditis, 68
clinical considerations, 58–59
diagnosis of, 69
and hyperthyroidism, 55

Thyroiditis—*Continued*
  MEN syndrome, 264
  radioactive iodine uptake in, 66
Thyroid-stimulating hormone. *See*
    Thyroid function tests; Thyro-
    tropin
Thyrotoxicosis, 69
  clinical considerations, 54–55
  galactorrhea with, 30
  and gynecomastia and feminization,
    227
  MEN syndromes, 264
  therapy, TSH levels in, 64
  triiodothyronine in, 54, 67, 73
Thyrotropin, 15, 60. *See also* Thyroid
    function tests
  alpha subunit, 18
  assays, 64
  in diagnosis, 69
  goiter and, 73
  in hypopituitarism, 24, 25, 26
  in hypothyroidism, 55–56, 57
  intracranial pressure and, 16
  lithium and, 71
  in short stature, 46
  stimulation of, 23, 61
  thyroid adenoma and, 54–55
  and thyroid nodules, 74
  thyrotrope cell hyperplasia and, 19
Thyrotropin-releasing hormone. *See*
    also Thyroid function tests
  in acromegaly, 38
  assays, 64–65
  in hyperthyroidism, 68
  with insulin tolerance test, 132, 135,
    136
  in pituitary disorders, acromegaly,
    36
  prolactin stimulation, 22, 28, 29
Thyrotropin-releasing hormone infu-
    sion test, drugs interfering
    with, 304
Thyrotropin-releasing hormone-
    mediated TSH release, in
    hypothyroidism, 65
Thyroxine, 59, 62, 68. *See also* Thy-
    roid function tests
  free, 62, 68
  goiter and, 73
  growth hormone therapy and, 48
  and growth retardation, 47
  in hyperprolactinemia, 30, 31
  in hypopituitarism, 24–25, 26
  in hypothyroidism, 57

index, 63
propylthiouracil and, 67
in thyroid disorder diagnosis, 69
Thyroxine-binding globulin, 61, 63–
    64, 68, 69, 70
  exogenous estrogens and, 301
  in hyperthyroidism, 68, 69
  liver disease and, 298
  phenytoin and, 300
  and thyroid hormone levels, 55, 71
Tolbutamide infusion test, 6, 287
Toxicosis, triiodothyronine, 68
Transcortin, exogenous estrogens
    and, 301
Transfusions, and hypocalcemia, 99,
    102
Trauma
  and glucose tolerance, 3
  and hypopituitarism, 17, 20
  and hypothyroidism, 57
  and male hypogonadism, 225
TRH. *See* Thyroid function tests;
    Thyrotropin-releasing hor-
    mone
Triethylenemelamine, and gonadal
    function, male, 233
Triglycerides, 247–248
  assays, 255
  and cardiovascular disease, 256
  in chylomicronemia syndrome, 253
  decreased catabolism, 252
  in differential diagnosis, 256, 257
  endogenous, excess input of, 251–
    252
Triiodothyronine. *See also* Thyroid
    function tests
  in hypothyroidism, 55–56, 57
  resin uptake
    drugs interfering with, 304
    exogenous estrogens and, 301
  reverse, 57, 60
Trousseau's sign, 99
TSH. *See* Thyroid function tests;
    Thyrotropin
Tumors. *See also* Multiple endocrine
    neoplasia (MEN) syndromes;
    Pheochromocytomas
  ACTH producing, 146
  adrenal, and hirsutism, 212
  and adrenal insufficiency, second-
    ary, 127
  adrenal scintiscan with, 182, 185,
    187
  AVP-producing, 112, 113

and Cushing's syndrome, 144, 145,
    153–154
and dexamethasone suppression
    test, 155
and diabetes insipidus, 110
growth hormone-secreting, 33–35
and gynecomastia and feminization,
    227
hCG-secreting, 239
and hirsutism, 217, 218, 219
and hypercalcemia, 82, 83–89
and hyperthyroidism, 54–55
and hypocalcemia, 102
and hypoglycemia, 281, 289, 291
and hypopituitarism, 20
and hypothyroidism, 57
ovarian, and hirsutism, 212
parathyroid, 83, 88–89
pituitary, 16–19
and primary aldosteronism, 175,
    176, 177
and prolactin levels, 28, 29–33
and reproductive disorders
    female, 196–199, 204
    male, 242, 243
and short stature, 40, 41
and thyrotoxicosis, 55
Turner's syndrome
    amenorrhea with, 192–193, 197, 206
    and premature menopause, 199
    and short stature, 42

Ulcers. See Peptic ulcer disease
Ultrasound
    adrenal, 150
    insulinoma localization, 287
    in ovarian disorders, 202, 204
    in pheochromocytoma, 166, 169
    thyroid, 72, 75, 76
Uremia. See Kidney disease
Uric acid, in hypertriglyceridemia,
    familial, 251
Urinalysis
    in familial hypercalciuric hypercal-
        cemia, 85
    glycosuria, 5, 8, 9–10
    in polyuria, 119
    in short stature, 42
Urinary catecholamines, in pheo-
    chromocytoma, 162–163
Urinary steroids. See also specific
        hormones
    in adrenal insufficiency, 133–134
    in Cushing's syndrome, 147, 151

in hirsutism, 213, 214
in MEN-IIa syndrome, 273
pregnancy and, 299
Urine, sulfonylurea metabolites, 286
Uterine disease, and amenorrhea,
    196, 200

Vanillylmandelic acid, 162, 167, 303
Varicocele, and male infertility, 226,
    231
Vascular collapse, phentolamine and,
    165
Vascular disorders. See also Cardio-
        vascular disease
    acromegaly and, 34–35
    and hypopituitarism, 17
    and impotence, 226
    pituitary, 20
Vasodepressor test, in pheochromo-
        cytoma, 164–165
Vasopressin. See Arginine vasopres-
        sin; Diabetes insipidus and
        SIADH
Vena cava sampling, for catechol-
        amines, 169
Venography
    adrenal, 182, 185, 186, 187
    in hypercalcemia, 88
    in pheochromocytoma, 166, 169
Venous sampling, adrenal, 181–182,
    185
Viral infections. See Infections
Virilization
    with amenorhhea, 204, 206
    Cushing's syndrome and, 145
Visual disturbances, 41. See also
        Retina
    pituitary disorders and, 21, 26, 31
    Turner's syndrome and, 193
Vitamin D
    and calcium metabolism, 81–82,
        97–98
    hypercalcemia, 87, 89
    hypocalcemia, 99, 101–102
    phenytoin and, 302
Volume depletion
    and hypercalcemia, 85
    and hyponatremia, 112
    pheochromocytoma and, 159, 166
    and renin measurement, 179
    in SIADH, 121, 123
Volume disorders. See also Diabetes
        insipidus and SIADH
    diagnosis, 118–123

Volume disorders—*Continued*
  hyponatremia with, 112

Water clearance, free, 118
Water deprivation test, 115–116, 120,
  121
Water drinking, compulsive, 109, 110,
  111, 116, 120, 121, 122
Water intoxication, and hyponatremia, 113
Water loading, 117–118, 123
Water metabolism, regulation of,
  108–109. *See also* Diabetes
  insipidus and SIADH
WDHA syndrome, 264, 270
Wermer's syndrome. *See* Multiple endocrine neoplasia (MEN) syndromes

Xanthelasmas, 251, 255
Xanthomas
  in chylomicronemia syndrome, 253
  in differential diagnosis, 257, 258

in familial hypercholesterolemia,
  251
with hyperlipidemia, 248
in lipoprotein lipase deficiency, 252
X-rays. *See also* Radiology
  in acromegaly, 37, 38
  in Cushing's syndrome, 154
  in MEN syndromes, 270
  skull, 21
XYY syndrome, and male hypogonadism, 225

Y chromosome, in amenorrhea, 206

Zollinger-Ellison syndrome, 263–264,
  271. *See also* Peptic ulcer disease
Zuckerkandl, organ of, 161, 163